ALLE · ZEIT · WACH · 1842

T. M. Schroeder-Kurth A. D. Auerbach
G. Obe (Eds.)

Fanconi Anemia

Clinical, Cytogenetic and Experimental Aspects

With 69 Figures in 122 Separate Illustrations

Springer-Verlag Berlin Heidelberg New York
London Paris Tokyo

Professor Dr. med. Traute M. Schroeder-Kurth
Institut für Humangenetik und Anthropologie
der Universität Heidelberg
Im Neuenheimer Feld 328
D-6900 Heidelberg 1
Federal Republic of Germany

Arleen D. Auerbach, Ph. D.
Laboratory for Investigative Dermatology
The Rockefeller University
1230 York Avenue
New York, NY 10021-6399, USA

Professor Dr. Günter Obe
Universität Gesamthochschule Essen
Fachbereich 9 Genetik
Universitätsstraße 5
D-4300 Essen 1
Federal Republic of Germany

ISBN-13: 978-3-642-74181-4 e-ISBN-13: 978-3-642-74179-1
DOI: 10.1007/978-3-642-74179-1

Library of Congress Cataloging-in-Publication Data
Fanconi anemia : clinical, cytogenetic, and experimental aspects / T. M. Schroeder-Kurth, A. D. Auerbach, G. Obe (eds.). p. cm. Includes index.
(U.S.)
1. Fanconi's anemia. I. Schroeder-Kurth, T. M. (Traute M.), 1930- II. Auerbach, A. D. (Arleen D.), 1937- . III. Obe, G. RC641.7.F36F36 1989 616.1'52--dc19 88-38914 CIP

Softcover reprint of the hardcover 1st edition 1989

2127/3145-543210 - Printed on acid-free paper

Our work is dedicated
to our patients
and their parents.

Preface

Sixty years ago, G. Fanconi published a paper entitled: *"Familiäre infantile perniziosaartige Anämie (perniziöses Blutbild und Konstitution)"*, in which he reported that this type of severe aplastic anemia represents a hereditary disease distinct from other pancytopenias of childhood (Fanconi 1927). Later this syndrome was named Fanconi anemia (FA; van Leeuwen 1933). A more recent study of the genetics of FA confirmed that the syndrome is inherited in an autosomal recessive manner (Schroeder et al. 1976). Prenatal diagnosis in FA families showed that about 25% of fetuses are affected (Auerbach et al. 1985, 1986).

In 1964, Schroeder et al. discovered high frequencies of chromosomal aberrations in cultured peripheral blood lymphocytes from patients with FA. Schuler et al. (1969) reported that cells from FA patients are particularly sensitive to the chromosome-breaking activity or clastogenic effect of a polyfunctional alkylating agent. Since that time, studies of baseline and induced frequencies of chromosomal aberrations have been used for the identification of patients with FA. There is now a large body of data concerning the possible mechanism(s) underlying the hypersensitivity of FA cells to DNA cross-linking agents, the biochemical basis for which is still unknown.

Complementation analysis, using cells from different FA patients, has demonstrated genetic heterogeneity in the syndrome. The new methods of gene technology are presently being applied to the study of FA in an attempt to isolate and sequence the FA gene(s). Unfortunately, we still have little knowledge of the molecular basis of the syndrome. Until a molecular probe is available for use in diagnosis, there will continue to be difficulties in ascertaining and differentially diagnosing FA.

Five years ago, an International Fanconi Anemia Registry (IFAR) was organized to provide a centralized computer database for clinical, hematologic, and genetic information on FA patients. Patients with clinical features of FA are registered, and then classified according to their cellular sensitivity to DNA cross-linking agents. In the absence of a molecular probe, this is the best available marker for the syndrome.

Recently it has been shown that in some cases the anemia in FA patients can be cured by bone marrow transplantation. Thus FA represents one of the riare inherited diseases which can be treated successfully.

This book is intended to give an overview of our current knowledge of FA, both clinical and experimental. We hope it will be useful not only for specialists in the field, but also for others who are interested in human genetic diseases.

We thank Springer-Verlag, particularly Dr. J. Wieczorek, and Mrs. R. Till from the Institute of Human Genetics and Anthropology for their help in producing this book.

Heidelberg — T. M. Schroeder-Kurth
New York — A. D. Auerbach
Essen — G. Obe

References

Auerbach AD, Sagi M, Adler B (1985) Fanconi anemia: prenatal diagnosis in 30 fetuses at risk. Pediatrics 76: 794-800

Auerbach AD, Zhang M, Ghosh R, Pergament E, Verlinsky Y, Nicholas H, Boué J (1986) Clastogen-induced chromosomal breakage as a marker for first trimester prenatal diagnosis of Fanconi anemia. Hum Genet 73: 86-88

Fanconi G (1927) Familiäre infantile perniziosaartige Anämie (perniziöses Blutbild und Konstitution). Jahrb Kinderheilkd 117: 257-280

Schroeder TM, Anschütz F, Knopp A (1964) Spontane Chromosomenaberrationen bei familiärer Panmyelopathie. Humangenetik 1: 194-196

Schroeder TM, Tilgen D, Krüger J, Vogel F (1976) Formal genetics of Fanconi's anemia. Hum Genet 32: 257-288

Schuler D, Kiss A, Fabian F (1969) Chromosomal peculiarities and "in vitro" examinations in Fanconi's anemia. Humangenetik 7: 314-322

van Leeuven HC (1933) Ein Fall von "konstitutioneller infantiler perniziosaähnlicher Anämie" (Fanconi) Folia Haematol (Leipz) 49: 434-443

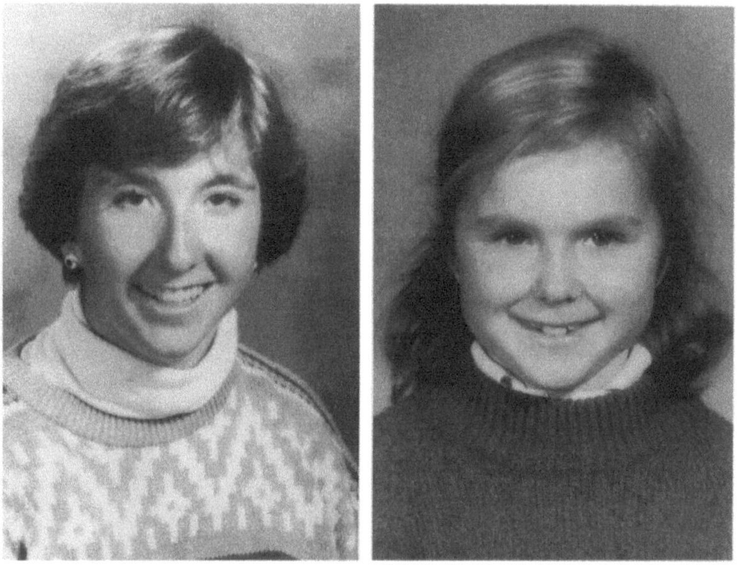

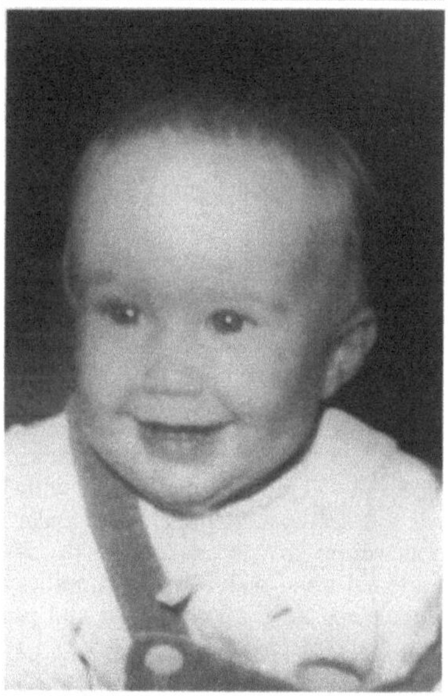

Fig. 1. Three children affected with Fanconi anemia

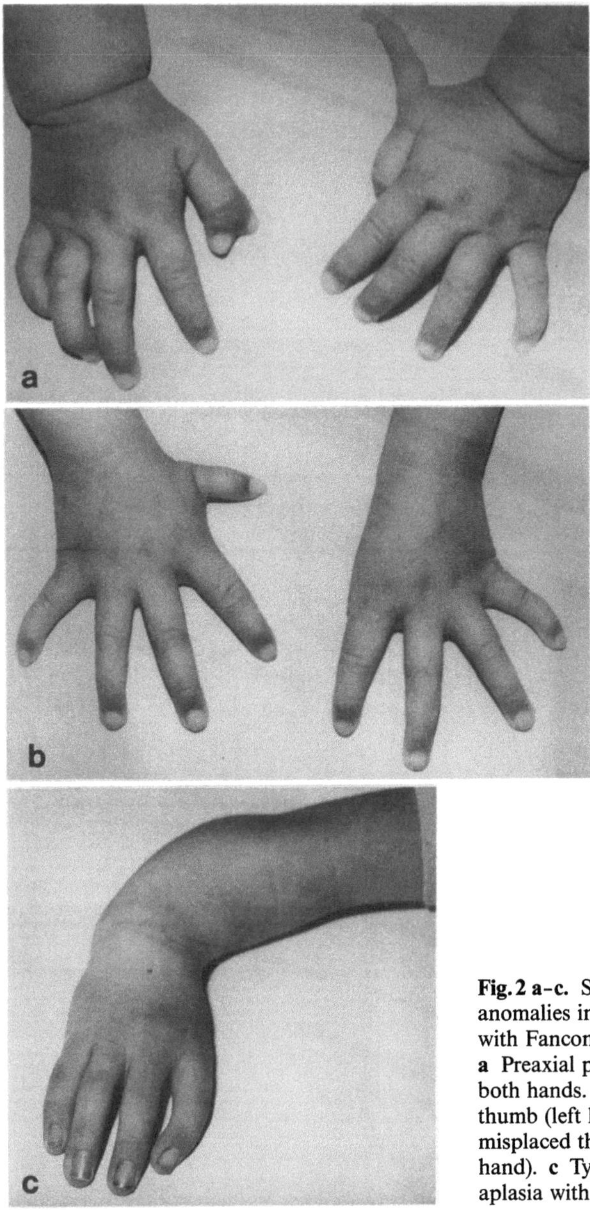

Fig. 2 a–c. Some radial anomalies in three children with Fanconi anemia. **a** Preaxial polydactyly on both hands. **b** Missing thumb (left hand) and short, misplaced thumb (right hand). **c** Typical radial aplasia with absent thumb

Fig. 3 a–d. Three-year-old female with Fanconi anemia. The physical findings are: low-set ears, stenotic ear canals, hearing loss (**a**), multiple café-au-lait spots, severe growth retardation (**b**), absent left thumb and radius, bowed and shortened ulna, with scar from pollicization of index finger; right thumb pedunculated, treated by removal and pollicization of index finger (**c**), bilateral second and third toe syndactyly (**d**). Large hematoma and ecchymoses between eyes from a recent fall

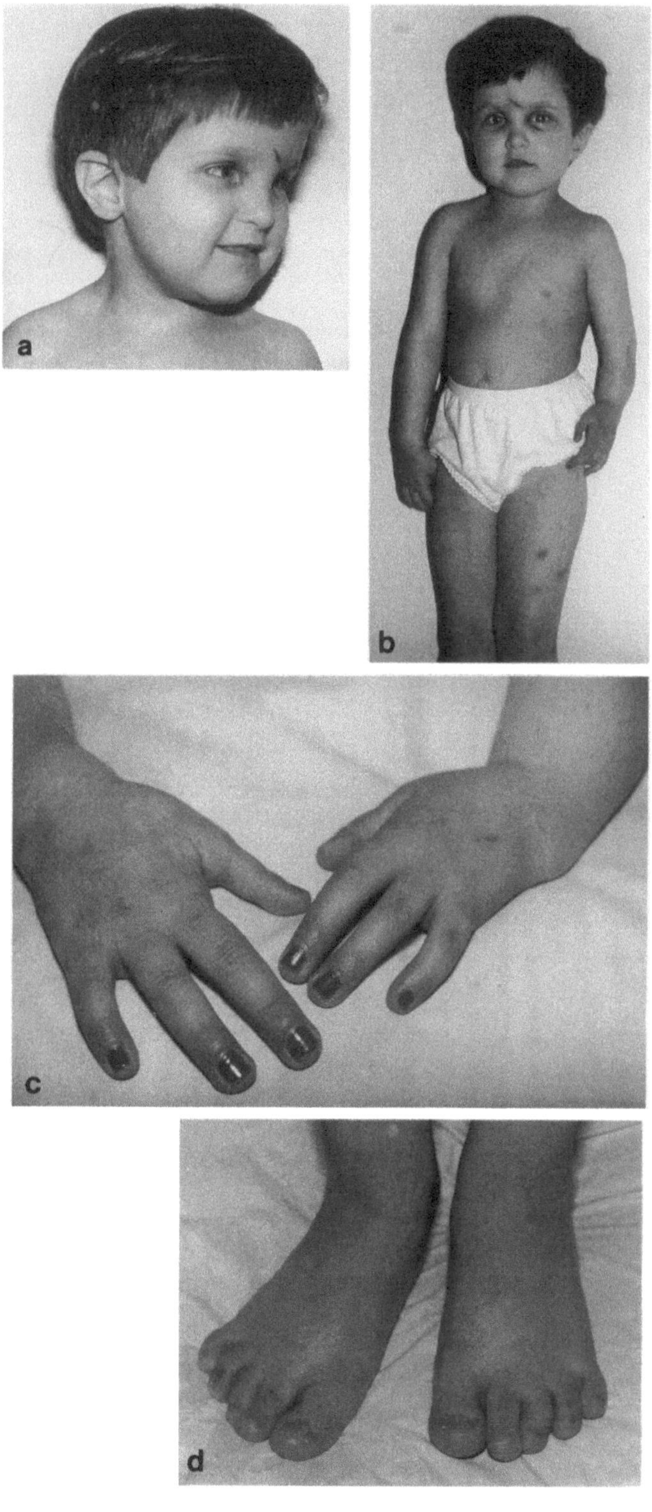
a
b
c
d

Table of Contents

List of Contributors

Arwert, F.
Institute of Human Genetics, Free University, P.O. Box 7161, 1007 MC Amsterdam, The Netherlands

Auerbach, A. D.
Laboratory for Investigative Dermatology, The Rockefeller University, 1230 York Avenue, New York, NY 10021-6399, USA

Averbeck, D.
Institut Curie-Biologie, 26 rue d'Ulm, 75231 Paris Cédex 05, France

Berger, R.
Laboratoire d'Oncologie et d'Immunohématologie (L. O. I., C. N. R. S.) and Unité INSERM U 301, Hôpital Saint-Louis, 1 Av. Claude Vellefaux, 75475 Paris Cédex 10, France

Buchwald, M.
Research Institute, The Hospital for Sick Children, 555 University Avenue, Toronto, Ontario M5G 1X8, Canada, and Department of Medical Genetics and Medical Biophysics, University of Toronto, Ontario, Canada

Chiorazzi, N.
Department of Medicine, North Shore University Hospital, 300 Community Drive, Manhasset, NY 10030, USA

Clarke, C.
Research Institute, The Hospital for Sick Children, Toronto, Ontario M5G 1X8, Canada

Le Coniat, M.
Laboratoire d'Oncologie et d'Immunohématologie (L. O. I., C. N. R. S.) and Unité INSERM U 301, Hôpital Saint Louis, 1 Av. Claude Vellefaux, 75475 Paris Cédex 10, France

Dallapiccola, B.
Department of Public Health and Cell Biology, 2nd University,
Via Orazio Raimondo, 00173 Rome, Italy

Devergie, A.
Bone Marrow Transplantant Unit, Hôpital Saint-Louis, 1,
rue Claude Vellefaux, 75475 Paris Cédex 10, France

Digweed, M.
Institut für Humangenetik, Freie Universität Berlin,
Heubnerweg 6, D-1000 Berlin 19, Federal Republic of Germany

Diatloff-Zito, C.
Institut Curie-Biologie, 26 rue d'Ulm, 75231 Paris Cédex 05,
France

Duckworth-Rysiecki, G.
Research Institute, The Hospital for Sick Children,
Toronto, Ontario M5G 1X8, Canada

Dutreix, J.
Radiotherapy Department, Institut Gustave Roussy, 39,
avenue Camille Desmoulins, 94800 Villejuif, France

Ebell, W.
Kinderklinik der Medizinischen Hochschule,
Konstanty-Gutschow-Str. 8, D-3000 Hannover 61,
Federal Republic of Germany

Fleischer, B.
Institut für Humangenetik und Anthropologie
der Universität Heidelberg, Im Neuenheimer Feld 328,
D-6900 Heidelberg, Federal Republic of Germany

Friedrich, W.
Kinderklinik II, Universität Ulm, Prittwitzstr. 43,
D-7900 Ulm, Federal Republic of Germany

Frohnmayer, D.
FA Support Group, 2875 Baker Blvd., Eugene, Oregon 97403,
USA

Frohnmayer, L.
FA Support Group, 2875 Baker Blvd., Eugene, Oregon 97403,
USA

Ghosh, R.
Laboratory for Investigative Dermatology,
The Rockefeller University, 1230 York Avenue, New York,
NY 10021-6399, USA

Gille, J. J. P.
Institute of Human Genetics, Free University,
Van der Boechorststraat 7, 1081 BT Amsterdam, The Netherlands

Gluckman, E.
Bone Marrow Transplantant Unit, Hospital Saint-Louis, 1,
rue Claude Vellefaux, 75475 Paris Cédex, France

Gök, M.
Institut für Humangenetik und Anthropologie
der Universität Heidelberg, Im Neuenheimer Feld 328,
D-6900 Heidelberg, Federal Republic of Germany

Hoehn, H.
Institut für Humangenetik, Universität Würzburg,
Koellikerstr. 2, D-8700 Würzburg, Federal Republic of Germany

Hong, Y.
Tongyi Medical University, Xiehe Hospital,
Department of Pediatrics, Wuhan, People's Republic of China

Joenje, H.
Institute of Human Genetics, Free University,
Van der Boechorststraat 7, 1081 BT Amsterdam, The Netherlands

Kohne, E.
Kinderklinik II, Universität Ulm, Prittwitzstr. 43,
D-7900 Ulm, Federal Republic of Germany

Koorse, R. E.
Laboratory for Investigative Dermatology,
The Rockefeller University, 1230 York Avenue, New York,
NY 10021-6399, USA

Kubbies, M.
Institut für Humangenetik, Universität Würzburg,
Koellikerstr. 2, D-8700 Würzburg, Federal Republic of Germany

Kuyt, L. P.
Vrije Universiteit, Antropogenetisch Instituut, Postbus 7161,
1007 MC Amsterdam, The Netherlands

Kwee, M. L.
Vrije Universiteit, Antropogenetisch Instituut, Postbus 7161,
1007 MC Amsterdam, The Netherlands

Marx, M. P.
Department of Human Genetics, Faculty of Medicine,
University of Stellenbosch, P.O. Box 63, Tygerberg 7505,
Republic of South Africa

Moustacchi, E.
Institut Curie-Biologie, 26 rue d'Ulm, 75231 Paris Cédex 05,
France

Natarajan, A. T.
Department of Radiation Genetics and Chemical Mutagenesis,
State University of Leiden, Wassenaarseweg 72, AL 2333 Leiden,
The Netherlands

Ng, J.
Research Institute, The Hospital for Sick Children
and Departments of Medical Genetics and Medical Biophysics,
University of Toronto, Toronto, Ontario M5G 1XB, Canada

van Niekerk, C. H.
Department of Pediatrics and Child Health, Medical School,
University of the Orange Free State, Bloemfontein,
Republic of South Africa

Obe, G.
Universität Gesamthochschule Essen, Fachbereich 9 Genetik,
Universitätsstraße 5, D-4300 Essen, Federal Republic of Germany

Papadopoulo, D.
Institut Curie-Biologie, 26 rue d'Ulm, 75231 Paris Cédex 05,
France

Pollio, P. C.
Laboratory for Investigative Dermatology,
The Rockefeller University, 1230 York Avenue, New York,
NY 10021-6399, USA

Poot, M.
Institut für Humangenetik, Universität Würzburg,
Koellikerstr. 2, D-8700 Würzburg, Federal Republic of Germany

Porfirio, B.
Department of Public Health and Cell Biology, 2nd University,
Via Orazio Raimondo, 00173 Rome, Italy

Rabinovitch, P. S.
Department of Pathology, University of Washington,
NE Pacific St, Seattle, WA 98195, USA

Rogatko, A.
Department of Epidemiology and Biostatistics,
Memorial Sloan-Kettering Cancer Center, 1275 York Ave.,
New York, NY, USA

Schindler, D.
Institut für Humangenetik, Universität Würzburg,
Koellikerstr. 2, D-8700 Würzburg, Federal Republic of Germany

Schroeder-Kurth, T. M.
Institut für Humangenetik und Anthropologie der Universität
Heidelberg, Im Neuenheimer Feld 328, D-6900 Heidelberg 1,
Federal Republic of Germany

Smith, S.
Department of Pediatrics and Child Health, Medical School,
University of the Orange Free State, Bloemfontein,
Republic of South Africa

Sperling, K.
Institut für Humangenetik, Freie Universität Berlin,
Heubnerweg 6, D-1000 Berlin 19, Federal Republic of Germany

Venkatraj V. S.
Laboratory for Investigative Dermatology,
The Rockefeller University, 1230 York Avenue, New York,
NY 10021-6399, USA

Vijayalaxmi
MRC Clinical and Population Cytogenetics Unit,
Western General Hospital, Edinburgh, United Kingdom

Vossen, J. M. J. J.
Department of Pediatrics, Academic Hospital,
University of Leiden, AL 2333 Leiden, The Netherlands

van Weel-Sipman, M. H.
Department of Pediatrics, Academic Hospital,
University of Leiden, AL 2333 Leiden, The Netherlands

Weksberg, R.
Research Institute, The Hospital of Sick Children,
Toronto, Ontario M5G 1X8, Canada

Westphal, I.
Institut für Humangenetik und Anthropologie
der Universität Heidelberg, Im Neuenheimer Feld 328,
D-6900 Heidelberg 1, Federal Republic of Germany

Wunder, E.
Institut Jacques Monod, CNRS, Université Paris VII, Tour 43,
2 place Jussieu, 75252 Paris Cédex 05, France

Zakrzewski-Lüdcke, S.
Institut für Humangenetik, Freie Universität Berlin,
Heubnerweg 6, D-1000 Berlin 19, Federal Republic of Germany

Zhang, M.
Laboratory for Investigative Dermatology, The Rockefeller
University, 1230 York Avenue, New York, NY 10021-6399, USA

Zhu, T.H.
Institute for Molecular Biology, Nan-Kai University,
94 Weijin Road, Tianjin, People's Republic of China

Part I

Clinical and Therapeutical Aspects

International Fanconi Anemia Registry: First Report*

A. D. Auerbach, A. Rogatko, and T. M. Schroeder-Kurth

Introduction

Progress has been made in the elucidation of the basic mechanisms that underlie both developmental abnormalities and malignancy through careful studies of heritable diseases that predispose persons to these problems. Fanconi anemia (FA), ataxia-telangiectasia, xeroderma pigmentosum, and Bloom syndrome are a few examples of such rare disorders, which are of interest in their own right but have even more significance because of their relevance to cancer predisposition and the interaction of genetic and environmental factors in cancer risk. Registries for surveillance of cancers have been established for Bloom syndrome (German et al. 1984), ataxia-telangiectasia (Spector et al. 1978) and xeroderma pigmentosum (Lambert 1987). In order to study a large number of FA patients with the full spectrum of the diverse features of the disease, the International Fanconi Anemia Registry (IFAR) was established at The Rockefeller University in 1982. The registry serves as a central repository for clinical, hematologic, and genetic information on FA patients. The large clinical database generated by the IFAR and cellular material stored from IFAR patients and their families provide an important resource which should enable us to better define the disorder.

It has recently been recognized that the FA phenotype, originally characterized by progressive pancytopenia, diverse congenital abnormalities, and increased predisposition to malignancy (Fanconi 1967; Schroeder et al. 1976; Swift 1971), is so variable that diagnosis on the basis of clinical manifestations alone is difficult and often unreliable (Glanz and Fraser 1982; Alter and Potter 1983). Literature reports of FA are undoubtedly biased toward the most severe clinical cases, since our concept of the syndrome is based on the cases originally described, which showed many congenital malformations, and cases that do not conform to this preconceived picture will not be diagnosed. FA patients without congenital malformations who were previously described as having the Estren-Dameshek syndrome

* This work was supported in part by Basil O'Connor Starter Research Grant No. 5-446 from the March of Dimes Birth Defects Foundation (A. D. A.), by PHS Grant No. HL32987 from the National Institutes of Health (A. D. A.), by a General Clinical Research Center Grant RR00102 from the National Institutes of Health to The Rockefeller University Hospital, by support from the Pew Memorial Trust to the Laboratory for Investigative Dermatology, by PHS Grant No. GM36295 from the National Institutes of Health (A. R.), and by the Deutsche Forschungsgemeinschaft (T. M. S.-K.).

T. M. Schroeder-Kurth A. D. Auerbach G. Obe (Eds.)
Fanconi Anemia, Clinical, Cytogenetic and Experimental Aspects

(Estren and Dameshek 1947; Dallapiccola et al. 1980) are found in the same sibships as classical FA patients (Glanz and Fraser 1982), indicating that phenotypic diversity cannot be accounted for by genetic heterogeneity alone.

Although the molecular basis of the syndrome is unknown, hypersensitivity to the clastogenic effect of DNA cross-linking agents provides a unique marker for the FA genotype (Sasaki and Tonomura 1973; Auerbach and Wolman 1976, 1978). This cellular characteristic can be used to identify preanemic cases as well as patients with aplastic anemia or leukemia who do not show the physical features characteristic of the syndrome (Auerbach et al. 1981; Cervenka et al. 1981; Duckworth-Rysiecki et al. 1984). It is useful for prenatal as well as postnatal diagnosis of FA (Auerbach et al. 1985, 1986). For purposes of the IFAR, we have classified patients as FA or non-FA, based on their sensitivity to the clastogenic effect of diepoxybutane (DEB), a difunctional alkylating agent, or to other DNA cross-linking agents such as mitomycin C (MMC).

Patients

Ascertainment of Patients

The primary source of case material for the IFAR was voluntary reporting by physicians. Announcements in hematology and genetics journals, posters at national meetings, and approaches to physicians at medical centers known to specialize in the treatment of aplastic anemia have led to the reporting of possible cases by interested physicians. Patients were ascertained on the basis of the presence of congenital malformations known to be associated with FA, hematologic manifestations such as aplastic anemia or leukemia, both aplastic anemia and malformations, or family screening. Once a potential case was identified, an IFAR questionnaire form was completed by the referring physician and copies of laboratory reports and other patient records were obtained (see Appendix 1 for IFAR questionnaire). Whenever possible, patients were examined by one of us. Chromosome breakage studies including testing for hypersensitivity to the clastogenic effect of the DNA cross-linking agent DEB were performed (Auerbach et al. 1981, 1985, 1986). Patients were classified as FA or non-FA on the basis of the sensitivity of cultured peripheral blood lymphocytes to DEB-induced chromosomal breakage. Blood specimens from siblings of FA patients were also tested.

Diagnosis of Fanconi Anemia

Of a total of 222 patients with completed IFAR questionnaires, 162 were classified as FA and 60 as non-FA. Cells from FA patients exhibited multiple chromatid breaks and exchanges after exposure to a concentration of DEB that had little clastogenic effect on normal cells; considerable variation in the response of cells from different FA patients was found. In FA patients, the mean frequency of baseline chromosomal breakage was 0.25 breaks per cell (range, 0.02–0.8 mean chromosome breaks per cell), and the mean frequency of DEB-induced chromosomal breakage was 9.2 breaks per cell (range, 1.06–23.9 mean chromosome breaks per

Table 1. DEB-induced chromosomal breakage in lymphocytes from FA patients with two cell populations

Case	Sex	Age	Mean chromosome breaks/cell	Cells with breaks (%)	Mean chromosome breaks/aberrant cell
1[a]	F	10	2.10	19	11.10
2	M	2	1.34	24	5.58
3[b]	M	21	1.60	36	4.44
4[b]	F	20	1.60	38	4.21
5	M	7	1.06	19	5.58
6	M	12	2.57	32	8.03
7	M	16	1.60	40	4.00
Means			1.70	29.7	6.13

[a] This patient has a sister with typical FA breakage.
[b] These patients are siblings and have a brother with typical FA breakage and another affected brother who died prior to our ascertainment of the family.

cell). There was no significant difference in chromosomal instability between male and female FA patients. While most FA patients exhibited typical chromosomal breaks and exchanges in most or all cells analyzed after DEB exposure, seven patients appeared to have two populations of cells (Table 1). In these individuals, the majority (between 60% and 81%) of DEB-treated cells examined appeared to have no chromosomal breakage, while the remainder of cells examined in each case exhibited the high number of breaks and exchanges typical of FA patients. The mean DEB-induced breakage in these seven patients ranged from 1.06–2.57, a frequency at least five times that of patients diagnosed as non-FA, while the mean breakage frequency calculated as breaks per aberrant cell was 6.13. Three of these cases were from multiplex sibships in which the proband exhibited typical FA breakage. Thus this phenomenon of two cell populations does not seem to be related to genetic heterogeneity in FA. It is important to note that false-negative diagnoses would probably be obtained in these FA patients with two cell populations if diagnostic tests for FA based on differential inhibition of cell growth when FA and normal lymphocytes are co-cultured in a medium containing MMC are used (German et al. 1987; Arwert and Kwee, this volume). Patients with some clinical manifestations of FA, diagnosed as nonaffected on the basis of our DEB test, exhibited a mean baseline breakage frequency of 0.03 breaks per cell (range, 0–0.12 breaks per cell) and a mean DEB-induced breakage frequency of 0.06 breaks per cell (range, 0–0.26 breaks per cell).

Constitution of Patient Sample

The constitution of the sample consisting of the 222 patients with completed IFAR questionnaires, classified by sex, is shown in Table 2. There was no significant difference in the sex ratio in either of the two groups ($\chi_1^2=0.25$, $p=0.62$). The clinical manifestations of the FA patients were highly variable, and many non-FA patients showed some clinical features associated with FA. Table 3 shows

Table 2. Constitution of the IFAR sample by DEB sensitivity and sex

Group	Sex					
	Male		Female		Total	
	(*n*)	(%)	(*n*)	(%)	(*n*)	(%)
FA	79	35.6	83	37.4	162	73
Non-FA	27	12.2	33	14.9	60	27
Total	106	47.7	116	52.3	222	100

Table 3. Basis of diagnosis of FA and non-FA

Aplastic anemia	Malformations					
	No		Yes		Total	
	(*n*)	(%)	(*n*)	(%)	(*n*)	(%)
FA						
No	8	4.9	39	24.1	47	29
Yes	43	26.5	72	44.4	115	71
Total	51	31.5	111	68.5	162	100
Non-FA						
No	0	0	18	30	18	30
Yes	33	55	9	15	42	70
Total	33	55	27	45	60	100

the presence or absence of hematologic manifestations and congenital malformations at the time of diagnosis in both the FA and non-FA patient groups. Both hematologic abnormalities and congenital malformations were the basis for diagnosis in only 44% of FA patients; 51% had only malformations or hematologic symptoms and 5% had neither. This latter group was comprised of siblings of probands who were diagnosed as affected on the basis of a DEB test with a positive result. These eight patients all developed hematologic manifestations of FA after the chromosome breakage studies were performed. Our sample differs from that obtained by a review of the literature, as most reports in the literature required both hematologic manifestations and congenital malformations to be present for a diagnosis of FA to be made. Among the non-FA patients, 85% had only hematologic manifestations or malformations resembling those associated with FA, while 15% had both features. The total number of congenital abnormalities found in patients with any given abnormality is shown in Tables 4–6. A comparison of the FA and non-FA groups shows that many of the patients from both groups have overlapping phenotypes. When FA males and females are compared, it is seen that the total sum of abnormalities in males tends to be greater than in females. Abnormalities which occurred with significantly greater frequency in FA males than in FA females were growth retardation, microphthalmia, and malformations of the heart or kidney.

Table 4. Congenital abnormalities in FA males

Abnormality	Total number of abnormalities											
	0	1	2	3	4	5	6	7	8	9	10	11
Birthmarks		3	1	6	8	3	8	5	4	4	1	2
Thumb and radius		0	1	3	8	9	11	6	4	3	1	2
Other skeletal		0	0	1	2	2	5	5	2	4	1	2
Kidney and urinary		1	0	1	2	1	8	6	1	4	1	2
Genital		0	1	1	3	6	6	4	4	4	1	1
Cardiac		0	0	1	2	4	4	4	1	2	0	2
Ear, deafness		0	0	1	4	1	2	3	4	1	1	1
Microphthalmia		0	1	3	3	2	6	7	5	3	0	2
Microcephaly		0	0	2	6	10	8	6	5	3	1	2
Growth retardation		2	2	4	10	10	12	8	5	4	1	2
Learning disabilities		1	0	0	1	3	3	3	1	1	1	2
Other		0	0	1	7	4	5	6	4	3	1	2
Total	2	7	3	8	14	11	13	9	5	4	1	2

Table 5. Congenital abnormalities in FA females

Abnormality	Total number of abnormalities										
	0	1	2	3	4	5	6	7	8	9	10
Birthmarks		5	11	8	7	6	2	7	3	0	1
Thumb and radius		1	7	3	8	4	3	8	4	1	1
Other skeletal		0	1	2	6	4	3	7	3	1	0
Kidney and urinary		1	5	5	3	2	2	5	3	1	1
Genital		0	0	0	0	0	0	1	0	0	0
Cardiac		0	0	2	1	0	1	3	1	1	1
Ear, deafness		0	0	1	3	1	0	7	3	0	1
Microphthalmia		0	0	1	4	4	3	10	4	1	1
Microcephaly		0	2	2	5	3	3	10	4	1	1
Growth retardation		0	9	5	8	5	3	10	4	1	1
Learning disabilities		1	1	0	1	1	1	4	1	1	1
Other		0	2	4	7	4	3	5	2	1	1
Total	4	8	19	11	13	7	4	11	4	1	1

Discriminant Analysis

Two sets of categorical variables were analyzed for the DEB-positive (DEB$^+$) and DEB-negative (DEB$^-$) patient groups: hematologic manifestations and congenital abnormalities (see Appendix 1, IFAR form, questions 6 and 12). The basic question to be answered is whether the DEB$^+$ and DEB$^-$ cases may be considered as belonging to distinct clinical groups, and if so, which are the variables that provide the best discrimination between these groups. In order to test the clinical basis of the classification of patients by the DEB sensitivity test, a stepwise multivariate logistic regression was applied (Dixon et al. 1981). The dependent variable was group (DEB$^+$ or DEB$^-$), and the predictors were the five types of hematologic

Table 6. Congenital abnormalities in non-FA males and females

Abnormality	Total number of abnormalities									
	0	1	2	3	4	5	6	7	8	9
Birthmarks		1	5	1	3	1	2	1		1
Thumb and radius		4	0	2	2	1	2	2		1
Other skeletal		2	0	5	4	1	1	2		1
Kidney and urinary		1	1	0	1	0	0	1		0
Genital		0	0	2	0	1	0	1		0
Cardiac		0	0	1	1	0	0	1		1
Ear, deafness		0	0	1	1	2	1	2		1
Microphthalmia		0	0	1	1	0	0	0		1
Microcephaly		0	2	1	4	1	1	1		1
Growth retardation		1	5	4	5	2	1	1		0
Learning disabilities		1	4	3	3	1	2	0		1
Other		1	1	3	3	0	2	2		1
Total	18	11	9	8	7	2	2	2		1

Table 7. Probability of belonging to FA group based on the simplified score

Simplified score	FA (n)	Non-FA (n)	(p)
−1	0	3	0
0	5	12	0.29
1	19	32	0.37
2	43	10	0.81
3	43	3	0.93
4 or > 4	52	0	1

manifestations scored (low red cell counts, low white cell counts, low platelet counts, preleukemia, or leukemia) and the 12 congenital abnormalities scored (see Tables 4-6). Each variable was coded for presence or absence.

The eight variables that best discriminate between the two groups are: (1) microphthalmia, (2) birthmarks, (3) kidney and urinary abnormalities, (4) growth retardation, (5) learning disabilities, (6) absence of radius and/or thumb, (7) other skeletal abnormalities, and (8) low platelet count (Auerbach et al. 1989). The fit of the data to the logistic model is very good ($p = 0.998$). Thus it is possible to determine the probability of a patient ascertained through the usual procedures of the IFAR (see the section on "Ascertainment of Patients") being DEB^+ or DEB^-, taking into account only the presence or absence of these eight selected clinical markers. Therefore, the DEB^+ and DEB^- groups of patients ought to be considered as belonging to distinct clinical entities.

Instead of using the logistic model to classify a patient, a simplified score was derived (Auerbach et al. 1989). Although these eight abnormalities are all found with a higher frequency in FA patients than in the general population, markers 1, 2, 3, 4, 6, and 8 are more indicative of the DEB^+ group, while markers 5 and 7 are more indicative of the DEB^- group. By adding one point for the presence of each of the first set of abnormalities (markers 1–8, except 5 and 7), and subtracting one point for the presence of each of the second set (markers 5 and 7), one can predict the probability of a patient belonging to the DEB^+ or DEB^- groups. The greater the score, the higher the probability of belonging to the DEB^+ group. The distribution of this score is given in Table 7. In the IFAR sample, if the score is equal to or greater than 4, the discrimination is absolute; all such patients were DEB^+ in the chromosome breakage analysis.

Segregation Analysis

A segregation analysis was performed on the IFAR sibships in order to study the mode of inheritance and to test the homogeneity of the FA (DEB^+) and non-FA (DEB^-) groups, which had sample sizes of 88 and 31 probands with siblings, respectively. The segregation probability (p) and the probability of being a sporadic case (x) are the parameters of interest (Morton 1959), and are expected to be $p = 0.25$ and $x = 0$ in a simple autosomal recessive mode of inheritance. In order to make inferences about these two parameters a Bayesian approach was developed, since the ascertainment of the sample was uncertain (Rogatko and Auerbach 1988).

The results of the analysis are presented in Figs. 1 and 2, which show the distributions of p and x respectively, for the two groups, with the modal values and the 95% credible intervals. A 95% credible interval (or Bayesian confidence interval) means that the true value of the parameter has a probability of 0.95 of belonging to this interval (Rogatko et al. 1986). The credible intervals of the two groups include the values of $p = 0.25$ and $x = 0$. Therefore the two groups can be considered as homogeneous with respect to these two parameters and the inheritance follows a monogenic autosomal recessive mode. However, the modal values suggest that the frequency of sporadic cases might the greater in the non-FA group ($x = 0.399$)

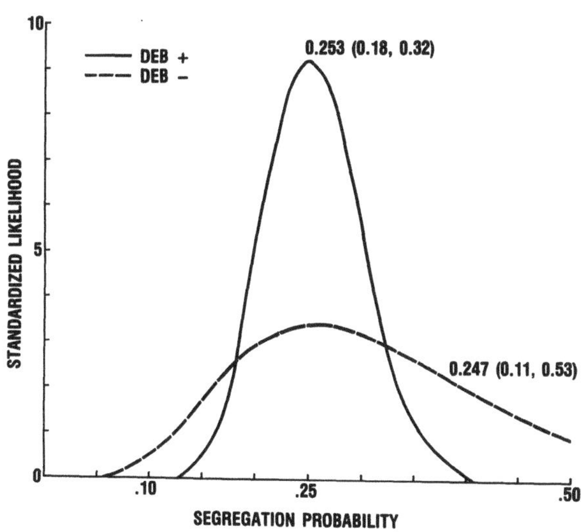

Fig. 1. Marginal distributions of p (segregation probability) for DEB^+ and DEB^- groups with modal values and credible intervals in parentheses

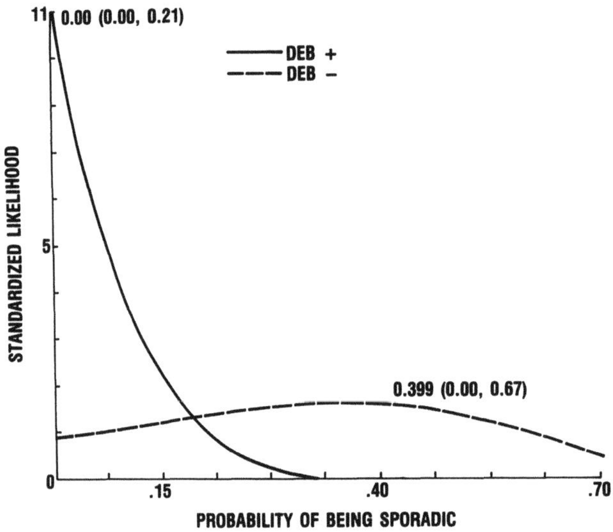

Fig. 2. Marginal distributions of x (probability of being a sporadic case) for DEB^+ and DEB^- groups with modal values and credible intervals in parentheses

than in the FA group ($x=0$), although the difference between the two groups was not significant at the 5% level. It is likely that the non-FA group is highly heterogeneous and comprises a variety of genetic and nongenetic entities.

Preliminary Analysis of the Fanconi Anemia Group

Although the number of patients in the FA group is currently too small to enable us to draw definitive conclusions regarding questions related to the clinical course of the disease, a statistical analysis of some of the age-related data ascertained on the FA patients may be useful. There was a negative correlation between the age of hematologic onset and the number of congenital abnormalities present. Males have more congenital abnormalities and a younger age of onset of hematologic manifestations than females. There was no significant correlation between the age of onset of hematologic manifestations and the duration of disease (age at death minus age of onset of hematologic manifestations). There were no significant sex differences in the age of death and duration of the disease.

Heterogeneity within the FA group was determined by studying multiplex sibships, of which there were 16 in the IFAR. The age of onset of hematologic manifestations showed a very high heritability (1.0 ± 0.34) indicating that the great differences between sibships in this variable are due to genetic heterogeneity. On the other hand, analysis of the number of congenital abnormalities found within sibships showed lower heritability (0.61 ± 0.36); thus modifier genes or other factors probably play a role in the etiology of the malformations.

Conclusion

The IFAR serves as a worldwide referral center for FA patients. Information on patients is furnished to us by physicians, who submit a completed IFAR questionnaire, as well as copies of laboratory reports and other patient records. Our current database consists of 222 patients who have been tested for sensitivity of peripheral blood lymphocytes to the clastogenic effect of DNA cross-linking agents such as DEB. Results of a discriminant analysis of the IFAR database indicate that patients with DEB^+ and DEB^- results belong to discrete groups which should be considered as being clinically distinct. For purposes of the registry, these groups will be designated as FA and non-FA.

The results of a segregation analysis performed on the IFAR sibships show that for both the FA and non-FA groups the inheritance follows a monogenic autosomal recessive mode. However, the analysis suggests that the two groups differ in that the frequency of sporadic cases was much lower in the FA than in the non-FA group. It seems likely that the non-FA group is highly heterogeneous, consisting of a variety of genetic and nongenetic entities.

Data currently gathered indicate that the clinical diversity in FA patients is much more widespread than previously recognized. In approximately 30% of the patients who had positive results in the DEB test there was no evidence of any congenital abnormalities. These patients have all developed hematologic manifestations typical of FA. An analysis of the multiplex sibships in the registry shows that some of these patients have siblings exhibiting the classical FA phenotype. Therefore, there is no longer any basis for the distinction between the classical and the Estren-Dameshek forms of the syndrome. We suggest that all patients under the age of 25 with aplastic anemia of unknown etiology need to be tested for DEB sensitivity in order to rule out a diagnosis of FA.

We are continuing to enter patients in the IFAR and expect that a larger database followed up for a longer period of time will result in additional new and interesting information. A larger sample size should enable us to better characterize the non-FA group of patients. Questions relating to diagnosis, natural history of the disease, prognosis, treatment, and cancer incidence in FA will be addressed in the future. We need to gather more information on the age-related variables in order to better predict the life expectancy of FA patients. These are all questions which FA families and their physicians are continually asking, and it is expected that the IFAR will serve as a valuable resource in finding answers.

References

Alter BP, Potter NU (1983) Long term outcome in Fanconi's anemia: description of 26 cases and review of the literature. In: German J (ed) Chromosome mutation and neoplasia. Liss, New York, pp 43-62

Auerbach AD, Wolman SR (1976) Susceptibility of Fanconi's anaemia fibroblasts to chromosome damage by carcinogens. Nature 261: 494-496

Auerbach AD, Wolman SR (1978) Carcinogen-induced chromosome breakage in Fanconi's anaemia heterozygous cells. Nature 271: 69-71

Auerbach AD, Adler B, Chaganti RSK (1981) Prenatal and postnatal diagnosis and carrier detection of Fanconi anemia by a cytogenetic method. Pediatrics 67: 128-135

Auerbach AD, Sagi M, Adler B (1985) Fanconi anemia: prenatal diagnosis in 30 fetuses at risk. Pediatrics 76: 794-800

Auerbach AD, Zhang M, Ghosh R, Pergament E, Verlinksy Y, Nicholas H, Boué J (1986) Clastogen-induced chromosomal breakage as a marker for first trimester prenatal diagnosis of Fanconi anemia. Hum Genet 73: 86-88

Auerbach AD, Rogatko A, Schroeder-Kurth TM (1989) International Fanconi Anemia Registry: relation of clinical symptoms to diepoxybutane sensitivity. Blood 73: 391-396

Cervenka J, Arthur D, Yasis C (1981) Mitomycin C test for diagnostic differentiation of idiopathic aplastic anemia and Fanconi anemia. Pediatrics 67: 119-127

Dallapiccola B, Alimena G, Brinchi V, Isacchi G, Gandini E (1980) Absence of chromosome heterogeneity between classical Fanconi's anemia and the Estren-Dameshek type. Cancer Genet Cytogenet 2: 349-360

Dixon WD, Brown MB, Engleman L, Frane JW, Hill MA, Hennrich RI, Toporek JD (eds) (1981) BMDP statistical software 1981. University of California Press, Los Angeles

Duckworth-Rysiecki G, Hulten M, Mann J, Taylor AMR (1984) Clinical and cytogenetic diversity in Fanconi's anaemia. J Med Genet 21: 197-203

Estren S, Dameshek W (1947) Familial hypoplastic anemia of childhood. Report of eight cases in two families with beneficial effect of splenectomy in one case. Am J Dis Child 73: 671-687

Fanconi G (1967) Familial constitutional panmyelocytopathy, Fanconi's anemia (FA). I. Clinical aspects. Semin Hematol 4: 233-240

German J, Bloom D, Passarge E (1984) Bloom's syndrome XI. Progress report for 1983. Clin Genet 25: 166-174

German J, Schonberg S, Caskie S, Warburton D, Falk C, Ray JH (1987) A test for Fanconi's anemia. Blood 69: 1637-1641

Glanz A, Fraser FC (1982) Spectrum of anomalies in Fanconi anaemia. J Med Genet 19: 412-416

Lambert WC (1987) Genetic diseases associated with DNA and chromosomal instability. Dermatol Clin 5: 85-108

Morton NE (1959) Genetic tests under incomplete ascertainment. Am J Hum Genet 11: 1-16

Rogatko A, Auerbach AD (1988) Segregation analysis with uncertain ascertainment: application to Fanconi anemia. Am J Hum Genet 42: 889-897

Rogatko A, Pereira CAB, Frota-Pessoa O (1986) A Bayesian method for the estimation of penetrance: application to mandibulofacial and frontonasal dysostoses. Am J Med Genet 24: 231-246

Sasaki MS, Tonomura A (1973) A high susceptibility of Fanconi's anemia to chromosome breakage by DNA cross linking agents. Cancer Res 33: 1829-1836

Schroeder TM, Tilgen D, Krüger J, Vogel F (1976) Formal genetics of Fanconi's anemia. Hum Genet 32: 257-288

Spector BD, Perry GS, Kersey JH (1978) Genetically determined immunodeficiency disease (GDID) and malignancy. Report from the Immunodeficiency-Cancer Registry. Clin Immunol Immunopathol 11: 12-29

Swift M (1971) Fanconi's anaemia in the genetics of neoplasia. Nature 230: 370-373

Appendix 1

Leave Blank

Patient IFAR ______
Physician Code ______
Date received ______
Date of follow-up ______

International Fanconi Anemia Registry (IFAR)

(This information is confidential and for research purposes only)

1. Referring physician:
   a. Name______
   b. Address ______
   street city state zip
   c. Telephone______ d. Specialty______
   e. Date of report______
2. a. Patient's name______
   b. Address______
   street city state zip
   c. Telephone______
   d. Sex______ e. Date of birth______
   f. Place of birth ______
   city state country
   g. If deceased, date of death______
3. Date of diagnosis of Fanconi anemia______ Age at diagnosis______
   Place of diagnosis______
4. Ascertainment: aplastic anemia □ malformations □ family screening □ genetic counseling □ leukemia or cancer □ other______
5. Basis of diagnosis: aplastic anemia □ malformations □ family history □ cytogenetic studies □ leukemia or cancer □ other______
6. Does the patient have hematologic manifestations? Yes □ No □ Red cells □ white cells □ platelets □ Preleukemia □ Leukemia □
   If yes, date of onset of hematologic manifestations______ Age______
   Antecedent illness or medication______
   ______
   ______
   Treatment ______
   ______
   ______
   (Please send copies of hematology, bone marrow aspirate, and bone marrow biopsy reports, and bone marrow smear and biopsy slides (for a comparative study, if possible. All slides will be returned.)
7. Has the patient been reported in the literature? Yes □ No □. If yes, give reference or enclose reprint______
   ______
8. Has the patient had cytogenetic studies? Yes □ No □. If yes, please give date, laboratory, and result (please enclose a copy of the report, if available)
   ______
   ______
9. Have cells from the patient been tested for sensitivity to mutagens?
   Yes □ No □. If yes, please give date, laboratory, chemical used, and results.______
   ______
   ______

10. Have cultured cell lines been established from the patient?
    Yes □ No □. If yes, please give laboratory, and cell line designation.
    ____
    ____

11. Birth history:
    a. Full term □ Premature □ Gestational age______
    b. Complications during pregnancy______________________________
    ____
    c. Type of delivery______________________________
    d. Measurements at birth: weight______ (%ile___) length______ (%ile___)
    head circumference______ (%ile___).
    e. APGAR score______________ f. General status at birth______________
    ____

12. Summary of medical history (please give description, treatment, date):
    a. Abnormalities noted at birth or in childhood:
        1. Birthmarks, moles, café-au-lait spots______________________
        2. Thumb and radius______________________
        3. Other skeletal______________________
        4. Kidney and urinary tract______________________
        5. Genital______________________
        6. Cardiac______________________
        7. Ear, deafness______________________
        8. Eye (such as microphthalmia)______________________
        9. Microcephaly______________________
        10. Growth retardation, failure to thrive______________________
        11. Learning disabilities______________________
        12. Other______________________
        ____
        ____
    b. Hospitalizations or surgery:
        1.______________________
        2.______________________
        3.______________________
        4.______________________
    c. Acquired illnesses (heart, liver, kidneys, blood, bone, cancer, chronic conditions)__________
    ____
    ____
    d. Allergies ______________________
    e. Frequent infections______________________
    f. If deceased, please provide information and autopsy report if available__________
    ____
    ____
    ____

13. Growth and development:
    a. Age when walked__________ talked__________
    b. Were developmental "milestones" normal? Yes □ or delayed □
    If delayed, comment______________________
    ____
    c. Was the onset of puberty and secondary sexual development normal?
    Yes □ No □ Not applicable □ If no, comment______________________
    ____
    d. Has menstruation started? Yes □ No □
    If yes, age at onset______________________
    e. Current weight______ (%ile___) height ______ (%ile___)
    Head circumference______ (%ile___) Date of measurements__________

14. Family History: If a pedigree is available, please enclose a copy. (Medical history should include history of birth defects, short stature, anemia, leukemia, cancer, diabetes).

a. Mother's name____________________ Date of birth__________
Height________ National origin____________________
Medical history______________________________

b. Father's name____________________ Date of birth__________
Height________ National origin____________________
Medical history______________________________

c. Parental consanguinity (are the parents of the patient related)?
Yes ☐ No ☐. If yes, please specify____________________

d. Please indicate the ancestral groups to which the parents belong. Answer as many as apply. (P: paternal, M: maternal).

P M		P M		P M	
____	British Isles	____	Polish	____	African (Negro)
____	Scandinavian	____	Russian	____	American Indian
____	German	____	Ashkenazi Jewish	____	Mexican
____	French	____	Sephardic Jewish	____	Other Latin America
____	Spanish	____	Other Jewish	____	Japanese
____	Italian	____	Middle Eastern	____	Chinese
____	Greek	____	North African	____	Other Asian
____	Turkish	Other (please specify)__________			

e. Siblings: Number (full)____ (half)____
List below, in order of pregnancy, all full and half siblings of the patient. Please include deceased siblings, stillbirths and abortuses. For additional information, use space provided on next page.

Name	Sex	Date of Birth	Full or half	Medical History
1.____				
2.____				
3.____				
4.____				
5.____				
6.____				
7.____				
8.____				

Use this space for additional information on any of the above individuals, or if more than 8 siblings.____________________

f. Have HLA studies been done in this family? Yes ☐ No ☐. If yes, please enclose a copy of the results.

g. Other family history or any other information you think may be helpful.
(Include relatives with malformations, anemia, leukemia, or cancer).

____
____
____
____
____
____
____
____
____
____
____

Please return to nearest IFAR center.

Arleen D. Auerbach, Ph. D.
Assistant Professor
Laboratory for Investigative Dermatology
The Rockefeller University
1230 York Avenue
New York, New York 10021-6399
USA
(212) 570-7533

Traute M. Schroeder-Kurth
Professor Dr. med.
Institute of Human Genetics
University of Heidelberg
Im Neuenheimer Feld 328
6900 Heidelberg
West Germany
06221-563877

These data may be published in summary form, with proper acknowledgement.

____
Signature of physician

Appendix 2

Leave Blank

Patient IFAR ______
Physician Code ______
Date received ______
Date of follow-up ______

International Fanconi Anemia Registry (IFAR)
Follow-Up Questionnaire
(This information is confidential and for research purposes only)
(will be sent out annually)

1. a. Patient's name______________________________
   b. Sex______ c. Date of birth______________
2. Has the patient been reported in the literature since entered in IFAR?
   Yes □ No □. If yes, please give reference or enclose report______________________
   ____
3. Is the patient deceased? Yes □ No □
   If deceased, date of death______________
   Cause of death______________________________________
   (Please provide autopsy report if available)

4. Does the patient have hematologic manifestations?
   Status as of_____ Yes ☐ No ☐ Red cells ☐ White cells ☐
   Platelets ☐ Preleukemia ☐ Leukemia ☐
   Current status: Yes ☐ No ☐ Red cells ☐ White cells ☐
   Platelets ☐ Preleukemia ☐ Leukemia ☐
   Date of onset of hematologic manifestations__________ Age________
   Antecedent illness or medication____________________

   Treatment____________________

   (Please send copies of hematology, bone marrow aspirate, and bone marrow biopsy reports.)
5. Medical follow-up since________
   a. Hospitalizations and surgery ____________________

   b. Acquired illnesses ____________________

   c. Growth and development ____________________

6. Family History: Additional medical information relating to anemia, leukemia, cancer, diabetes etc. in close relatives.

7. Are there additional siblings born since________
   Yes ☐ No ☐

	Name	Sex	Date of Birth	Full or Half	Medical history
1.					
2.					

8. Any other information or questions:____________________

Thank you

Arleen D. Auerbach, Ph. D.
Assistant Professor
Laboratory for Investigative Dermatology
The Rockefeller University
1230 York Avenue
New York, New York 10021-6399
U.S.A.
(212) 570-7533

Traute M. Schroeder-Kurth
Professor Dr. med.
Institute of Human Genetics
University of Heidelberg
Im Neuenheimer Feld 328
6900 Heidelberg
West Germany
06221-563877

____
Signature of physician

Fanconi Anemia in The Netherlands

M. L. Kwee and L. P. Kuyt

Introduction

Fanconi anemia (FA), first described by Fanconi in 1927, is an autosomal recessive disease characterized by aplastic anemia (pancytopenia with bone marrow hypoplasia) and associated with a variety of congenital anomalies, increased risk of malignancy, and chromosomal instability (Schroeder et al. 1964). The basic defect is still unknown. The congenital malformations may vary in site and severity and some patients do not have any malformation at all (Alter and Potter 1983; Glanz and Fraser 1982). The age of onset of pancytopenia is also variable. This variability in symptoms causes problems in the early diagnosis of the disease. The aims of this study were:

1. To evaluate the intrafamilial and interfamilial variability of the clinical, hematological, and cytogenetic findings in the patients
2. To determine the most useful diagnostic symptoms and signs postnatally as well as prenatally
3. To test the data for the presumed autosomal recessive inheritance
4. To study the genealogical aspects of FA families

Material and Methods

In the Netherlands there is not yet a registry of birth defects. Sources of our study were:

1. The Departments of Pediatrics and Hematology of the eight academic hospitals, and two Pediatric Departments of regional and local hospitals in the Netherlands. They provided data on 20 probands and 11 affected sibs. The Department of Pediatrics of the Academic Hospital of the State University of Leiden is the only center for bone marrow transplantation for children in the Netherlands and contributed a relatively high number of FA cases.
2. Centers for Clinical Genetics and Cytogenetics affiliated to the eight universities in the Netherlands. The cooperation of five centers resulted in data on four probands and three affected sibs.
3. Referrals from a regional hospital for cytogenetic evaluation in our specialized laboratory. This resulted in data on one proband and one affected sib.

T. M. Schroeder-Kurth A. D. Auerbach G. Obe (Eds.)
Fanconi Anemia, Clinical, Cytogenetic and Experimental Aspects

In total, these sources provided us with data on 25 Dutch probands (16 males and nine females), diagnosed in the past 29 years (1957–1986), and on 15 affected sibs (seven males and eight females).

The probands were born between 1945 and 1986, the affected sibs between 1951 and 1984. Only in two cases were the medical records not available. In one of these cases, the medical records of a subsequently affected sib described the clinical history of the previously affected proband (which had led to the diagnosis of both cases). Therefore these two cases and their sibship were included in the analysis. In the other case, no clinical or cytogenetic data could be obtained, for which reason we excluded that particular sibship, leaving 39 patients (24 probands and 15 affected sibs) and their sibships for analysis. Cases of foreign origin were not studied because of inadequate information about family history. The following diagnostic criteria were used:

1. Clinical symptoms relevant to FA and chromosomal instability, or
2. Clinical symptoms relevant to FA and a sib with FA as described above, or
3. Chromosomal instability and a sib with FA as described above.

Therefore cases or sibships with symptoms resembling FA but without proven chromosomal instability were excluded from this study.

Results

Patients are referred to in the tables by case number. If there is more than one affected child in one sibship, the letter a is used for the proband, and b, c, etc., for the affected sibs. Data regarding pregnancy and birth of the patients are presented in Table 1. Low birthweight was noticed in six probands and one affected sib. Two of them had been born prematurely. Head measurements were available in only a small proportion of cases.

Congenital Anomalies

The anomalies found in the probands and their affected sibs as noted in medical records are described in Table 2. These two groups are compared in Table 3. Usually the proband had more malformations than the affected sib within the same sibship. Four probands and four affected sibs had no congenital malformation besides pigment spots (in four of them, Table 2: 12a, 12b, 13c, 19b). Congenital hydrocephaly was found in one proband and his affected sib. Their stillborn nephew had phocomelia of the arms, a renal anomaly, and esophageal atresia with tracheoesophageal fistula (Hustinx et al. 1987). This nephew was not included in our study because there had been no chromosomal investigation, his parents were not related to each other, and their heterozygosity could not be proven.

A variety of renal anomalies was found in the patients (Table 4). Undescended testicles were uni- or bilateral. Anomalies of the anus were either atresia, malpositioned anus, rectourethral fistula, or a persisting cloaca. One patient had vaginal atresia, a uterine anomaly, a streak ovary, and an anal anomaly. In some cases the

Table 1. Birth data of patients with FA

Case no.	Sex	Pregnancy (weeks)	Birth weight (kg)	Length (cm)	Head circumference (cm)
1	M	ND	3.5	ND	ND
2	M	at	3.5	ND	ND
3	M	42	2.7	46	ND
4	F	37	2.6	45	ND
5a	F	at	2.5	ND	ND
5b	M	ND	ND	ND	ND
6a	F	ND	ND	ND	ND
6b	F	ND	3.5	40	ND
7a	M	ND	ND	ND	ND
7b	M	ND	ND	ND	ND
8a	M	ND	ND	ND	ND
8b	F	ND	ND	ND	ND
9	F	at	2.8	50	ND
10	M	38	2.5	46	ND
11a	M	40	2.34	46	ND
11b	M	40	2.78	ND	ND
12a	F	ND	ND	ND	ND
12b	F	ND	ND	ND	ND
13a	M	36	1.05	33	27
13b	M	42	3	47	37
13c	M	ND	ND	ND	ND
14	M	36	2.02	48	ND
15	M	at	2.9	49	ND
16	M	at	3	51	35
17	M	at	3	52	ND
18a	F	at	2.35	48	ND
18b	M	ND	2.5	48	ND
18c	F	ND	2	ND	ND
19a	M	ND	ND	ND	ND
19b	M	ND	ND	ND	ND
20a	M	ND	2.7	ND	ND
20b	F	at	2.2	ND	ND
21a	F	ND	3.6	ND	ND
21b	F	ND	3.2	ND	ND
22	F	36	2.18	45	31.5
23a	M	ND*	ND	ND	ND
23b	F	ND	ND	ND	ND
24a	M	38	2.24	42	ND
24b	F	ND	ND	ND	ND

a, b, c, patients from one sibship (a, proband); M, male; F, female; ND, no data; *twin pregnancy; at, at term

ear was malformed and the external ear canals narrowed or atretic. Eye anomalies include microphthalmia, strabismus, epicanthal folds, or deep-set eyes. Congenital heart defects described in these patients were ventricular septal defect, persisting ductus Botalli, peripheral pulmonary stenosis. Anomalies of the radius, the first metacarpal, and the thumb were mild or severe, with or without shortening of the ulna, and uni- or bilateral. Foot anomalies were redressable clubfoot or toe syndactylia. Vertebral anomalies mentioned in some of these cases were hemivertebrae, fusion defects of vertebral arch, or torsion of the vertebrae. For some pa-

Table 2. Symptoms of FA patients

Type of malformation	Case no.																																						
	1	2	3	4	5a	b	6a	b	7a	b	8a	b	9	10	11a	b	12a	b	13a	b	c	14	15	16	17	18a	b	c	19a	b	20a	b	21a	b	22	23a	b	24a	b
Skin pigment anomaly	+	+	+	+	+	+			+		ND		+		+	+	+	+				+	+	+	+	+	+		+		+	+	+						
Microcephaly					+	+					ND				+	+									+														
Hydrocephaly											ND								+	+																			
Renal anomaly			+	+	+	+	+				ND		+	+	+	+			+	+				+			+								+			+	
Hypospadia						+					ND								+	+											+								
Undescended testicle	+								+		ND			+	+				+	+		+		+					+										
Anal anomaly											ND		+						+	+															+				
Vaginal anomaly											ND																								+				
Uterine anomaly											ND																								+				
Mental retardation				+	+						ND		+		+										+														
Ear anomaly											ND					+			+	+																			
Deafness					+						ND					+																							
Eye anomaly				+	+						ND		+		+				+	+					+		+		+									+	
Heart defect											ND								+	+						+		+							+		+		
Radius and thumb anomaly					+						ND		+						+	+							+								+				
Thumb hypo-/aplasia				+		+					ND			+					+			+		+		+		+										+	
Extra thumb											ND			+																									
Ulnar hypoplasia											ND								+								+								+				
Hip dislocation											ND	+							+	+																			
Foot anomaly											ND		+							+																			
Vertebral anomaly	+										ND					+									+														
Rib anomaly											ND		+																			+			+				
Annular pancreas							+				ND																												
Esophageal atresia and tracheoesophageal fistula											ND																	+											
Duodenal atresia											ND			+																									
Short stature (<P3)			+		+						ND					+																							

+, Symptom present
ND, No data

Table 3. Congenital anomalies of probands with FA and affected sibs

Type of abnormality	Probands (16 M, 8 F)	Affected sibs (7 M, 8 F)
Skin pigment anomaly	17	5
Microcephaly	3	2
Hydrocephaly	1	1
Renal anomaly	11	4
Hypospadia	3	2
Undescended testicle	8	1
Anal anomaly	3	1
Vaginal anomaly	1	–
Uterine anomaly	1	–
Mental retardation	5	–
Ear anomaly	1	2
Deafness	1	1
Eye anomaly	8	2
Cardiovascular	3	3
Radius and thumb anomaly	4	2
Thumb hypo-/aplasia	7	2
Extra thumb	1	–
Ulnarhypoplasia	2	1
Hip dislocation	1	2
Foot anomaly	1	1
Vertebral anomaly	2	1
Rib anomaly	2	2
Annular pancreas	1	–
Esophageal atresia and tracheoesophageal fistula	–	1
Duodenal atresia	1	–
Short stature (< P3)	2	1

Table 4. Renal anomalies in FA patients

Anomaly	Patients ($n = 39$)
Aplasia	8
Duplication of pelvis and/or ureter	2
Ectopic or pelvic kidney	2
Horseshoe kidney	2
Hydronephrosis	2
Congenital renal cysts	2

tients described as small and slenderly built, exact measurements were not available. There was mild or severe mental retardation, but some patients had normal intelligence.

Hematological Symptoms

The usual presenting features were pallor and hematomas due to anemia and thrombocytopenia. The onset of pancytopenia was gradual without clinical symptoms of pancytopenia. The anemia was macrocytic, with poikilo- and anisocytosis and reticulocytopenia. The bone marrow was hypocellular; sometimes hypercellularity was found in the early stages of pancytopenia. Increased fetal hemoglobin concentration was observed in all patients. Two probands had leukemia, one had acute myeloblastic leukemia (AML) (Roozendaal and Nelis 1984), and the other acute lymphoblastic leukemia (ALL) as the first hematological manifestation of the disease.

Cytogenetic Analysis

Cytogenetic studies of peripheral lymphocytes of patients with FA showed normal karyotype, with an increased number of spontaneous chromatid and isochromatid breaks and gaps, rearrangements, chromatid interchange figures, and endoreduplications compared to the cultures of healthy controls. Aberrations were found in 10%-70% of the patients' cells and in less than 10% of the controls' cells. These chromosomal anomalies were found prior to the onset of pancytopenia in five patients (case nos. 4, 13, 18b, 22, 24a).

Culture of patients' cells (obtained from peripheral lymphocytes or skin fibroblasts) in the presence of clastogens (DNA-alkylating agents, e.g., mitomycin C, diepoxybutane, or *cis*-platinum in concentrations not toxic for the healthy controls' cells) showed a clear increase in the number of chromosomal breaks and rearrangements compared to unexposed cells (Auerbach and Wolman 1976; Auerbach et al. 1981; Cervenka et al. 1981; Kwee et al. 1983; Poll et al. 1982; Sasaki and Tonomura 1973). This method is used as a diagnostic test for FA (Cervenka et al. 1981). We performed these tests with different concentrations of clastogens in four of these patients from three different sibships (cases nos. 18b, 22, 23a, b). At concentrations of clastogens that hardly affected normal cells, three of the four patients exhibited a concentration-dependent increase in the number of cells with aberrant chromosomes, with a concomitant increase in the number of chromosomal aberrations per aberrant cell. The fourth patient (an adult affected sib who has congenital anomalies and only mild hematological symptoms, case no. 18b) was exceptional because with all three clastogens only 40% of his cultured cells exhibited a typical concentration-dependent response, while 60% of his cells responded like those from normal healthy controls (Kwee et al. 1983). This investigation was repeated three times at 1-year intervals with similar results. Later on, these tests were also done on two other adult FA patients of one sibship (cases nos. 12a, b), but they showed the same response as cases nos. 22, 23a and b mentioned before.

The cytogenetic method for diagnosis of FA is also used in second trimester prenatal diagnosis using amniotic cells obtained by amniocentesis in the 16th week of pregnancy, or in first trimester prenatal diagnosis using trophoblastic cells obtained by chorionic villi sampling in the 9th week of pregnancy (Auerbach et al. 1981, 1985, 1986; Shipley et al. 1984). The cytogenetic method was used in four pregnancies; it allowed the identification of three affected sibs, which was followed by termination of pregnancy. One fetus was unaffected. The diagnosis was confirmed postnatally.

Diagnosis

Most of the patients were diagnosed at the time when pancytopenia developed, which was between the ages of 5 and 10 years. The median age of probands at diagnosis was 4.5 years in females and 8 years in males (Table 5). Three patients were diagnosed at a relatively late age (13, 18, and 26 years). Four patients were diagnosed shortly after birth or in the preanemic phase of the disease because of the typical skeletal anomalies or multiple congenital malformations and chromo-

Table 5. Sources of data, general data, and year FA was diagnosed in patients in our sample

Probands				Affected sibs			
Case no.	Sex	Year of birth	Year of diagnosis	Case no.	Sex	Year of birth	Year of diagnosis
Groningen							
1	M	1957	1969				
2	M	1959	1969				
3	M	1958	1974				
4	F	1983	1986				
5a	F	1945	1957	5b	M	1951	1957
6a	F	1962	1969	6b	F	1963	1974
7a	M	1969	1979	7b	M	1981	1981[a]
8a	M	1968	?[b]	8b	F	1981	1981
Nijmegen							
9	F	1976	1980				
10	M	1980	1984				
	F	1956	?[b]				
11a	M	1976	1981	11b	M	1979	1983
12a	F	1968	1981	12b	F	1956	1982
13a	M	1982	1982	13b	M	1980	1982
				13c	M	1984	1984[a]
Leiden							
14	M	1971	1975				
15	M	1969	1976				
16	M	1973	1983				
17	M	1975	1983				
18a	F	1962	1967	18b	M	1960	1968
				18c	F	1951	1968
19a	M	1969	1974	19b	M	1978	1982
20a	M	1969	1975	20b	F	1966	1980
21a	F	1970	1977	21b	F	1962	1980
Amsterdam							
22	F	1979	1979				
23a	M	1968	1981	23b	F	1971	1981
Utrecht							
24a	M	1984	1984				
Rotterdam							
				24b	F	1986	1986[a]

a, b, c, patients from one sibship (a, proband); M, male; F, female; ND, no data.
[a] Prenatally diagnosed.
[b] Excluded from further analysis because of lack of information.

somal instabilities. An important factor in the early diagnosis is also how well the pediatrician is acquainted with this rare disease. Affected sibs were usually diagnosed shortly after the probands, because of similar phenotype and/or related clinical symptoms. In some cases, a sib was only found to be affected when he or she was investigated for bone marrow transplantation donorship. Two affected sibs were diagnosed retrospectively post mortem (Table 5: case nos. 13 b and 18 c), after the diagnosis had been made in the younger proband based upon family history, congenital malformation, hematological problems, and cytogenetic results. Patients with radius and thumb anomalies were diagnosed at an earlier age than those without these anomalies. Fetal ultrasound studies of skeletal anomalies supported the prenatal cytogenetic diagnosis.

Course of the Disease

Some probands showed progressive pancytopenia whereas others were chronically anemic. Affected sibs usually had fewer symptoms and a milder course of the disease. Some of them did not need therapy at all. One affected sib also had chronic renal failure (case no. 5 b). Besides leukemia in two probands (cases nos. 17 and 23 a) no other malignancy was found. Patient no. 23 a recovered and is still in remission (Roozendaal and Nelis 1984).

Therapy

Treatment of patients with progressive pancytopenia consisted of supportive therapy, e.g., transfusions of red cells, platelets, or white cells. Therapy androgens and corticosteroids resulted in improvement in some patients (Table 6). These drugs have virilizing side effects. Liver toxicity or hepatomas were not reported in our cases. Two probands and one affected sib (case nos. 1, 6 b, and 21 a) received bone marrow transplants (Vossen 1984).

Age and Cause of Death

In general, the prognoses of FA patients are poor. Most of the patients died from severe pancytopenia, hemorrhage, sepsis, or a combination of these (Table 6). One proband died of leukemia. Two patients died of graft-versus-host disease after bone marrow transplantation. Eleven patients died between the ages of 5 and 13 years, about 2-9 years after diagnosis. The oldest patient alive is 30 years old (case no. 12 b). Three patients died shortly after birth because of severe congenital malformations. An autopsy was performed in case nos. 6 a and 13 a. Besides the known symptoms, hyperplasia of the liver with no sign of malignancy was found in case no. 6 a. The three cases diagnosed prenatally showed no physical abnormalities.

Obligate Heterozygotes: Parents of Probands

Assuming autosomal recessive inheritance in all FA patients and a very small chance, with normal paternity, of spontaneous mutation of a normal gene into an FA gene, all parents of FA patients are obligate heterozygotes. Anomalies or dis-

Table 6. Cytogenetic studies, treatment, and causes of death

Cytogenetic results	Case no.																																						
	1	2	3	4	5a	b	6a	b	7a	b	8a	b	9	10	11a	b	12a	b	13a	b	c	14	15	16	17	18a	b	c	19a	b	20a	b	21a	b	22	23a	b	24a	b
Increased spontaneous chromosomal breakage	+	+	+	+			+	+	+	+	ND	+	+	+	+	+	+	+	+		+	+	+	+	+	+	+		+	+	+	+	+	+	+	+	+	+	+
Increased sensitivity to:																																							
Mitomycin C				+					+		ND	+	+	+	+	+	+	+					+	+	+		+		+		+	+	+	+	+	+	+	+	+
Diepoxybutane										+	ND																+								+	+	+	+	+
Cis-platinum											ND																+								+	+	+		
Not investigated					+	+					ND									+								+											
Therapy																																							
Transfusions	+				+	+	+		+		ND						+									+			+	+			+			+			
Corticosteroids									+		ND				+	+						+	+			+							+						
Androgens	+	+	+		+		+		+		ND				+	+							+						+				+						
Bone marrow transplant	+							+			ND																						+						
Cytostatics											ND														+											+			
None				+							ND	+						+	+	+							+				+	+		+	+			+	
Cause of death																																							
Pancytopenia					+	+	+															+				+			+	+	+								
Hemorrhage	+					+																+								+			+						
Graft-versus-host disease	+																																+						
Congenital abnormalities																			+	+								+											
Leukemia																									+														
Sepsis																																	+						
Abortion										+											+																		

ND, no data

eases of the parents mentioned in the medical records of the probands were: unilateral ureteropelvic obstruction in the mother (nine relatives of this mother have urinary tract anomalies) and small pelvic kidney in the father (case nos. 11 a, b; Hamel 1986); uterus bicornis bicollis and epidermolysis bullosa in the mother (case no. 2); and neurofibromatosis in the father (case no. 4). There were no parents with radial ray anomalies, anemia, or malignancy. Cytogenetic studies were done by us in the parents of case no. 23 only; the results were not significantly different from those of healthy controls.

Table 7. Data of sibships in FA families

	Sibship		Sibs					Abortion	Parental consanguinity
	No.	Size	Affected		Nonaffected		Ratio		
			M	F	M	F	Aff.: Nonaff.		
A	5	3	1	1	0	1	2 : 1	–	+
	6	8	0	2	4	2	2 : 6	–	–
	7	3	2	0	1	0	2 : 1	1[a]	–
	8	5	1	1	3	0	2 : 3	–	+
	11	2	2	0	0	0	2 : 0	1	–[b]
	12	4	0	2	1	1	2 : 2	–	+
	13	3	3	0	0	0	3 : 0	1[a]	
	18	4	1	2	1	0	3 : 1	1	–[c]
	19	3	2	0	1	0	2 : 1	–	–
	20	3	1	1	1	0	2 : 1	–	–
	21	4	0	2	1	1	2 : 2	–	+
	23	3	1	1	1	0	2 : 1	–	–
	24	2	1	1	0	0	2 : 0	1[a]	–
Total		47	15	13	14	5	28 : 19	5	4
B	1	9	1	0	5	3	1 : 8	–	–
	2	4	1	0	2	1	1 : 3	–	+
	3	4	1	0	2	1	1 : 3	–	–
	4	2	0	1	1	0	1 : 1	–	–
	9	1	0	1	0	0	1 : 0	3	–[b]
	10	2	1	0	0	1	1 : 1	1	–[c]
	14	3	1	0	1	1	1 : 2	–	–
	15	2	1	0	0	1	1 : 1	–	–
	16	4	1	0	3	0	1 : 3	–	–
	17	3	1	0	1	1	1 : 2	–	–
	22	3	0	1	0	2	1 : 2	–	–
Total		37	8	3	15	11	11 : 26	4	1
Total *A+B*		84	23	16	29	16	39 : 26	6+3[a]	5

A, Sibships with more than one affected member; *B*, sibships with only one affected member
[a] Prenatally diagnosed affected fetus.
[b] Common ancestor six generations back.
[c] Common ancestor four or five generations back.

Sibships

Only four of the 45 nonaffected sibs were investigated cytogenetically. Most of the nonaffected sibs were considered not to have the disease because they had no hematological problems and no congenital malformations typical of FA. In total, 13 sibships had more than one affected child and 11 sibships had only one affected child (Table 7). There were in total six spontaneous abortions among the mothers mentioned in the medical records of the probands; these were not investigated.

Genealogical Studies

Data for pedigree analysis were obtained from the parents of 24 families/sibships. Genealogical data were collected from state and local archives. The information was based upon population records, civil registration (instituted during the French occupation in 1810 and maintained and developed since then), parish records with the registration of births, marriages and deaths, notarial records, and the registration of death duties.

The 24 pedigrees, made up to the eighth and mostly ninth generation, showed a remarkable concentration of the descent of the ancestors in the provinces of Friesland, Groningen, Drenthe and Overijssel, i. e., the northern and north eastern part of the Netherlands (Fig. 1). Interestingly, this particular concentration of ancestral birthplaces does not correlate with the distribution of the general population of the Netherlands, which is more concentrated in the provinces located in the western part of the country. Only a few ancestors were found in the south western part of the Netherlands. Parental consanguinity was proven in five of the 24 pedigrees (Fig. 2), which is more frequent than would be expected. Four FA sibships are related to each other (Fig. 3). Other pedigrees showed a kind of relationship based upon common ancestral birthplaces, mostly small villages with peasants and day laborers. The degree of correlation between ancestral consanguinity and the close geographical relationship of their birthplaces is not yet known, and is a matter for further study.

Segregation Analysis

The 24 FA sibships collected (N) comprise a total of 84 children (T) of whom 39 are recessives (R) (Table 7). The hospital or physicians' records contain only those patients who come for treatment, and therefore only their families are known to the investigator. The chance of an affected sibship being ascertained is probably proportional to the number of affected persons within a sibship. The sample is therefore not representative of the true distribution of FA families in the general population. We therefore used Li's method (Li 1954), subtracting one recessive member from each sibship in our analysis. The corrected estimate of the recessive proportion in such families is:

$$b = \frac{R-N}{T-N} = \frac{39-24}{84-24} = \frac{15}{60} = 0.2500$$

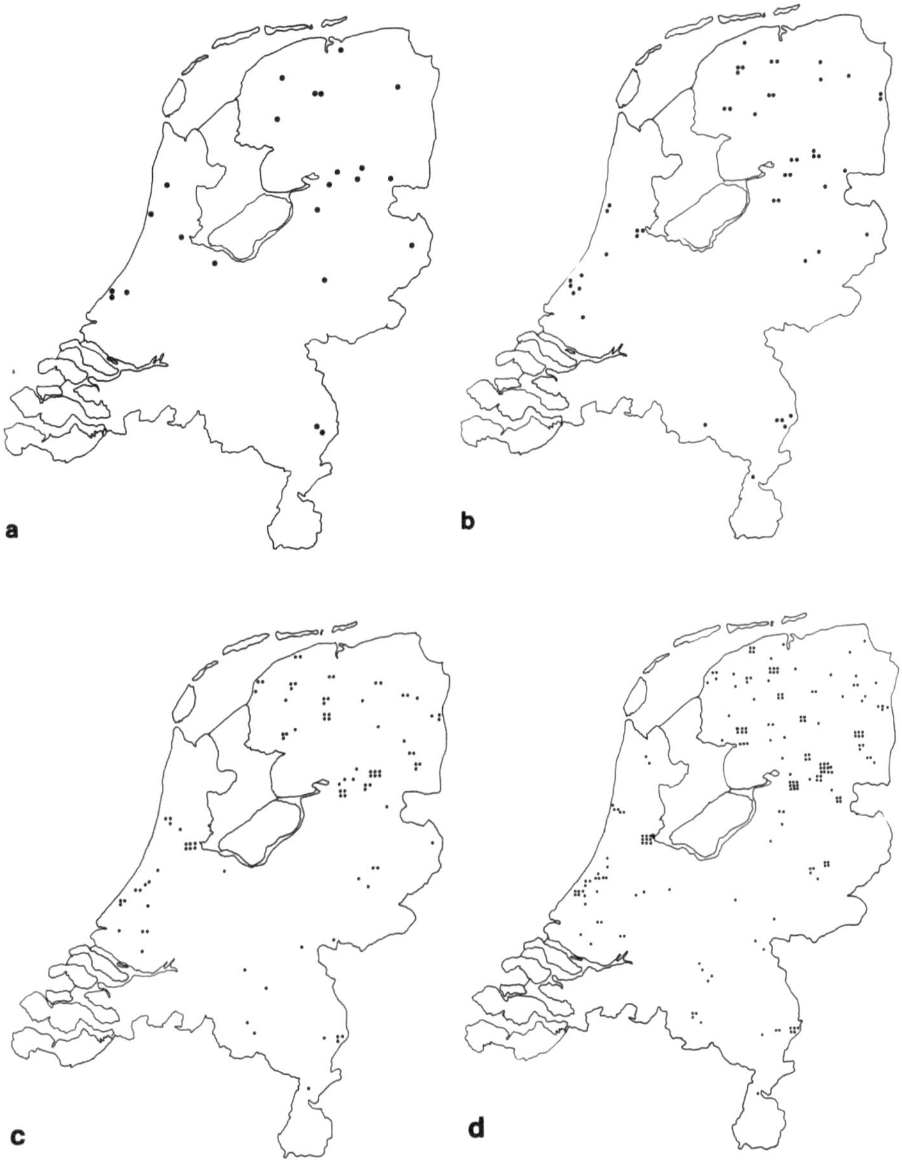

Fig. 1. a–d. Birthplaces of **a** probands, **b** their parents, **c** their grandparents, and **d** their great-grandparents

$$\text{with variance } v(b) = \frac{ab}{T-N} = \frac{3/4 \times 1/4}{84-24} = \frac{0.1875}{60} = 0.003125$$

$v(b) = 0.003125$, standard error of $b = \sqrt{0.003125} = 0.0559$

($a = 1 - b$, a being the probability that a child will be normal given that it has two normal heterozygote parents).

The total numbers are too small for truncate analysis.

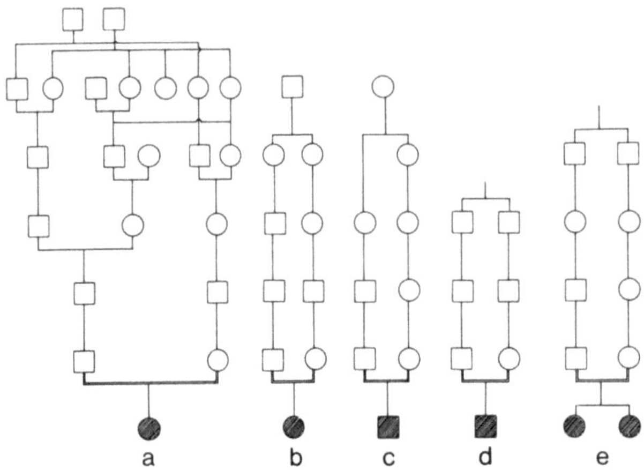

Fig. 2

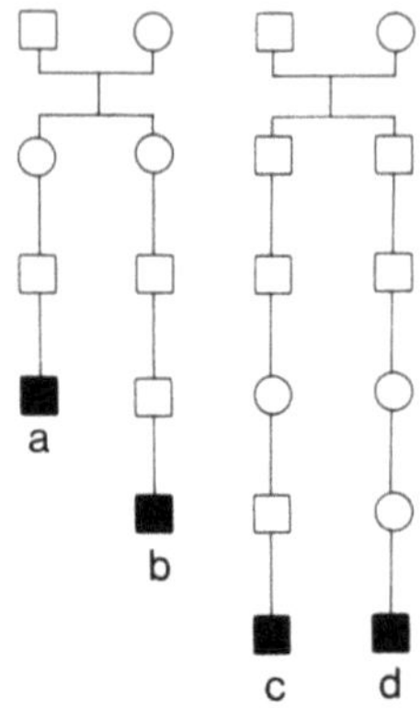

Fig. 3

Fig. 2. Parental consanguinity in pedigree of patients with FA in case nos. 5 (*a*), 22 (*b*), 2 (*c*), 8 (*d*), and 12 (*e*)

Fig. 3. Relation between FA sibships in case nos. 18 (*a*), 10 (*b*), 11 (*c*), 9 (*d*)

Discussion

The variability of congenital anomalies in the patients with FA is inter- as well as intrafamilial. Usually, the affected sibs have fewer anomalies than the proband of the same sibship. There is no clear difference in severity of the congenital anomalies or age of onset of pancytopenia between the sexes. Four probands and four affected sibs had no congenital anomalies besides a skin pigment anomaly (in four of them, Table 2: 12a, 12b, 18 c, 19b. There is no correlation between the severity of the anomalies and the course of the disease. FA patients with several anomalies and especially those with radial ray defects were diagnosed earlier than those patients without anomalies.

The sex ratio among probands shows a (nonsignificant) male preponderance, in accordance with previous reports (Alter and Potter 1983). This suggests a better ascertainment of affected male probands, since the sex ratio among affected sibs is close to 1:1. A better ascertainment of male probands cannot be explained since there are no FA-specific genital abnormalities: cryptorchidism is the only sex-linked anomaly which is easily identified and frequently observed on physical examination but no indication for FA. Anomalies of the female genital tract were never the presenting sign leading to the diagnosis FA but were only observed as an additional feature. Furthermore, the sex ratio among all presumably nonaffected sibs also shows a male preponderance for unknown reasons.

It was mentioned in the medical records of most patients that their other sibs and parents were healthy and without congenital anomalies. However, full investigations including physical examination, hematological investigation, intravenous pyelography, radiography of the forearms, wrists, and hands, body measurements, and cytogenetic studies especially are required to rule out the disease.

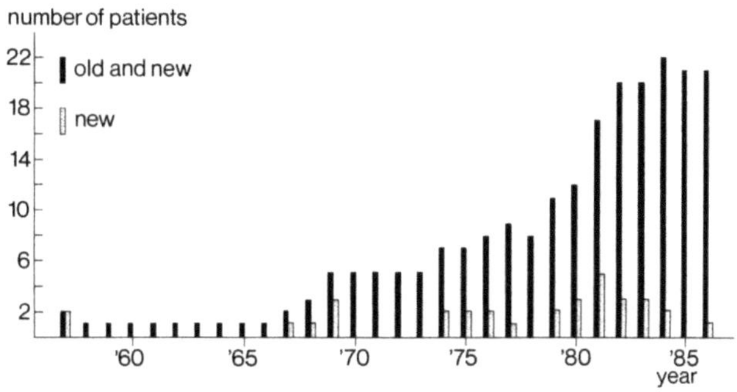

Fig. 4. Number of known FA patients alive 1957–1986

The congenital anomalies mentioned in this article are not specific for FA, which has to be differentiated from several syndromes (genetic as well as nongenetic) like Baller-Gerold syndrome (Anyane-Yeboa et al. 1980), the VACTERL association (Quan and Smith 1973), TAR syndrome (Hall et al. 1969), Holt-Oram syndrome (Holt and Oram 1960), the IVIC syndrome (Arias et al. 1980), Aase syndrome (Aase and Smith 1969), WT syndrome (Gonzalez et al. 1977), syndromes with a combination of radial ray defects and renal abnormalities (Siegler et al. 1980), dyskeratosis congenita (Sirinavin and Trowbridge 1975), Schwachman syndrome (Aggett et al. 1980), other chromosomal syndromes (Butler et al. 1982; Gardner et al. 1984; Haspeslagh et al. 1984), etc. The aplastic anemia present in FA should be differentiated from other constitutional aplastic anemias (Cervenka et al. 1981; Griffiths 1983; Zaizov et al. 1969), and from the acquired form of aplastic anemia, as the genetic implications are vital.

The hematological course showed intra- as well as interfamilial variability in age of onset and course of the disease. Again, the proband is usually the most severely affected in any one sibship, probably due to selection, as diagnosis was made on more significant anomalies or symptoms. As the anomalies and the onset of the hematological symptoms are variable, the most useful diagnostic tool to be applied in FA postnatally as well as prenatally is the cytogenetic investigation. The presence of mosaicism in peripheral lymphocyte-sensitivity to clastogens was seen in one adult male patient with FA, who has a radial ray defect and only mild hematological symptoms. We did not find this mosaicism in two other adult female patients with FA. Cytogenetic methods have not yet proved reliable for the detection of heterozygotes. Early diagnosis of the first affected child makes it possible to offer to the parents first- or second-trimester prenatal diagnosis in subsequent pregnancies and may prevent the birth of another affected child.

This study confirmed the mode of autosomal recessive inheritance of FA; the proportion of recurrence was within the expected one-quarter (0.2500 + 0.0559). The sex ratio of the patients was not significantly different from 1:1; FA in parents was absent, and parental consanguinity frequent. In applying Li's method (Li 1954), we assumed incomplete ascertainment of cases. There may have been an underrepresentation of cases with a typical symptomatology and sibships with single cases. The increase in the prevalence of FA in recent years (Fig. 4) is probably due to the improvement in diagnostic methods so that more cases are detected at an earlier age, and mild cases are also diagnosed.

Genetic heterogeneity could not be investigated with the material available. The high proportion of sibships with common ancestors or ancestors born in a similar region in the Netherlands suggests the same single gene defect for the FA cases ascertained.

Acknowledgements. The authors acknowledge the contributions of Drs. F. Arwert, F. A. Beemer, A. S. P. M. Breed, J. H. M. Bollen, J. O. van Hemel, T. W. J. Hustinx, H. Joenje, J. de Koning, J. J. P. van de Kamp, D. Lindhout, L. Meertens, C. van Oostrom, K. J. Roozendaal, G. A. M. de Vaan, E. T. van't Veer-Korthof, J. A. de Vries, C. M. R. Weemaes, and Professors A. W. Eriksson, G. B. Humphrey, G. B. A. Stoelinga, J. M. J. J. Vossen. We thank Dr. D. Lindhout for critical comments on the manuscript, Mrs. D. Boden, A. Oostra, and A. H. Wanamarta for technical assistance, and Mr. G. J. Lijnzaad for preparing the illustrations.

References

Aase JM, Smith DW (1969) Congenital anemia and triphalangeal thumbs: a new syndrome. J Pediatr 74: 471-474

Aggett PJ, Cavanagh NPC, Matthew DJ, Pincott JR, Sutcliffe J, Harries JT (1980) Schwachman's syndrome. Arch Dis Child 55: 331-347

Alter BP, Potter NU (1983) Long term outcome in Fanconi's anemia. Description of 26 cases and review of the literature. In: German J (ed) Chromosome mutation and neoplasia. Liss, New York, pp43-62

Anyane-Yeboa K, Gunning L, Bloom AD (1980) Baller-Gerold syndrome. Clin Genet 17: 161-166

Arias S, Penchaszadeh VB, Pinto-Cisternas J, Sarrausi S (1980) The IVIC syndrome: a new autosomal dominant complex pleiotropic syndrome with radial ray hypoplasia, hearing impairment, external ophthalmoplegia and thrombocytopenia. Am J Med Genet 6: 25-59

Auerbach AD, Wolman SR (1976) Susceptibility of Fanconi's anaemia fibroblasts to chromosome damage by carcinogens. Nature 261: 494-496

Auerbach AD, Alder B, Chaganti RSK (1981) Prenatal diagnosis and carrier detection of Fanconi anemia by cytogenetic method. Pediatrics 67: 128-135

Auerbach AD, Sagi M, Adler B (1985) Fanconi anemia: prenatal diagnosis in 30 fetuses at risk. Pediatrics 76: 794-800

Auerbach AD, Zhang M, Ghosh R, Pergament E, Verlinsky Y, Nicolas H, Boué J (1986) Clastogen induced chromosomal breakage as a marker for first trimester prenatal diagnosis of Fanconi anemia. Hum Genet 73: 86-88

Butler MG, Russel LJ, Palmer CG, Bull M, Hodes ME (1982) A child with radius aplasia, cleft of lip and palate, microcephaly and unusual chromosome findings. Am J Med Genet 13: 369-372

Cervenka J, Arthur D, Yasis C (1981) Mitomycin C test for diagnostic differentiation of idiopathic aplastic anemia and Fanconi anemia. Pediatrics 67: 119-127

Fanconi G (1927) Familiäre infantile perniziosaartige Anaemie (perniziöses Blutbild und Konstitution). Jahrb Kinderheilkd 117: 257-280

Gardner RJM, Grindley RM, Chewings WE, Clarkson JE (1984) Ring chromosome 1 associated with radial ray defect. J Med Genet 21: 400

Glanz A, Fraser FC (1982) Spectrum of anomalies in Fanconi anaemia. J Med Genet 19: 412-416

Gonzalez CH, Durkin-Stamm MV, Geimer NF, Shahidi NT, Schilling RF, Rubira F, Opitz JM (1977) The WT syndrome - a "new" autosomal dominant pleiotropic trait of radial/ulnar hypoplasia with high risk of bone marrow failure and/or leukemia. Birth Defects Orig Artic Ser XIII (3 B): 31-38

Griffiths AD (1983) Constitutional aplastic anaemia: a family with a new X-linked variety of amegakaryocytic thrombocytopenia. J Med Genet 20: 361-364
Hall JG, Levin J, Kuhn JP, Ottenheimer LJ, van Berkum KAP, McKusick VA (1969) Thrombocytopenia with absent radii (TAR). Medicine (Baltimore) 48: 411-439
Hamel BCJ (1966) Urinary tract abnormalities in a family with Fanconi Anaemia (Abstract). In: 7th International Congress of Human Genetics, Berlin, Part II, p 699
Haspeslagh M, Fryns JP, Moerman Ph (1984) Severe limb malformations in 4p deletion. Clin Genet 25: 353-356
Holt M, Oram S (1960) Familial heart disease with skeletal malformations. Br Heart J 22: 236
Hustinx TWJ, Scheres JMJC, Bollen JHM, Taalman RDFM, van Eyk R, Weemaes CMR (1987) Clinical variability in Fanconi's anaemia: examples of the extremes. Am Univ Sarav Med (Suppl) 7: 152-154
Kwee ML, Poll EHA, van de Kamp JJP, de Koning H, Eriksson AW, Joenje H (1983) Unusual response to bifunctional alkylating agents in a case of Fanconi anaemia. Hum Genet 64: 348-387
Li CC (1954) Some methods of studying human genetics. Methods Med Res 6: 1-38
Poll EHA, Arwert F, Joenje H, Eriksson AW (1982) Cytogenetic toxicity of antitumor platinum compounds in Fanconi anemia. Hum Genet 611: 228-230
Quan L, Smith DW (1973) the VATER association, Vertebral defects, Anal atresia, T-E fistula with esophageal atresia, Radial and Renal dysplasia: a spectrum of associated defects. J Pediatr 82: 104
Roozendaal KJ, Nelis KOAH (1984) Leukemia in a case of Fanconi's anaemia (Abstract). Clin Genet 25: 208
Sasaki MS, Tonomura A (1973) A high susceptibility of Fanconi's anemia to chromosome breakage by DNA crosslinking agents. Cancer Res 33: 1829-1836
Schroeder TM, Anschütz F, Knopp A (1964) Spontane Chromosomenaberrationen bei familiärer Panmyelopathie. Humangenetik 1: 194-196
Shipley J, Rodeck CH, Garrett C, Galbraith J, Gianelli (1984) Mitomycin C induced chromosome damage in fetal blood cultures and prenatal diagnosis of Fanconi's anaemia. Prenat Diagn 4: 217-221
Siegler RL, Larsen P, Buehler BA (1980) Upper limb anomalies and renal disease. Clin Genet 17: 117-119
Sirinavin C, Trowbridge A (1975) Dyskeratosis congenita: clinical features and genetic aspects. J Med Genet 12: 339-354
Vossen JMJJ (1984) Experience with bone marrow transplantation in Fanconi's anemia (Abstract). Clin Genet 25: 209
Zaizov R, Matoth Y, Mamon Z (1969) Familial aplastic anaemia without congenital malformations. Acta Paediatr Scand 58: 151-156

Clinical Aspects of a Cluster of 42 Patients in South Africa* with Fanconi Anemia

S. Smith, M. P. Marx, C. J. Jordaan, and C. H. van Niekerk

Introduction

Fanconi anemia (FA) is one of the chromosomal instability syndromes, a group of disorders with diverse etiologies and different clinical manifestations.

FA is an autosomal recessive disorder, characterized by bone marrow hypoplasia, usually beginning with thrombocytopenia and later on developing into pancytopenia; it is associated with a variety of phenotypic abnormalities. The hematological features of the disease usually appear between the ages of 5 and 9, but can become apparent at any time between the ages of 17 months and 22 years (Schroeder et al. 1976; Glanz and Clarke Fraser 1982). In 1927 Fanconi described three siblings with anemia, skin pigmentation, microcephaly, strabismus, hyperreflexia, and genital hypoplasia. Subsequently other abnormalities were added to the list (Beard et al. 1973; Nilson 1960; Gmyrek and Syllm-Rapoport 1964).

Phenotypic abnormalities may be present in one or more of the following: the skeleton, the skin, the renal and central nervous systems, the cardiovascular, ocular, and auditory systems (Glanz and Clarke Fraser 1982; Gözdasöğlu et al. 1980). The abnormalities vary from patient to patient, and some cases may even show no abnormality at all. A few cases of familial hypoplastic anemia without associated congenital anomalies - the Estren-Dameshek variant of FA (Estren and Dameshek 1947) - have been documented. This variability in expression of the disease, however, makes firm diagnosis of FA on clinical grounds alone almost impossible. Cytogenetic studies (Auerbach et al. 1981; Marx et al. 1983; Cervenka and Hirsch 1983) have demonstrated chromosomal abnormalities in both affected homozygous persons and the heterozygous carriers.

The diagnosis of FA can be confirmed by cytogenetic methods. The lymphocyte and bone marrow cultures of FA homozygotes show a high frequency of spontaneous chromosomal breaks. Diepoxybutane (DEB) is a difunctional alkylating agent which seems to be specific for the cellular defect in FA (Auerbach and Wolman 1976, 1978; Marx et al. 1983; see also Schroeder-Kurth et al., this volume). DEB stress causes a drastic increase in chromosomal damage in FA cells. Cells from patients with FA show a ten- to 30-fold increase in chromosomal damage when subjected to DEB in vitro. Cells from heterozygous FA gene carriers do

* This work was supported in part by grants from the South African Medical Research Council and by the Central Research Fund UOFS

T. M. Schroeder-Kurth A. D. Auerbach G. Obe (Eds.)
Fanconi Anemia, Clinical, Cytogenetic and Experimental Aspects

not demonstrate an increase in the number of spontaneous chromosomal breaks, but a three- to five-fold increase in the number of chromosomal breaks is caused by DEB stress in such cells. Using this method, we were able to clearly differentiate FA homozygotes, FA heterozygotes, and normal controls (Marx et al. 1983).

The pathogenesis of FA is still unexplained, although chromosomal instability, including spontaneous and induced chromosomal breaks (Schroeder et al. 1976; Schroeder 1982; Cervenka and Hirsch 1983; Auerbach et al. 1981), may be related to subsequent neoplastic change (Jacobs and Karabus 1983; Potter et al. 1983). Treatment remains controversial; anabolic androgens stimulate the erythropoiesis to maintain a reasonable hemoglobin concentration and allogenec bone marrow transplantation is a method currently in use (Gluckman et al. 1984; Deeg et al. 1983; see also Ebell et al., this volume; Gluckman et al., this volume). We report here on our experience with a large cluster of 42 FA patients in 31 families.

Material and Methods

During the period from October 1979 to August 1986, 42 patients with an increased frequency of chromosomal breaks, pancytopenia and other features described as consistent with FA were studied. These patients were registered with the Hematology Service at the Bloemfontein Teaching Hospital of the University of the Orange Free State. In addition, 52 obligate heterozygotes were identified. The majority of these patients were diagnosed after presenting with some feature of bone marrow failure; some were diagnosed as a result of having an affected family member. All patients underwent a complete physical examination, as did all relatives who could be located.

At the Pediatric Hematology Clinic, 30 patients who presented with pancytopenia and varying phenotypic abnormalities were diagnosed as having FA. From 1982 onwards, all available family members of an affected individual were studied. The families of the 30 probands were examined physically, hematologically, and cytogenetically. This resulted in the screening of 178 blood relatives and the identification of another 12 FA homozygotes and 95 FA heterozygotes. Five of the 12 FA homozygotes showed some form of bone marrow failure, while the other seven were hematologically normal at the time of diagnosis. Since diagnosis, three of these seven FA homozygotes have developed hematological symptoms and now require therapy.

Initially all FA patients underwent the following routine investigations: a full blood count, bone marrow aspiration and histology, chromosomal analysis, intravenous pyelography, serum chemistry analysis, ferrokinetic studies, and chest X-ray. Later on during the study, additional investigations were carried out on all new patients and patients attending the follow-up clinic, i.e., homologous leukocytic antibody (HLA) typing, electrocardiography (ECG), electroencephalography (EEG), hemoglobin electrophoresis, and T cell subpopulation studies.

A physical examination was performed on 47 heterozygotes attending our clinic. They were related to the probands as follows: nine fathers, 12 mothers, six brothers, eight sisters, two uncles (mothers' brothers), four aunts (mothers' sisters), four cousins, and two maternal grandmothers. These relatives also underwent chromosomal analysis. HLA typing, intravenous pyelography (ten patients), full blood count and serum chemistry analysis.

Cytogenetic studies were carried out on peripheral blood lymphocytes and bone marrow cultures utilizing DEB, according to the method described elsewhere (Marx et al. 1983; see also Marx and Smith, this volume). Therapy for patients with FA was started as soon as problems secondary to bone marrow failure were encountered and consisted of daily administration of an oxymetholone preparation and prednisolone. This report will concentrate on the clinical aspects of our population, and certain selected findings of special investigations pertaining to literature reports.

Results

Description and Frequency of Anomalies

From our group of 47 patients, we listed the phenotypic abnormalities present in the 42 probands (Table 1). There were 14 males and 28 females, giving a male : female ratio of 1:2. Skin changes were the most frequent physical features (79%), these being hyperpigmentation, including café au lait spots, and hypopigmented

Table 1. Phenotypic abnormalities

Abnormality	Affected patients (%) ($n=42$)
Growth retardation	57
Skin changes	
Hyperpigmentation (café au laut)	79
Hypopigmentation	31
Microcephaly	48
Skeletal abnormalities	
Thumb - absence/hypoplasia	55
Fingers - polydactyly/syndactyly	17
Feet - pes cavus	7
Cardiovascular abnormalities	
Absent or displaced radial artery	19
Heart defects	12
Renal anomalies	7
Eye abnormalities	
Microphthalmia	43
Ptosis	26
Strabismus	29
Central nervous system	
Mental retardation	2
Learning disorders	19
Hyperreflexia	55
Hypogonadism	5

areas varying in size and shape but always numbering more than seven per patient. This confirms the frequency of hyperpigmentation already reported for patients with FA. Hypopigmentation, however, was found in 31% of our patients, which is more than previously reported. Growth retardation was present in 57% of patients. Another parameter of growth, head circumference, was below the third percentile for age in 48% of cases. Skeletal abnormalities consisted mainly of thumb abnormalities, with rudimentary thumbs and proximal displacement or absence of the thumb in 55% of the patients (Fig. 1). Thumb abnormalities or a hypoplastic thenar eminence were always associated with abnormalities of the radial artery. Infrequently encountered skeletal abnormalities were polydactyly in 17%, and foot abnormalities, which were even less common. Although often described as part of the classical picture of FA (Glanz and Clarke Frazer 1982; Gmyrek and Syllm-Rapoport 1964), radial abnormalities were not clinically detectable in any of our FA homozygous patients. X-rays, performed on 23 of our FA patients with clinically demonstrable thumb abnormalities, showed slight radial hypoplasia in only two cases (Fig. 1).

The facial features of all our patients, present despite prior androgen therapy (Fig. 2), were quite striking, resembling elfin facies with relative hypertrichosis. Microphthalmia was found in 43% and strabismus in 29% of the cases. The pres-

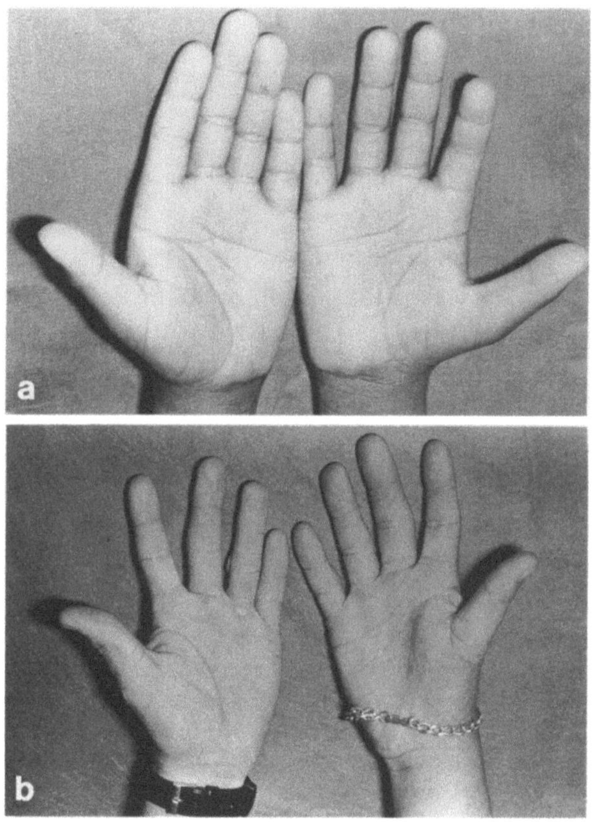

Fig. 1 a, b. Abnormalities of the thumb and hands in patients with FA

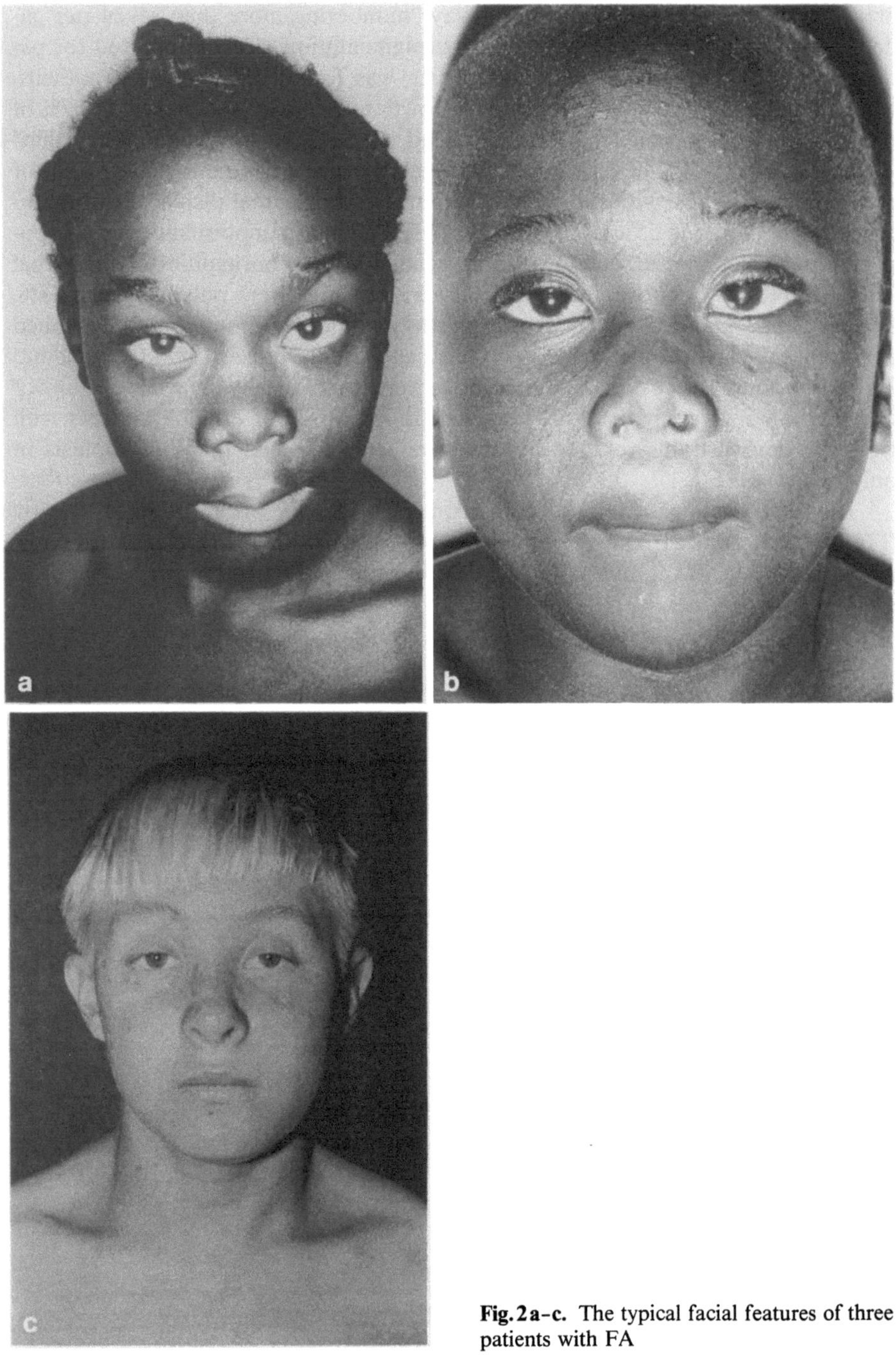

Fig. 2 a–c. The typical facial features of three patients with FA

ence of bilateral ptosis (in 26% of the patients) together with the other features mentioned made a quite typical facies.

The cardiovascular abnormalities found were displaced or missing radial arteries, either unilateral or bilateral, mostly in conjunction with abnormalities of the thumb. Five of our patients had heart defects: three a ventricular septal defect, one a pulmonary valve stenosis, and one a patent ductus arteriosus. Only the last condition required corrective surgery.

Central nervous system involvement consisted of (a) microcephaly (48%), (b) poor performance in school or need of special education, but not mental retardation (2%; only three patients were not in school at the time of this report), and (c) increased deep tendon (stretch) reflexes (55%). This last finding was especially noticeable on eliciting the knee jerk. Hyperreflexia demonstrated in tendon reflexes, especially at the knees, was fairly prominent, but hyporeflexia in at least one tendon was also demonstrated in 12% of our patients with FA.

No specific correlation could be found between the number of congenital abnormalities per patient and the age of onset of hematological problems. This seems to suggest that gross physical abnormalities are not an indication of the severity of the hematological manifestation of FA. One patient presented at the age of 6 months with unresponsive macrocytic anemia, and FA with primary lymphoma of bone was subsequently diagnosed. Another patient presented at the age of ten with a tendency to bleeding - no cause was established at that stage, but a splenectomy was performed. This patient developed acute lymphoblastic leukemia at the age of 45, and the diagnosis of FA was then cytogenetically confirmed.

Intravenous pyelography was a standard investigation in all our patients. In only three patients was an abnormality detected: ectopic kidneys in two instances and a horseshoe kidney with hydronephrosis in one.

Hematological Findings

The majority of our patients had complications secondary to bone marrow failure, usually from the age of five onwards; the average age of onset was 6 years and 7 months. The blood picture in the preanemic phase was normal with a tendency towards macrocytic hemopoiesis. The first noticeable abnormality in the peripheral blood was thrombocytopenia followed by leukopenia, with a predominance of lymphocytes, and later on macrocytic anemia. The histology of bone marrow aspiration in all the patients was compatible with hypoplastic anemia and showed depressed erythropoiesis and myelopoiesis and usually an absence of megakaryocytes. Ferrokinetic studies with ^{59}Fe revealed a slow plasma clearance of iron as seen in aplastic anemias (Retief et al. 1978; Barosi et al. 1978).

Cytogenetic Findings

Results are given in Table 2 and illustrated in Figs. 3 and 4. The spontaneous and DEB-induced mean chromosomal breakage rates in lymphocyte cultures were significantly higher in FA homozygous patients than in controls ($p < 0.001$). Spontaneous chromosomal breakage in FA heterozygotes did not differ statistically from that in the control group ($p < 0.5$). Treatment of cells with DEB, however,

Table 2. Chromosome breakage per 100 metaphases in lymphocyte cultures of FA homozygotes, FA heterozygotes, and controls

Genotype	Individuals Studied (*n*)	Spontaneous Breakage		DEB					
				0.01 μg/ml		0.10 μg/ml		1 μg/ml	
		Mean	Range	Mean	Range	Mean	Range	Mean	Range
FA homozygotes	44	0.8	0.46-1.28	1.76	1.20-1.96	2.68	2.14-2.95	6.11	4.25-7.9
FA heterozygotes	56	0.065	0.019-0.071	0.338	0.2-0.52	0.993	0.73-1.05	1.341	0.97-1.36
Controls	46	0.017	0.01-0.05	0.025	0.01-0.04	0.048	0.01-0.07	0.077	0.051-0.08

differentiated the two groups: at DEB concentrations of 0.01, 0.1, and 1 μg/ml there was a highly significant ($p < 0.001$) increase in the breakage rate in the group with FA compared with that among the controls. It is evident that the chromosomal breakage rate was at least ten times higher in the FA heterozygotes than in the control group (see Marx and Smith, this volume; Table 2, Figs. 3 and 4).

Discussion

Considering our findings of varying degrees of phenotypic abnormalities in FA homozygotes, it seems that the incidence of many congenital abnormalities associated with the disease has been overestimated. No single entity is pathognomonic for FA and the clinical presentation varies widely. What is surprising is that in our study, many anomalies generally thought to be an integral part of FA were not found as frequently as expected.

The hereditary and familial basis of FA are well illustrated in this series. More than one sibling was affected with FA in five families. We agree with Glanz et al. (1982) that the diagnosis of FA should not be ruled out in an anemic patient with chromosomal breaks even in the absence of dysmorphic features. This was well illustrated in one of our own patients as well as in the cases presented by Estren and Dameshek (1947).

The majority of the patients presented with a history of increasing pallor, easy bruising, and recurrent nose bleeds; recurrent respiratory tract infections were also common. A few patients had had excessive hemorrhage after a surgical procedure.

The mean age of our patients at first presentation was in accordance with literature reports (Fanconi 1967; Schroeder et al. 1976). In previous studies it was stated that there is a preponderance of males among patients with FA, i.e., 2:1 male:female ratio (Fanconi 1967). Glanz et al. (1982) and Gözdasǒğlu et al. (1980) also reported an excess of males. In our study, however, the male:female ratio was 1:2.

The two most common markers for the diagnosis of FA are hematological and cytogenetic anomalies. However, a multitude of phenotypic abnormalities which occur in patients with FA have been documented. In our study, a patient who presented with pancytopenia associated with short stature and skin changes was con-

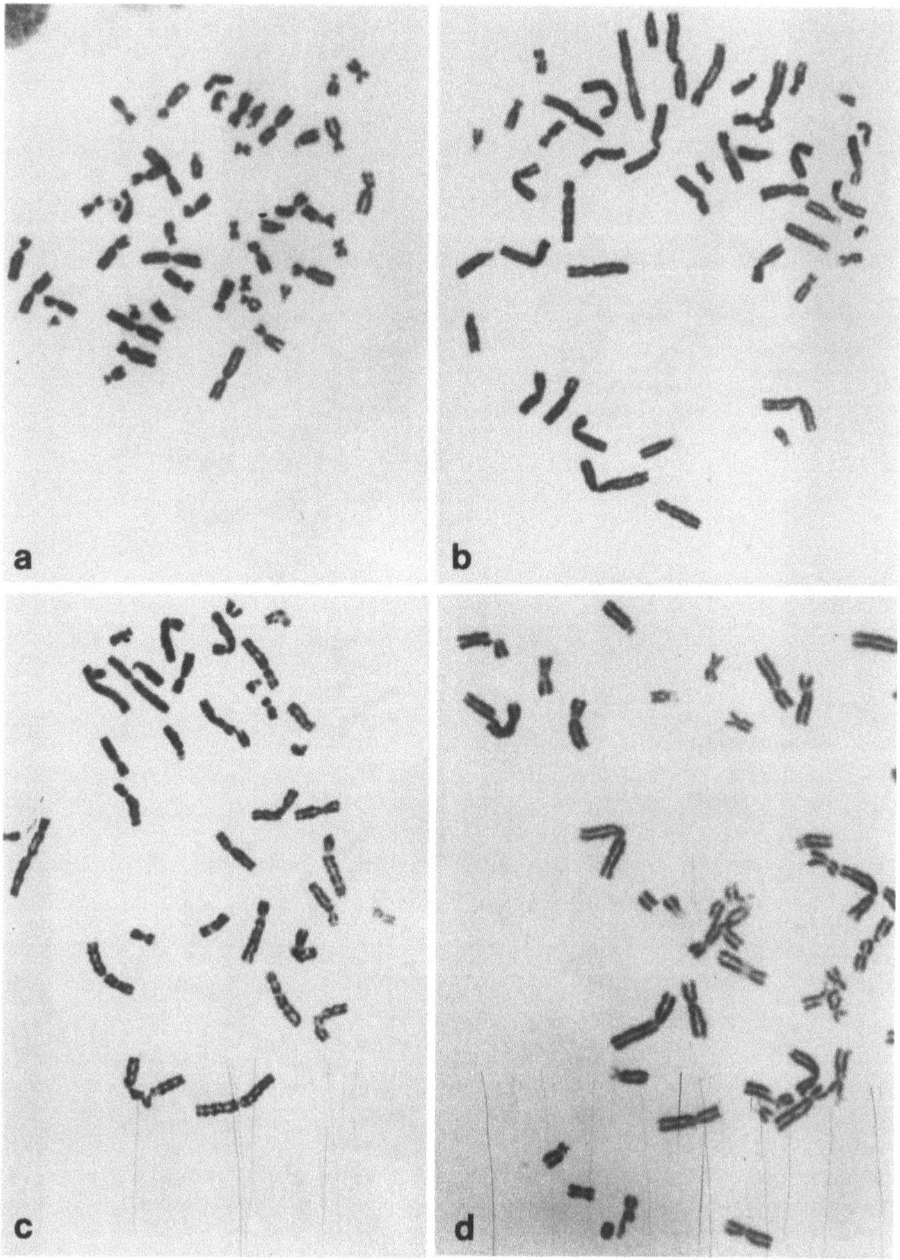

Fig. 3. **a** Metaphase spread from a lymphocyte culture from an FA homozygote showing spontaneous chromosomal damage. **b** Metaphase spread from a lymphocyte culture of an FA homozygote showing chromosomal damage after treatment with 0.01 μg/ml DEB. **c** Metaphase spread from a lymphocyte culture of an FA homozygote after treatment with 0.1 μg/ml DEB. **d** Methaphase spread from a lymphocyte culture of an FA homozygote after treatment with 1.0 μg/ml DEB

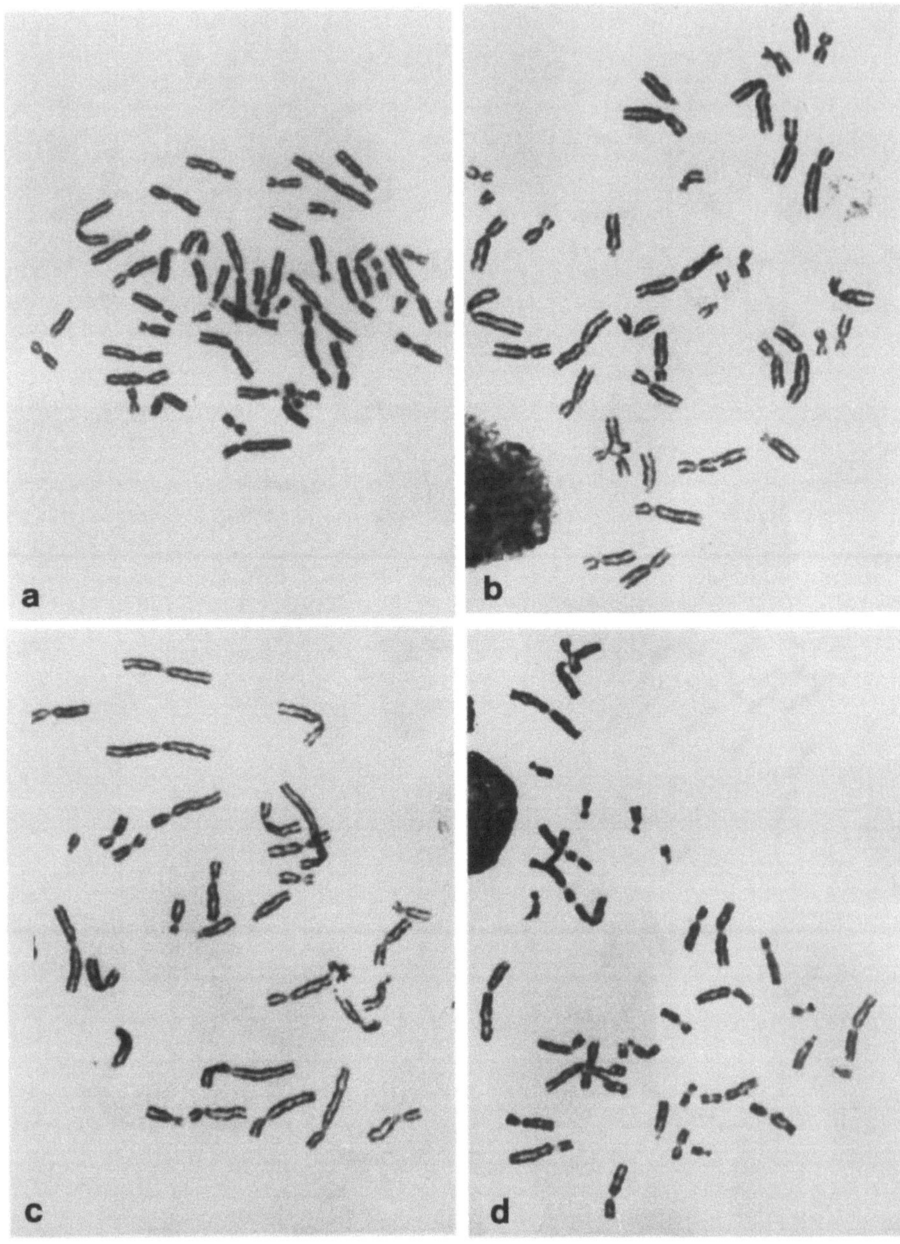

Fig. 4. a Spontaneous chromosome damage in lymphocyte culture from an FA heterozygote. **b** Chromosome damage after treatment of a lymphocyte culture from an FA heterozygote with 0.01 μg/ml DEB. **c** Chromosome damage after treatment of a lymphocyte culture from an FA heterozygote with 0.10 μg/ml DEB. **d** Chromosome damage after treatment of a lymphocyte culture from an FA heterozygote with 1.0 μg/ml DEB

sidered to have FA until proven otherwise by cytogenetic studies. Thumb abnormalities served to strengthen the clinical diagnosis of FA; they were usually associated with an absent or displaced radial artery, but forceful ulnar pulses. No patient had clinical or radiographic evidence of abnormalities of the radius. The incidence of renal, cardiovascular, and urogenital abnormalities, however, was considerably less than that in series reported elsewhere. Genital abnormalities were also infrequent. Growth acceleration or retardation following institution of therapy was not significant.

Skin changes, either hyperpigmentation or hypopigmentation, were consistent with those reported in the literature. Growth failure (affecting all parameters) and microcephaly were also very common, and together with the skin changes made the diagnosis of FA on clinical grounds almost a certainty. The growth failure seen in FA does not appear to be secondary to endocrine insufficiency (Stubbe and Prindull 1975) and treatment of these patients with growth hormones has been unsuccessful (Gleadhill et al. 1975; Costin et al. 1972; Schärer and Baumann 1964). In a study of four children with FA, Aynslee-Green et al. (1978) concluded that growth hormone deficiency associated with other hormonal defects is a common but not constant feature of FA.

Quite a striking feature which has not been emphasized to any great extent in the literature is the presence of hyperreflexia of the deep tendon reflexes. EEGs were frequently abnormal without any symptoms and treatment was not required.

The Department of Pediatrics and Child Health of the University of the Orange Free State serves an estimated population of 2.45 million, who live in the Orange Free State and Northern Cape areas of South Africa. The population in these areas comprises the following ethnic groups: 450000 Caucasians, 1650000 Negroids, mainly South Sothos, 375000 mixed Caucasian-Negroids and 2000 Asians. In the total population of this area, the incidence of FA is calculated as 0.018 per 1000. It is estimated that 40% of the population of the Republic of South Africa is 15 years of age or younger. FA is usually expressed in the first decade of life and is regarded as a disease of childhood. If extrapolated to the childhood population in our areas, the incidence of FA becomes 0.045 per 1000 children aged 15 years or younger. This is probably one of the highest incidences of FA in the world.

Considering all the causes of both aplastic and hypoplastic anemia, the predominance of FA in our population is startling. Aplastic anemia (AA) is subdivided according to etiology. About 70% is acquired or idiopathic and the remainder (±30%) is constitutional, including FA (Lipton and Nathan 1980; Alter et al. 1978). A total of 51 patients with AA registered for the hematology service at our institution. Only four of these patients have acquired or ideopathic AA, giving a 92% incidence for FA.

The very high incidence of FA may be attributed to the following influencing factors: (a) a restricted white gene pool due to a relatively small population, and (b) restriction of the gene pool in the black population by tribal customs and grouping which, because of marriage between members of the same tribe, creates a homogenous population. The majority of our patients reside in the gold and diamond mining areas as well as areas of intense maize production. Exogenous factors may thus also be involved. Consanguinity was established in 13% of the families studied.

The mean age of onset of hematological problems in our study was 6 years 7 months which correlates well with reports in the literature. No correlation was found between the number of congenital abnormalities per patient and the age of onset of hematological problems, suggesting that gross physical abnormalities are not indicative of the severity of bone marrow decompensation.

McDonald (1962) and Shahidi and Diamond (1961) reported on the treatment of both acquired and congenital AA with anabolic androgens. Following diagnosis of FA, we treated all our patients with an oxymetholone preparation (maximum dose 5 mg/kg) and prednisolone daily. The majority responded to this protocol and it was possible to maintain an adequate peripheral blood picture. The most troublesome problems during follow-up were recurrent nose bleeds, resistance to treatment, or progressive irreversible bone marrow failure. These patients became more and more transfusion-dependent with the development of transfusion siderosis, and infectious episodes, i.e., septicemia. We did not encounter any hepatic dysfunction secondary to therapy. A certain percentage of patients seem to go into spontaneous remission, not requiring any further treatment. Therapy can usually be discontinued at or about the time of puberty. As this stage of human development is associated with marked hormonal changes, it is possible that the bone marrow responds to endogenously produced hormones. FA is thus not a uniformly fatal disease as reported, although there has not been enough long term follow-up of these patients and we do not know enough about the eventual outcome.

Death in 17 of our patients was due to fatal hemorrhage, septicemia, and progressive bone marrow failure. Five patients developed malignancies, i.e., carcinoma of the vulva, acute myeloblastic leukemia (3 patients), and acute lymphoblastic leukemia. The development of leukemia was preceded by the development of several aneuploid and polyploid cell lines.

In two studies (Potter et al. 1983; Swift et al. 1980), no increased risk of cancer or high level of cancer deaths in the families of patients with FA or in FA heterozygotes was found. The risk of acute leukemia is markedly increased among patients with FA (Alter 1987). It remains to be seen whether the longer survival made possible by the use of anabolic steroids has facilitated the emergence of malignancy or contributed to its pathogenesis.

In this study, we have highlighted features of FA not reported before. The phenotypic features were limited to a few outstanding anomalies, whereas features stated as being frequent in FA were infrequently encountered in our patients. Contrary to other studies, we documented an excess of females over males. The majority of our patients responded to an androgen and adrenocorticosteroid regimen; it was possible to discontinue therapy in a number of patients. FA was the overwhelming cause of AA in our population, and the incidence in our pediatric population is probably the highest in the world.

Much has been written about the genetic heterogeneity of FA (Schroeder et al. 1976; Zakrzewski and Sperling 1982; Dallapiccola et al. 1980; Duckworth-Rysiecki et al. 1986), but the question whether this genetic heterogeneity applies to our population remains unanswered. Considering our patients, it does seem that a strong argument in support of this can be made.

References

Alter BP, Potter NU, Li FP (1978) Classification and aetiology of the aplastic anaemias. Clin Haematol 7: 431-465
Alter BP (1987) The bone marrow failure syndromes. In: Nathan GD Oski FA (eds) Hematology of infancy and childhood. Saunders, Philadelphia, pp 159-241
Auerbach AD, Wolman SR (1976) Susceptibility of Fanconi's anaemia fibroblasts to chromosome damage by carcinogens. Nature 261: 494-496
Auerbach AD, Wolman SR (1978) Carcinogen-induced chromosome breakage in Fanconi's anaemia heterozygous cells. Nature 271: 69-70
Auerbach AD, Adler B, Chaganti RSK (1981) Prenatal and postnatal diagnosis and carrier detection of Fanconi anemia by a cytogenetic method. Pediatrics 67: 128-135
Aynslee-Green A, Zachmann M, Werder EA, Illig R, Prader A (1978) Endocrine studies in Fanconi's anaemia. Arch Dis Child 53: 126-131
Barosi G, Cazzola M, Marchi A, Morandi S, Perani V, Stefanelli M, Perugini S (1978) Iron kinetics and erythropoiesis in Fanconi's anemia. Scand J Haematol 21: 29-39
Beard MEJ, Young DE, Bateman CJT, McCarthey GT, Smith ME, Sinclair L, Franklin AW, Scott RB (1973) Fanconi's anaemia. Q J Med 166: 403-422
Cervenka J, Hirsch BA (1983) Cytogenetic differentiation of Fanconi anemia, "idiopathic" aplastic anemia and Fanconi anemia heterozygotes. Am J Med Genet 15: 211-223
Costin G, Kogut MD, Hyman CB (1972) Fanconi's anemia associated with isolated growth hormone deficiency. Clin Res 20: 253
Dallapiccola B, Alimena G, Brinchi V, Isacchi G, Gandini E (1980) Absence of chromosome heterogeneity between classical Fanconi's anemia and the Estren-Dameshek type. Cancer Genet Cytogenet 2: 349-360
Deeg HJ, Sterb R, Thomas ED, Appelbaum F, Buckner CD, Clift RA, Doney K, Johnson L, Sanders JE, Stewart P, Sullivan KM, Witherspoon RP (1983) Fanconi's anemia treated by allogeneic marrow transplantation. Blood 61: 954-959
Duckworth-Rysiecki G, Cornish K, Clarke CA, Buchwald M (1985) Identification of two complementation groups in Fanconi anemia. Somatic Cell Mol Genet 11: 35-41
Estren S, Dameshek W (1947) Familial hypoplastic anemia without congenital malformations. Am J Dis Child 73: 671-681
Fanconi G (1927) Familiäre infantile perniziosaartige Anämie (perniziöses Blutbild und Konstitution). Jahrb Kinderheilkd 117: 257-280
Fanconi G (1967) Familial constitutional panmyelocytopathy, Fanconi's anemia. I. Clinical aspects. Semin Hematol 4: 233
Glanz A, Clarke Fraser F (1982) Spectrum of anomalies in Fanconi anaemia. J Med Genet 19: 412-416
Gleadhill V, Bridges JM, Hadden DR (1975) Fanconi's aplastic anaemia with short stature. Absence of response to human growth hormone. Arch Dis Child 50: 318
Gluckman E, Berger R, Dutreix J (1984) Bone marrow transplantation for Fanconi anemia. Semin Hematol 21: 20-26
Gmyrek D, Syllm-Rapoport I (1964) Zur Fanconi-Anämie (FA): Analyse von 129 beschriebenen Fällen. Z Kinderheilkd 91: 297
Gözdasöğlu S, Cavdar AO, Arcasoy A, Babacan E, Anal Ö (1980) Fanconi's aplastic anemia, analysis of 18 cases. Acta Haematol (Basel) 64: 131-135
Jacobs P, Karabus C (1983) Fanconi's anemia. A family study with 20-year follow-up including associated breast pathology. Cancer 54: 1850-1853
Lipton JM, Nathan DG (1980) Aplastic and hypoplastic anemia. Pediatr Clin North Am 27 (2): 217-235
Marx MP, Smith S, Heyns A du P, van Tonder IZ (1983). Fanconi's anemia: a cytogenetic study on lymphocyte and bone marrow cultures utilizing 1,2:3,4-diepoxybutane. Cancer Genet Cytogenet 9: 51-60
McDonald R (1962) Drug-induced remission in hypoplastic anemia (Fanconi type). S Afr Med J 36: 310-312
Nilson LR (1960) Chronic pancytopenia with multiple congenital abnormalities (Fanconi's anaemia). Acta Paediatr Scand 49: 518

Potter NU, Sarmonsakis C, Li FP (1983) Cancer in relatives of patients with aplastic anemia. Cancer Genet Cytogenet 9: 61-66

Retief FP, Heyns A du P, Hurralde M, Lotter MG, Minnaar PC (1978) Ferrokinetiese studies en Prognose by aplastiese anemie. S Afr Med J 54: 235-238

Schärer K, Baumann T (1964) Die Behandlung der idiopathischen Panmyelopathien mit Steroiden und hypophysärem Wachstumshormon. Schweiz Med Wochenschr 94: 1322

Schroeder TM (1982) Genetically determined chromosome instability syndromes. Cytogenet Cell Genet 33: 119-132

Schroeder TM, Tilgen D, Krüger J, Vogel F (1976) Formal genetics in Fanconi's anemia. Hum Genet 32: 257-288

Shahidi NT, Diamond LK (1961) Testosterone induced remission in aplastic anaemia in both acquired and congenital types. Further observations in 24 cases. N Engl J Med 264: 953

Stubbe P, Prindull G (1975) Fanconi anemia. II. Are multiple endocrine insufficiencies a substantial part of the disease? Acta Paediatr Scand 64: 790-794

Swift M, Caldwell RJ, Chase C (1980) Reassessment of cancer predisposition of Fanconi anemia heterozygotes. JNCI 65: 863-867

Zakrzewski S, Sperling K (1982) Analysis of heterogeneity in Fanconi's anemia patients of different ethnic origin. Hum Genet 62: 321-323

Therapeutic Aspects of Fanconi Anemia*

W. Ebell, W. Friedrich, and E. Kohne

Introduction

Fanconi anemia (FA) is an autosomal recessive disorder defined by chromosomal instability, delayed-onset marrow failure, increased risk of neoplasia, and a variety of constitutional abnormalities and congenital malformations (Alter et al. 1981). Since this familial form of aplastic anemia was first described by Fanconi in 1927, it has been well recognized that the presence in these patients of constitutional symptoms such as malformations of the skin, the skeletal system, the central nervous system, the genitourinary tract, and others is highly variable. The exact diagnosis of FA therefore depends heavily on the recognition of chromosomal abnormalities, consisting of an increased rate of spontaneous and induced chromosomal breaks. These chromosomal findings clearly distinguish FA from other forms of constitutional and acquired aplastic anemia, as discussed in other chapters of this book.

Until recently, treatment has consisted largely of supportive care and attempts to stabilize and improve hemopoietic functions by administering androgens and steroids. Although such treatment was useful in prolonging the course of the disease in many patients, in the long run patients still died of the hematologic complications of the syndrome. Bone marrow transplantation (BMT) now offers a realistic chance for permanent correction of marrow failure in patients with FA and thus reversal of the otherwise fatal course of the disease. These and other therapeutic aspects of FA are reviewed in this chapter. Our results with BMT and the overall experience will be discussed first to emphasize that this approach is the therapy of choice today. However, BMT still depends on a suitable marrow donor being found, and is associated with potentially fatal risks. Therefore, conventional forms of treatment still need to be revised as an alternative therapy for patients for whom no marrow donor can be found. FA is a syndrome frequently characterized by malignancies in addition to marrow aplasia, and multiple organ malformations or dysfunctions, and some important aspects of these problems will be summarized in this chapter.

* Dedicated to Professor E. Kleihauer on the occasion of his 60th birthday

T. M. Schroeder-Kurth A. D. Auerbach G. Obe (Eds.)
Fanconi Anemia, Clinical, Cytogenetic and Experimental Aspects

Bone Marrow Transplantation in Fanconi Anemia

In patients with acquired severe aplastic anemia and for whom a human leukocyte antigen (HLA)-matched related donor has been found, BMT now provides a realistic chance of cure, especially for pediatric patients (Bacigalupo et al. 1985; Sanders et al. 1986). When this method was first used to treat patients with FA, the results were disappointing. With conditioning regimens similar to those used for acquired forms of aplastic anemia, namely high doses of cyclophosphamide (200 mg/kg) for immunosuppression, only about one-third of the patients survived (Gluckman et al. 1980; Deeg et al. 1983; Table 1). The post-transplant course was characterized by severe toxicity related to the conditioning chemotherapy and the complications of graft-versus-host disease (GvHD). Toxicity consisted of mucositis, diarrhea, hemorrhagic cystitis, cardiac failure, and fluid overload. On the other hand, graft rejection was unexpectedly rare, although most of the patients reported had been heavily transfused before transplantation. Furthermore, the few long-term survivors showed a stable hemopoietic reconstitution, with the longest follow-up being 14 years to date. From in vitro and in vivo studies, it became more and more evident that cells from patients with FA are highly susceptible to chromosomal damage by alkylating agents such as cyclophosphamide metabolites (Berger et al. 1980; Auerbach et al. 1983) and by high-dose irradiation (Gluckman et al. 1983). It therefore became obvious that it was necessary to modify the condi-

Table 1. Overall results of bone marrow transplantation in Fanconi anemia

Center	(*n*)	Conditioning regimen	No. of surviving patients	Ref.
HLA-identical, related donors				
High-dose CY				
Seattle	8	CY 150-200 mg/kg	4	Deeg et al. 1983
Paris	5	CY 150-200 mg/kg ± ATG	1	Gluckman et al. 1980
Other centers	11	CY 160-200 mg/kg ± ATG, Proc. or TLI 7.5 Gy	4	Deeg et al. 1983; Gluckman et al. 1984
Low-dose CY				
Paris	15	CY 20 mg/kg + TAI 4-5 Gy	11	Gluckman et al. 1987
London	7	CY 20 mg/kg + TBI 6 Gy	5	Durrant et al. 1987
Ulm	8	CY 20 mg/kg + TAI 5 Gy ± ARA-C	7	-
HLA-mismatched, related donors				
London	5	CY 20 mg/kg + TBI 6 Gy	2	Gordon-Smith et al. 1987
Ulm	2	CY 20 mg/kg + TAI 5 Gy or Proc., ATG, TBI 8 Gy	1	-
HLA-phenotypic matched, unrelated donors				
London	4	CY 20 mg/kg + TBI 6 Gy	1	Gordon-Smith et al. 1987

HLA, human leukocyte antigen; CY, cyclophosphamide; ATG, antithymocyte globulin; Proc., procarbazine; TLI, total lymphnode irradiation; TAI, thoracoabdominal irradiation; TBI, total body irradiation; ARA-C, cytosine arabinoside

tioning regimen in these patients, taking into account this cellular hypersensitivity, either by reducing the dose of the conventional conditioning regimen of cyclophosphamide and irradiation (Gluckman et al. 1984) or by introducing other agents such as procarbazine with less clastogenic effect in vitro (Auerbach et al.

Table 2. Results of bone marrow transplantation in ten patients with Fanconi anemia (University Children's Hospital, Ulm, FRG)

Patient	Conditioning regimen	Donor	Graft-versus host prophylaxis: T cell depletion	Graft-versus host prophylaxis: Chemo-prophylaxis	Graft	Survival (days)
EV	CY 4×5 mg/kg TAI 5 Gy	HLA-identical sibling	-	CSA	Sustained	>840
SS	CY 4×5 mg/kg TAI 5 Gy	HLA-identical sibling	-	CSA	Sustained	>360
RU	CY 4×5 mg/kg TAI 5 Gy	HLA-identical sibling	-	CSA	Sustained	>470
ME	CY 4×5 mg/kg TAI 5 Gy	HLA-identical sibling	-	CSA	Sustained	>240
MS	CY 4×5 mg/kg TAI 5 Gy	HLA-identical sibling	-	CSA	Sustained	>310
YA	CY 4×5 mg/kg TAI 5 Gy	HLA-identical sibling	E-rosetting	-	Sustained	>680
YD	1. CY 4×5 mg/kg TAI 5 Gy	HLA-identical sibling	E-rosetting	-	Rejected day 15	-
	2. Proc. 3×12.5 mg/kg ATG 3×40 mg/kg TBI 3 Gy	HLA-identical sibling	-	CSA	No take	died day 57, Candida sepsis
AM	1. CY 4×5 mg/kg TAI 5 Gy ARAC 2×200 mg/m^2	HLA-identical sibling	E-rosetting	-	Rejected day 33	
	2. Proc. 3×12.5 mg/kg ATG 3×40 mg/kg CY 4×10 mg/kg Campath I 25 mg	HLA-identical sibling	-	CSA	Sustained	>410
NA	CY 4×5 mg/kg TAI 5 Gy	1 antigen-mismatched cousin	-	CSA+MTX	Sustained	>180
YH	Proc. 3×12.5 mg/kg ATG 3×40 mg/kg TBI 4×2 Gy ATG 15 mg/kg day+5 until+31 every other day	1 haplotype-mismatched uncle	Lectin-separation+E-rosetting	-	No take	died day 42, Aspergillus sepsis

CY, cyclophosphamide; TAI, thoracicoabdominal irradiation; Proc., procarbazine; ATG, antithymocyte globulin; TBI, total body irradiation; ARA-C, cytosine arabinoside; CSA, cyclosporin A; MTX, methotrexate

1983). Gluckman et al. (1987) demonstrated, in a larger series of patients with FA, that the results of BMT improved with a conditioning protocol which combined a drastically lowered dose of cyclophosphamide (20 mg/kg) and thoracoabdominal irradiation at a moderate dose of 4-5 Gy. These results are presented in the next chapter in this book and represent a breakthrough in BMT for the treatment of patients with FA. Similar results have been reported from the Hammersmith Hospital in London, where HLA-identical BMT was successful in five of seven patients, using a combination of low-dose cyclophosphamide (20 mg/kg) and 6 Gy total body irradiation (Durrant et al. 1987) (Table 1).

The following describes our experience with BMT in patients with FA. Eight patients have received transplants from HLA-identical siblings. Seven of these have survived for between 4 and 26 months (mean 15 months) after grafting (Table 1). The detailed transplant data of each patient are shown in Table 2. Five patients received a conditioning regimen according to Gluckman et al. (1984), a full marrow transplant, and then cyclosporin A was administered for GvHD prophylaxis. All of them showed a rapid engraftment of hemopoietic cells (Table 3). In three additional patients, the marrow graft was depleted of T cells by E-rosetting, to prevent GvHD. Two of these patients rejected the marrow. A second transplant with unseparated marrow from the same donor was successful in one of these patients. Toxicity was relatively low, even when other agents had been added or when further treatment was necessary for retransplantation. Mucositis and esophagitis remained the major problems. The incidence of acute GvHD in our patients was 38% (25% grade I+II, 13% grade III+IV) and further 38% had chronic GvHD. Although the number of patients in our study was small, our results seem to be similar to those reported by others (Gluckman et al. 1984). It is therefore obvious that GvHD remains one of the problems of BMT in patients with FA and that further efforts are needed to reduce this complication. Graft rejection in the HLA-identical cases only occurred in two of three patients receiving T cell-depleted marrow. As observed by others (Deeg et al. 1983; Gluckman et al. 1984; Durrant et al. 1987), polytransfusion and sensitization were not risk factors for graft rejection. Major AB0 blood group differences have been a problem. In all three patients with major blood group differences a delayed erythropoietic reconstitution was observed, which was related to persisting host-type B cells (see below) and isohemagglutinins (Table 3). However, this did not appear to contribute to graft rejection because in the patient (AM) in whom retransplantation was successful the delayed erythropoietic reconstitution was again present, but the second

Table 3. Hemopoietic reconstitution following bone marrow transplantation in Fanconi anemia (University Children's Hospital, Ulm, FRG)

Patients	Peripheral blood cell counts		Days after transplantation
All with engraftment ($n=8$)	Neutrophils	>500/µl	13±1
	Platelets	>100000/µl	36±8
AB0-compatible ($n=6$)	Reticulocytes	>1%	11±2
AB0-incompatible ($n=2$)	Reticulocytes	>1%	42±8

graft was not rejected. The chimeric status was sequentially investigated in six patients with a sex-mismatched marrow donor using Y-body staining with quinacrine and Q-banding in phytohemagglutinin-stimulated lymphocytes. Usually all hemopoietic cells were of donor origin by 14 days after BMT. In contrast, a major population of host-type lymphocytes with the capacity to proliferate following in vitro stimulation with mitogens remained detectable for up to 4 months after BMT, regardless of whether or not a T cell depleted marrow was given. The majority of these cells showed the phenotype of T-suppressor cells, but there was also a significant fraction of host-type B cells, which remained during the early period.

Restricting the donors to HLA-identical siblings, and sometimes other HLA-identical relatives, remains a considerable limitation on marrow transplantation, not only in FA. Therefore, attempts have been made to overcome this limitation by using either HLA-identical, unrelated or HLA-mismatched, related marrow donors. In the Hammersmith series, one of four unrelated, HLA-phenotypic matched and two of five related, HLA-mismatched marrow grafts were successful (Hows et al. 1986; Durrant et al. 1987) (Table 1). We tried two HLA-mismatched BMTs. One transplant from a cousin, mismatched for one antigen, was successful. One haplotype-mismatched transplant in another patient failed to engraft (Table 2).

In conclusion, recent experience of BMT in FA clearly shows that bone marrow failure can be completely reversed by modifying the preparative regimen: toxicity can be significantly decreased. Polytransfusion before BMT appears not to be a major risk factor for rejection when a regimen with low-dose cyclophosphamide and irradiation of lymphoid tissues is used. T cell depletion seems to be related to an increased rate of graft failure. This has also been reported by others, and is found in non-FA transplants as well (Durrant et al. 1987; Poynton et al. 1987). Partially mismatched, related transplants and HLA-identical, unrelated transplants were also successful in a significant number of patients (Hows et al. 1986). Late-stage disease with complete bone marrow aplasia and unresponsiveness to androgens and steroids might be the appropriate time for a marrow graft to be performed. On the other hand, postponing BMT entails the risk of serious bleeding complications, severe infections, androgen side effects, and the development of malignancies. GvHD remains a significant risk. The prevention of this complication by T cell depletion appears feasible; however, further steps are required to prevent rejection. Similarly, optimal procedures to ensure engraftment in HLA-haploidentical transplants remain to be determined. The risk of malignancies in long-term survivors of BMT is a crucial question. This includes the risk of leukemia if the marrow donor is heterozygous for FA, although this is probably not a major consideration (Garriga and Crosby 1959; Swift 1971; Swift et al. 1980). The exact nature of the cancer risk in patients with FA has not been clearly established. Several factors, such as increased susceptibility to viral transformation, chromosomal instability, susceptibility to mutagens, defective DNA repair, and defects of the immune system have been discussed (Kaplan et al. 1985). The hope is that the newly established donor immune system in patients in whom BMT has been successful will provide more effective immunosurveillance for cancer.

Conventional Treatment of Marrow Insufficiency in Fanconi Anemia

Conventional therapy of marrow failure in FA includes transfusion support and the administration of androgens and steroids. This type of treatment is all that is currently available for patients without a suitable marrow donor. If a transplant can be considered, the question remains as to whether an attempt at remission induction should be made with such drugs before proceeding with a bone marrow graft. The clinical heterogeneity of the syndrome makes it difficult to determine what might be the right procedure for an individual patient, given the BMT-related risks and the mortality on the one hand, and the possibility of survival for several years with conventional treatment on the other. While at least partial responses to androgens or steroids in individual patients with FA are clearly documented, carefully randomized trials have never been reported. This makes it even more difficult to draw final conclusions with respect to response rates, the survival rate, and side effects of such treatment modalities. The question remains whether patients with FA will respond similarly or even better to this type of therapy than patients with forms of acquired aplastic anemia (Gardner 1985). There is not much controversy about the transfusion program in these patients. It is essentially the same as in patients with other forms of aplastic anemia. Necessary transfusions should not be withheld in view of a possible marrow transplant, because polytransfusion does not seem to influence engraftment. Infection prophylaxis in neutropenic patients is handled in the same way as for any neutropenic patient.

The largest series of androgen-treated patients with FA and a comprehensive survey of the literature were reported by Alter and Potter in 1983. According to this summary of early reports, only 20% of the patients with transfusion support alone survived for 2 years after diagnosis and almost none for 4 years. Later, through the improvement of supportive care alone it was possible to prolong survival without any other treatment (50% survival for 2.5 years, 20% survival for 8 years). Androgen treatment, however, further improved survival (50% survival for 8 years). Compared to these cases from the literature, which were possibly selected, Alter and Potter also presented their own results of androgen treatment in 26 patients at the Children's Hospital Medical Center in Boston, which was somewhat less effective (50% survival for 4 years, 20% survival for 12 years). The initial response rate to androgens is also of interest. As cited by the above-mentioned authors, the overall literature review suggests a response rate of 50%, confirmed by the Boston patients with a 54% response rate.

Androgen response almost always means a partial response with independence from regular blood transfusion and a gradual increase in the number of platelets and granulocytes. Usually patients who show an initial response to androgens remain therapy-dependent and finally become resistant to this treatment. Androgen therapy not only has the unpleasant side effects of virilization, especially in girls, but also other complications such as hepatic tumors (hepatocellular carcinomas, hepatomas, adenomas, and peliosis hepatitis; Obeid et al. 1980; Alter and Potter 1983). Most of the androgen regimens also contain a low-dose steroid treatment to increase vascular stability. There are no reports in the literature analyzing the therapeutic effect of high-dose steroids alone in such patients.

In the following we present an analysis of treatment responses in a group of 21

Table 4. Physical abnormalities in 21 patients with Fanconi anemia (University Children's Hospital, Ulm, FRG)

Abnormality	Patients	
	(*n*)	(%)
Pigment anomalies	20	95
Skeletal malformations	13	62
Growth retardation	8	38
Low birth weight	7	33
Kidney and urinary tract malformations	5	24
Cryptorchidism and/or hypogenitalism	3/8 (M)	38
Eye defects	4	19
Hypothyroidism	3	14
Congenital heart disease	1	5

M, male

patients whom we were able to evaluate at our institution. These patients were either diagnosed and followed up for a prolonged period at our hospital or were referred for consultation or BMT having been diagnosed and pretreated in other hospitals. The age of these 21 patients (13 girls, eight boys) at the time of diagnosis ranged from 3-15 years (mean 6.6 years). The clinical features are summarized in Table 4. All patients had characteristic chromosomal abnormalities with spontaneous and induced chromosomal breakage (tested by T. M. Schroeder-Kurth and coworkers at the Institute of Human Genetics in Heidelberg).

Of these 21 patients, 16 are still alive between 1 and 8.5 years (mean 3.5 years) after diagnosis. Eight of them remain on a conservative treatment regimen and eight eventually received a successful marrow graft. Five patients died, three due to the marrow failure, and two due to unsuccessful BMT.

The group of 21 patients can be divided into three groups according to the therapy they received. (a) Five patients received only transfusion support. (b) Nine patients were treated with androgens (usually oxymetholone 2-5 mg/kg per day) with or without low-dose steroids such as 10 mg prednisolone every other day. (c) Seven patients received exclusively steroids using prednisolone at doses of about 2 mg/kg per day. All patients receiving androgens or steroids were transfusion-dependent and thrombocytopenic at the time when the therapy was initiated. If the erythropoiesis was stabilized without red cell transfusion being necessary, and if there was a gradual increase of granulocytes and platelets without bleeding symptoms, the patient was judged to have responded to treatment. Using these criteria, about half the patients responded either to steroids or androgens, as shown in Figure 1. These partial remissions are ongoing in five of seven patients, while two patients died after 6 years due to progressive marrow failure with severe infections. On the other hand, in nine patients who showed no response to either steroids or androgens, six are still alive, the longest survival period so far being 8 years after diagnosis. In the supportive care group all five patients are still alive between 1 and 4 years after diagnosis.

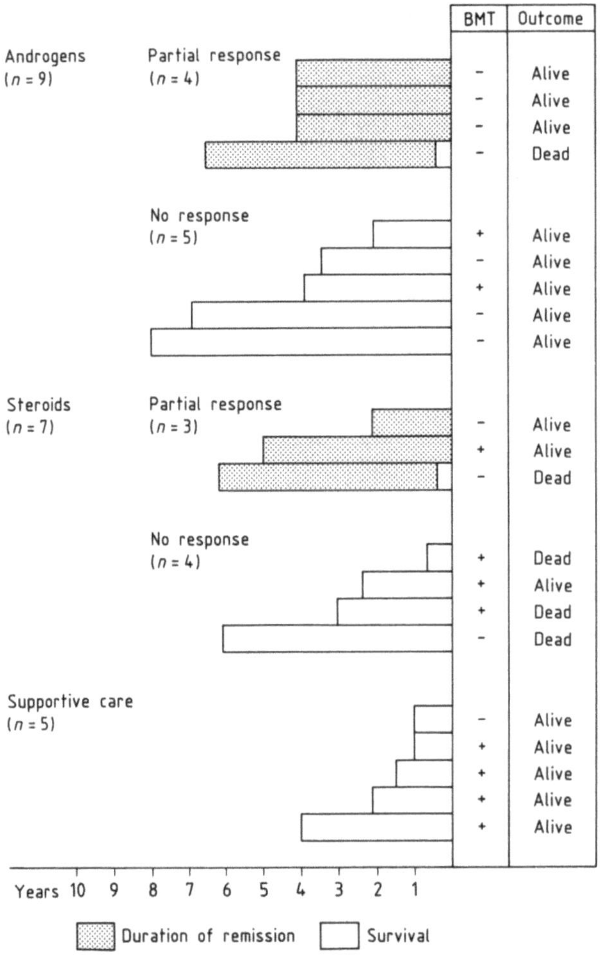

Fig. 1. Response rates to androgens or steroids and current survival in 21 patients with Fanconi anemia (University Children's Hospital, Ulm, FRG)

Our experience suggests that about 50% of patients respond to androgens, as cited in the literature (Alter and Potter 1983). The same percentage, however, also appears to respond to steroids alone, although we cannot judge how long these remissions will last. There were few side effects in the steroid-treated group. In the androgen-treated group, problems of virilization and, in one case, of peliosis hepatitis occurred. None of the 21 patients has developed leukemia or other malignant diseases. In some instances, severe bacterial infections occurred although the granulocyte counts were almost normal. The type of infections were similar to those described in patients with defective granulocyte function. We therefore analyzed five patients with bacterial infections and were able to demonstrate abnormalities of chemotaxis and phagocytosis in all of them. Two of them were treated with steroids, two with androgens, and one patient was not being treated at the time when the tests were performed. This is in contrast to previously reported results with regard to granulocyte functions (Pedersen et al. 1977; Hersey et al. 1982). However, several other impairments of the immune system have been described in the literature such as depressed mitogen responses (Pedersen et al. 1977; Johansson et al 1982), reduced, delayed-type hypersensitivity of the skin (Hersey et al. 1982; Johansson et al. 1982), and deficient natural killer cell activity (Hersey et al. 1982). Therefore, in order to define more exactly the disease status and risk factor in an individual patient, the evaluation of the residual lymphohemopoietic system also needs to include functional aspects. It is difficult to come to final conclusions from our study or the literature cases regarding the long-term outcome of androgen or steroid treatment in FA, due to the great variability of marrow failure in this disorder with respect to the age of onset, severity, and progression. In such a rare disease it is hard to find subgroups with similar features large enough to derive valid conclusions. Nevertheless, the careful consideration of disease status and side effects of the various therapeutic modalities should lead to the most effective and least harmful strategy. This should also help in the decision whether or not to proceed with a marrow transplant if a donor is available.

Finally, new therapeutic approaches did not lead to approved clinical treatment forms. The finding of decreased superoxide dismutase activity in erythrocytes and leukocytes in patients with FA (Joenje et al. 1978; Yoshimitsu et al. 1984), for example, led to the in vivo application of this radioprotective enzyme without long-lasting effect (Izakovic et al. 1985).

Treatment of Nonhematological Symptoms in Fanconi Anemia

In this section, we will briefly summarize some aspects of care of patients suffering from FA, related to associated malformations or organ dysfunctions. Since BMT now probably offers long-term survival to a significant number of patients, supportive care becomes even more important and requires the cooperation of various specialists such as surgeons, urologists, ophthalmologists, and endocrinologists. We will focus particularly on the endocrinological problems of these patients. A significant number of patients in our own series (14%), suffer from hypothyroidism which requires a life-long hormone substitution. About 30% of the boys have a cryptorchidism which should be corrected. Hypogonadism has been described in about 20% of males and females (Alter and Potter 1983; Berkovitz et al. 1984). This seems to be due to a gonadal defect rather than to an abnormality in the hypothalamic-pituitary axis (Berkovitz et al. 1984). About 40%-80% of the patients are of short stature, the reason being unknown in most patients; growth hormone deficiency has been reported in some (Pochedly et al. 1971; Zachmann et al. 1972). In a review by Nordan et al. (1979), three of six patients responded to growth hormone treatment; interestingly, the responders had a birth weight and length above the fifth percentile of the general population compared to the nonresponders. It is too early to comment on growth behavior following successful marrow transplantation. Finally, both homozygotes and heterozygotes for FA have an increased risk of diabetes mellitus (Morell et al. 1986), which should be considered, especially with respect to steroid treatment.

Management of Malignancies in Fanconi Anemia

FA is associated with an increased risk of malignancies, which is a well established observation. Acute leukemia has been the terminal event in about 5%-20% of patients with FA (Obeid et al. 1980; Alter and Potter 1983). The vast majority of these leukemias were acute nonlymphocytic leukemias, but acute lymphoblastic leukemia has also been observed, as well as one case of megakaryoblastic leukemia (Dharmasena et al. 1986). In some instances leukemia was the initial event leading to the diagnosis of FA (Auerbach et al. 1982), but usually there is an interval of several years (mean 5 years) from the onset of pancytopenia to the development of leukemia (Alter and Potter 1983). Besides these hematological malignancies, there is a substantial risk of hepatic tumors, which have been observed particularly in androgen-treated patients but also in at least one nontreated child (Cattan et al. 1974). Squamous cell carcinoma is another relatively frequent malignancy (Kennedy and Hart 1982; Reed et al. 1983; Wilkinson et al. 1984; Alter and Potter 1983). Other solid tumors have also been reported, for example, adenocarcinomas of the stomach or colon (Hill et al. 1981), and breast cancer (Jacobs and Karabus 1984). In addition, de Chadarevian et al. (1985) reported on one patient who had a medulloblastoma combined with a Wilms tumor. In a review of 300 reported cases, the overall incidence of solid tumors was estimated at about 2% (Obeid et al. 1980). The impression is that malignancies occur mainly in patients with late-onset marrow failure and longer survival, with or without androgen therapy (Kennedy and Hart 1982; Alter and Potter 1983). In addition, females have a higher cancer risk than males (Kennedy and Hart 1982; Reed et al. 1983; Wilkinson et al. 1984). Whereas a regression of androgen-related, presumably nonmalignant, hepatic tumors following marrow transplantation has been described (Schmidt et al. 1984), the overall outcome of malignant tumors in FA is very poor. The 22 patients with leukemia, reported by Alter and Potter (1983), all died within 1 year, most of them within a month. Only one of these patients showed a partial response to chemotherapy. For squamous cell carcinomas, the mean survival period is 1 year after diagnosis. Interestingly enough, patients do not seem to die as a result of their tumor but of sepsis due to the underlying disease or to high sensitivity to chemotherapy (Reed et al. 1983). As already discussed in the context of BMT, the predisposition of individuals who are heterozygous for FA to cancer is controversial. Early reports suggested such an increased cancer risk (Garriga and Crosby 1959; Swift 1971). However, more extensive studies, some from the same authors, did not confirm these earlier findings. Thus, Swift et al. (1980) revised their initial observations, denying a specific cancer risk in Fanconi relatives at least for leukemia, while a predisposition among FA heterozygotes to bladder, stomach, or breast cancer, at an early age, could not be completely excluded. Since malignancies in FA have such a poor prognosis, it is preferable to attempt to prevent such tumors. The hope is that BMT will have this prophylactic effect.

Conclusion

Although the exact genetic basis of FA remains unclear, the increasing knowledge about this disease has led to a significantly improved outlook for affected patients. BMT has become the therapy of choice because of its potential to correct the marrow failure and hopefully also prevent the late occurrence of malignancies. However, the problems of BMT-related risks, in particular, the limitation of finding suitable marrow donors, have to be solved in order to make full use of this therapeutic approach. Therefore, patients not eligible for marrow transplantation will continue to depend on conventional forms of treatment, and prospective trials are certainly needed to gain a better knowledge of the usefulness of androgens, steroids, or new approaches, as compared with supportive care alone. In the evaluation of such studies, response rates, survival, side effects, and cancer risk have to be very carefully considered. Finally, despite the promising results of marrow transplantation, genetic counseling and prenatal diagnosis still have an important role to play in combatting this disease (Auerbach et al. 1981, 1985).

References

Alter BP, Potter NU (1983) Long-term outcome in Fanconi's anemia: description of 26 cases and review of the literature. In: German J (ed) Chromosome mutation and neoplasia. Liss, New York, pp 43-61

Alter BP, Parkman R, Rappeport JM (1981) Bone marrow failure syndromes. In: Nathan DG, Oski FA (eds) Hematology of infancy and childhood, 2nd edn. Saunders Philadelphia, pp 168-249

Auerbach AD, Adler B, Chaganti RSK (1981) Prenatal and postnatal diagnosis and carrier detection of Fanconi anemia by a cytogenetic method. Pediatrics 67: 128-135

Auerbach AD, Weiner MA, Warburton D, Yeboa K, Lu L, Broxmeyer HE (1982) Acute myeloid leukemia as the first hematologic manifestation of Fanconi anemia. Am J Hematol 12: 289-300

Auerbach AD, Adler B, O'Reilly RJ, Kirkpatrick D, Chaganti RSK (1983) Effect of procarbazine and cyclophosphamide on chromosome breakage in Fanconi anemia cells: relevance to bone marrow transplantation. Cancer Genet Cytogenet 9: 25-36

Auerbach AD, Sagi M, Adler B (1985) Fanconi anemia: prenetal diagnosis in 30 fetuses at risk. Pediatrics 76: 794-800

Bacigalupo A, DiGiorgio F, Congiu M, Van Lint MT, Frassoni F, Daga MG, Gogioso L, Marmont AM (1985) Treatment of severe aplastic anemia in Europe 1970-1983. A report of the EBMT SAA Working Party. Exp Hematol 13 (Suppl 17): 56-57

Berger R, Bernheim A, Gluckman E, Gisselbrecht C (1980) In vitro effect of cyclophosphamide metabolites on chromosomes of Fanconi anaemia patients. Br J Haematol 45: 565-568

Berkovitz GD, Zinkham WH, Migeon CJ (1984) Gonadal function in two siblings with Fanconi's anemia. Horm Res 19: 137-141

Cattan D, Kalifat R, Wantier JL, Meignan S, Vesin P, Piet R (1974) Maladie de Fanconi et cancer du foie. Arch Fr Mal Appar Dig 63: 41-48

De Chadarevian JP, Vekemans M, Bernstein M (1985) Fanconi's anemia, medulloblastoma, Wilms' tumor, horseshoe kidney, and gonadal dysgenesis. Arch Pathol Lab Med 109: 367-369

Deeg HJ, Storb R, Thomas ED, Appelbaum F, Buckner CD, Clift RA, Doney K, Johnson L, Sanders JE, Stewart P, Sullivan KM, Witherspoon RP (1983) Fanconi's anemia treated by allogeneic marrow transplantation. Blood 61: 954-959

Dharmasena F, Catchpole M, Erber W, Mason D, Gordon-Smith EC (1986) Megakaryoblastic leukaemia and myelofibrosis complicating Fanconi anaemia. Scand J Haematol 36: 309-313

Durrant STS, Swirsky DM, Hows JM, Gordon-Smith EG (1987) Bone marrow transplantation of Fanconi anaemia: the Hammersmith experience. Bone Marrow Transplant 2 (Suppl 1): 104

Fanconi G (1927) Familiäre infantile perniziosaartige Anämie (perniziöses Blutbild und Konstitution). Z Kinderheilkd 117: 257-280
Gardner FM (1985) Anabolic steroids in aplastic anemia. Acta Endocrinol [Suppl] (Copenh) 271: 87-96
Garriga S, Crosby WH (1959) The incidence of leukemia in families of patients with hypoplasia of the marrow. Blood 14: 1008-1012
Gluckman E, Devergie A, Schaison G, Bussel A, Berger R, Sohier J, Bernard J (1980) Bone marrow transplantation in Fanconi anaemia. Br J Haematol 45: 557-564
Gluckman E, Devergie A, Dutreix J (1983) Radiosensitivity in Fanconi anemia: application to the conditioning regimen for bone marrow transplantation. Br J Haematol 54: 431-440
Gluckman E, Berger R, Dutreix J (1984) Bone marrow transplantation for Fanconi anemia. Semin Hematol 21: 20-26
Gluckman E, Devergie A, Meletis J, Traineau R, Vilmer E, Lehn P, Keable H, Bourrhis JH, Varrin F (1987) Bone marrow transplantation in severe aplastic anemia. Report of 100 consecutive cases. Bone Marrow Transplant 2 (Suppl 2): 101
Hersey P, Edwards A, Lewis R, Kemp A, McInnes J (1982) Deficient natural killer cell activity in a patient with Fanconi's anaemia and squamous cell carcinoma. Association with defect in interferon release. Clin Exp Immunol 48: 205-212
Hill LS, Dennis PM, Fairham SA (1981) Adenocarcinoma of the stomach and Fanconi's anaemia. Postgrad Med J 57: 404
Hows JM, Yin JL, Marsh J, Swirsky D, Jones L, Apperley JF, James DCD, Smithers S, Batchelor JR, Goldman JM, Gordon-Smith EC (1986) Histocompatible unrelated, volunteer donors compared with HLA nonidentical family donors in marrow transplantation for aplastic anemia and leukemia. Blood 68: 1322-1328
Izakovic V, Strbakova E, Kaiserova E, Krizan P (1985) Bovine superoxide dismutase in Fanconi anaemia. Therapeutic trial in two patients. Hum Genet 70: 181-182
Jacobs P, Karabus C (1984) Fanconi's anemia. A family study with 20-year follow-up including associated breast pathology. Cancer 54: 1850-1853
Joenje H, Eriksson AW, Frants RR, Arwert F, Houwen B (1978) Erythrocyte superoxide-dismutase deficiency in Fanconi's anaemia. Lancet i: 204
Johannson E, Niemi KM, Siimes M, Pyrhönen S (1982) Fanconi's anemia: tumor-like warts, hyperpigmentation associated with deranged keratinocytes, and depressed cell-mediated immunity. Arch Dermatol 118: 249-252
Kaplan MJ, Sabio H, Wanebo HJ, Cantrell RW (1985) Squamous cell carcinoma in the immunosuppressed patient: Fanconi's anemia. Laryngoscope 95: 771-775
Kennedy AW, Hart WR (1982) Multiple squamous-cell carcinomas in Fanconi's anemia. Cancer 50: 811-814
Morell D, Chase CL, Kupper LL, Swift M (1986) Diabetes mellitus in ataxia-telangiectasia, Fanconi anemia, xeroderma pigmentosum, common variable immune deficiency, and severe combined immune deficiency families. Diabetes 35: 143-147
Nordan UZ, Humbert JR, MacGillivray MH, Fitzpatrick JE (1979) Fanconi's anemia with growth hormone deficiency. Am J Dis Child 133: 291-293
Obeid DA, Hill FGH, Harnden D, Mann JR, Wood BSB (1980) Fanconi anemia. Oxymetholone hepatic tumors, and chromosome aberrations associated with leukemia transition. Cancer 46: 1401-1404
Pedersen FK, Hertz H, Lundsteen C, Platz P, Thomsen M (1977) Indication of primary immune deficiency in Fanconi's anemia. Acta Paediatr Scand 66: 745-751
Pochedly C, Collipp PJ, Wolman SR, Suwansirikul S, Rezvani I (1971) Fanconi's anemia with growth hormone deficiency. J Pediatr 79: 93-96
Poynton CH, MacDonald D, Byrom NA, Barett AJ (1987) Rejection after T cell depletion of donor bone marrow. Bone Marrow Transplantation 2 (Suppl 1): 153
Reed K, Ravikumar TS, Gifford RRM, Grage TB (1983) The association of Fanconi's anemia and squamous cell carcinoma. Cancer 52: 926-928
Sanders JE, Whitehead J, Storb R, Buckner CD, Clift RA, Mickelson E, Appelbaum FR, Bensinger WI, Stewart PS, Doney K, Sullivan K, Deeg HJ, Witherspoon RP, Thomas ED (1986) Bone marrow transplantation experience for children with aplastic anemia. Pediatrics 77: 179-186

Schmidt E, Deeg HJ, Storb R (1984) Regression of androgen-related hepatic tumors in patients with Fanconi's anemia following marrow transplantation. Transplantation 37: 452-455

Swift M (1971) Fanconi's anemia in the genetics of neoplasia. Nature 230: 370-373

Swift M, Caldwell RJ, Chase C (1980) Reassessment of cancer predisposition of Fanconi anemia heterozygotes. JNCT 65: 863-867

Wilkinson EJ, Morgan LS, Friedrich EG (1984) Association of Fanconi's anemia and squamous-cell carcinoma of the lower female genital tract with condyloma acuminatum. A report of two cases. J Reprod Med 29: 447-453

Yoshimitsu K, Kobayashi Y, Usui T (1984) Decreased superoxide dismutase activity of erythrocytes and leukocytes in Fanconi's anemia. Acta Haematol (Basel) 72: 208-210

Zachmann M, Illig R, Prader A (1972) Fanconi's anemia with isolated growth hormone deficiency. J Pediatr 80: 159-160

Bone Marrow Transplantation for Fanconi Anemia

E. Gluckman, A. Devergie, and J. Dutreix

Introduction

Fanconi anemia (FA) is an autosomal recessive inherited condition in which congenital malformations are associated with bone marrow failure. The most common abnormalities are skin pigmentation, microcephaly, short stature, skeletal defects, particularly of the lateral aspect of the forearms and hands, and kidney and cardiac malformations (Fanconi 1967; Beard 1976). Multiple abnormalities of peripheral blood lymphocyte chromosomes are almost always present. Left to follow its natural course, FA is always fatal, with death caused by progressive marrow aplasia or, less frequently, by development of acute leukemia (Swift 1976; Prindull et al. 1979). Bone marrow transplantation (BMT) has the potential to correct the stem cell defect. In the past, the outcome of transplantation in patients with FA has been poor because of the severe and prolonged toxicity of the pretransplantation conditioning regimen and subsequent graft-versus-host disease (Gluckman et al. 1980). The poor tolerance to alkylating agents has been related to a DNA repair defect leading to increased chromosomal instability. Recently, efforts have been made to modify the conditioning regimen according to cell sensitivity to alkylating agents and to irradiation.

Cytogenetic Analysis

Cytogenetic analysis is very important for confirming the diagnosis of FA and for predicting sensitivity to alkylating agents. In the case of BMT, it is mandatory to perform a complete cytogenetic analysis on the donor to determine if he or she is healthy, a heterozygote, or a homozygote for the FA gene. The classical cytogenetic analysis performed on the peripheral lymphocytes of FA patients at birth shows an increase in the chromosomal breakage rate with chromatid breaks, and dicentric and ring chromosomes. The type and frequency of chromosomal breaks vary markedly from patient to patient, and in the same patient when analyzed on different occasions. For this reason, more sensitive tests have been described. They utilize the sensitivity of lymphocytes to DNA cross-linking agents. Berger studied the effect of cyclophosphamide metabolites in FA (Berger et al. 1980a) and showed an increase in the frequency of chromosomal breaks in FA lymphocytes when they were incubated with low concentrations of sera from a cyclophospha-

T. M. Schroeder-Kurth A. D. Auerbach G. Obe (Eds.)
Fanconi Anemia, Clinical, Cytogenetic and Experimental Aspects

mide-treated patient. No effect was observed in cells from parents of these patients or from controls. A similar effect was observed by Auerbach et al. (1983). Furthermore, nitrogen mustard added at a final concentration of 0.085 μg/liter after 1 day of culture of phytohemagglutin (PHA)-stimulated lymphocytes drastically increased the level of chromosome breakage in the cells of patients with FA (Berger et al. 1980b). A clear distinction between patients and parents was possible, allowing the detection of heterozygotes: nitrogen mustard added to the cultures significantly increased sister chromatid exchange in FA heterozygotes compared with that in controls. Auerbach described the hypersensitivity of FA cells to the clastogenic effect of diepoxybutane (DEB) (Auerbach and Wolman 1976, 1978). This test was used for prenatal and postnatal diagnosis of FA (Auerbach et al. 1981), but there was too much overlap between normal and FA-heterozygote cells for accurate heterozygote detection.

Radiosensitivity in Fanconi Anemia

Lymphocytes from FA patients exposed to 1 Gy irradiation show a higher rate of chromosome breaks per cell than those from controls ($p<0.01$) (Higurashi and Conen 1971). An in vivo test of radiosensitivity and cell restoration as a predictor of the patient's response to irradiation for BMT conditioning has been described (Gluckman et al. 1983). The sensitivity of the skin to radiation was tested in two ways: in a first test to measure overall radiosensitivity, two areas of skin, 15 mm in diameter, on the anterior aspect of the thigh, were irradiated with a 50 kV X-ray source at 0.5 Gy/s. One area received 8 Gy, the other 10 Gy. The skin was examined every 2 weeks for evidence of pigmentation and desquamation. In a previous study of 20 normal controls, slight desquamation appeared 30-40 days after irradiation (Dutreix et al. 1973). Cell repair was evaluated by comparing the reaction of the skin to a single dose of irradiation with the reaction after irradiation given in two equal fractions separated by an interval of 3-4 hours. Fractions of 4 Gy, 5 Gy, 6 Gy, or 7 Gy were given. Cell repair was considered normal when the reaction of the skin to a single 10 Gy dose was similar to that of a 2 × 6 Gy fractionated dose. The results are shown in Table 1. Before BMT, 12 patients were studied for skin radiosensitivity in order to predict their reaction to the irradiation used for conditioning. The most constant abnormality was a delay in the peak skin reaction, ranging from 40 to 55 days in comparison with 30 days for the 20 controls. This observation could be related to an increased transmission time from the basal layer to the surface layer of the skin. The second abnormality observed in ten patients was an increased sensitivity to a single dose of 10 Gy. The practical implication of the demonstration of increased radiosensitivity is proper adjustment of the irradiation dose given for conditioning. Absence of repair was demonstrated in only three cases, which can be related to the lack of sensitivity of the method or to the heterogeneity of the disease. Absence of repair implies that the relative protection expected from low-dose rate or fractionated irradiation of tissues exhibiting rapid repair such as those of the gut, mucosa, and lung, would not be furnished. Because of these results, we have chosen to lower the irradiation dose from 6 to 5 Gy given in a single fraction at a mean dose rate of 10 cGy/min.

Table 1. Skin radiosensitivity test in Fanconi anemia

Patients UPN	Delay of reaction peak (days)	Reaction at 10 Gy	Repair	Number of abnormalities
SLA 87	55	D_2	O	3
SLA 92	50	D_2	O	3
SLA 97	40	D_1	N	2
SLA 100	40	D_2	N	2
SLA 101	50	D_1	N	2
SLA 103	40	P_2	N	2
SLA 116	40	D_1	N	2
SLA 118	40	P	N	1
SLA 126	40	D_2	N	2
SLA 134	40	D_1	O	3
SLA 139	40	D_1	N	2
SLA 148	40	D_1	N	2

D, desquamation; P, pigmentation

The fields were calculated for complete protection of the lungs, part of the liver, testicles, head, and the lower two-thirds of the legs.

The predictive value of the radiosensitivity remains to be demonstrated. In our series of patients, we did not find any correlation between the results of this test, the severity of the disease, and the outcome of the graft.

Results of Bone Marrow Transplantation

A total of 21 patients with FA have received transplants in our unit. The first five patients were conditioned with high-dose cyclophosphamide (100-200 mg/kg given over 4 days). Details of the results are given in Table 2. Only one patient is still surviving; 8 years after BMT, her growth is normal and she shows signs of puberty. Her blood counts give normal results and chromosomal analysis shows no elevation of chromosomal aberrations (Berger et al. 1980c). The other patients died early after BMT. They all had toxic complications related to cyclophosphamide: hemorrhagic cystitis, cardiac failure, fluid overload, and severe mucositis with intestinal hemorrhages. These were always associated with an early take and severe grade III-IV graft-versus-host disease (GVHD). These results prompted us to modify the conditioning regimen according to in vitro tests of lymphocyte sensitivity to cyclophosphamide and to in vivo radiosensitivity skin tests.

A subsequent series of 16 patients received a modified conditioning regimen (Table 3) consisting of cyclophosphamide 20 mg/kg given at a daily dose of 5 mg/kg IV on days −6, −5, −4 and −3 followed on day −1 by 5 Gy thoracoabdominal irradiation (TAI). Details of this conditioning regimen have been published elsewhere (Gluckman et al. 1983); it mimics the 150 mg/kg cyclophosphamide and 6 Gy TAI (Gluckman et al. 1984a), currently used in our unit to prepare patients for BMT who have severe aplastic anemia due to other causes than FA. Cyclosporin A (CYA) was given as a prophylaxis against GVHD from day −1 until at least day 180 after transplantation. The initial dose was given according to a

Table 2. Bone marrow transplant results after conditioning with 100-200 mg/kg cyclophosphamide

Patient UPN	Age	Sex	Take	AGVHD Grade	CGVHD	Survival (and cause of death)
SLA 22	7	F	+	IV	O	>7 years, A/W
SLA 31	11	M	+	IV	NE	† 40 days, GVHD
SLA 35	11	M	+	IV	NE	† 48 days, GVHD
SLA 44	10	F	+	IV	NE	† 48 days, GVHD
SLA 50	7	F	+	III	NE	† 150 days, liver failure

† Death
AGVHD, acute graft-versus-host disease; CGVHD, chronic graft-versus-host disease; A/W, alive and well; NE nonevaluable; GVHD, graft-versus-host disease

Table 3. Bone marrow transplantation results after conditioning with 20 mg/kg cyclophosphamide and 5 Gy thoracoabdominal irradiation

UPN	Age	Sex	Take	AGVHD Grade	CGVHD	Survival (and cause of death)
SLA 87	15	M	+	O	O	>5 Years A/W
SLA 92	10	F	+	III	O	>4 Years A/W
SLA 97	15	M	+	O	Mild	>4 Years A/W
SLA 100	10	M	+	I	Mild	>4 Years A/W
SLA 101	13	M	+	III	Mild	† 996 Days acute liver failure sepsis
SLA 103	12	M	+	II	O	>4 Years A/W
SLA 116	5	F	+	II	O	>3 Years
SLA 118	14	M	+	III	NE	† 60 Days HUS
SLA 126	17	F	+	III	NE	† 104 Days CMV IP+GVHD
SLA 134	11	F	0	NE	NE	† 40 Days Candida sepsis
SLA 139	19	M	+	O	O	>2 Years A/W
SLA 141	11	M	+	II	Mild	>2 Years A/W
SLA 148	9	M	+	II	O	>18 Months A/W
SLA 165	12	M	+	II	O	>11 Months A/W
SLA 166	7	M	+	II	O	>11 Months A/W
SLA 180	6	M	+	NE	NE	>1 Month

† Death
AGVHD, acute graft versus host disease; CGVHD, chronic graft versus host disease; NE, nonevaluable; A/W, alive and well; HUS, hemolytic and uremic syndrome; CMV IP, cytomegalovirus interstitial pneumonia

preliminary individual pharmacokinetic study (RIA) in order to obtain a CYA plasma level of 100 ng/ml. Subsequently, the dose of CYA was adjusted to the results of weekly measurements of CYA plasma levels and to blood urea and creatinine dosages (Gluckman et al. 1984b). The mean age at the time of diagnosis was 6.6 years (range 2-17), the mean age at the time of transplantation was 11.5 years (range 5-19). All patients had typical malformations associated with FA, but in three patients there were only a few café au lait spots. Two patients had an affected sibling and in five other patients there were cases of early infant deaths, malformations, aplasia, or leukemia in the family history. In two families, there was proven consanguinity between parents. The geographical origin was: France, six cases (two from the French Basque country); Algeria, three cases; Italy, two cases; Tunisia, one case; Belgium, one case; Switzerland, one case; Portugal, one case; and Argentina, one case. All patients had been previously treated with androgens and corticosteroids; all except one had been given transfusions and eight patients were refractory to random platelet transfusions. One patient had multiple liver adenomas which had bled into the peritoneal cavity; they resolved spontaneously after transplantation. All patients had typical cytogenetic abnormalities the frequencies of which increased on incubation with nitrogen mustard. They received a bone marrow transplant from a healthy HLA-identical sibling. All donors were screened for absence of congenital malformations, normality of blood counts, and absence of chromosomal breaks in cytogenetic analysis. The patients received a mean cell dose of 4.9×10^8 nucleated cells/kg (range $2.3-9.8 \times 10^8$/kg). The conditioning regimen was well tolerated except in the first five patients who 2 months after transplantation developed severe esophagitis with strictures in three cases. Subsequently ranitidine was administered to all patients as preventive treatment. Severe esophagitis is quite unusual after BMT and it is postulated that FA patients may have esophageal abnormalities which become apparent after irradiation. None of the patients had hemorrhagic cystitis or any other sign of intolerance observed after high doses of cyclophosphamide.

Fifteen patients had a prompt take with a rise of peripheral blood counts starting around day 15. Engraftment failed to occur in only one patient, who died of *Candida* sepsis on day 40. GVHD was observed in 11/16 cases. Of these, seven patients had a grade I-II and four patients a grade III GVHD. Chronic GVHD was observed in four cases: it was limited, without progression to sclerosis. Currently, 12/16 patients are alive with a median follow-up period of 2 years. All the long-term survivors are doing well, with normal growth and a 100% Karnofsky score. All are back at school or work. Apparently the conditioning treatment had no long-term effect. One patient (SLA 116) was found to be seropositive for HIV infection but she has no opportunistic infections or subnormal immunological functions. One patient has focal epilepsy related to sequelae of a herpes encephalitis. Four patients died after BMT. One (SLA 101) had chronic liver GVHD; on day 906, he suddenly developed acute liver failure and died of peritonitis due to perforation of the Meckel's diverticulum. Starting on day 7, patient SLA 118 developed hemolytic and uremic syndrome with anuria; at the autopsy performed on day 60, signs of disseminated intravascular coagulation were found. Patient SLA 126 died on day 103 of acute GVHD associated with cytomegalovirus interstitial pneumonia. The overall results and complications of this series of patients do not vary markedly from those observed in patients who received transplants for aplastic anemia due to causes other than FA. The only difference is the relatively low figure of 20% of the patients with severe aplastic anemia (SAA) who had chronic GVHD. This difference could be due to the small number of patients or perhaps to an inability of FA fibroblasts to produce fibrosis through activation by donor lymphocytes.

Results Reported Elsewhere

Deeg et al. (1983) reported the results of their study of eight patients with FA given cyclophosphamide alone (seven patients) or combined with an antithymocyte globulin (one patient) followed by marrow grafts from HLA-identical siblings. Diagnosis of FA in the patients was not confirmed by DNA cross-link sensitivity studies. Seven developed acute GVHD and three chronic GVHD. Three patients died of GVHD and infectious complications (on days 19, 56 and 82) and one of intracerebral hemorrhage (day 540). This last patient had evidence of engraftment but required two additional infusions of marrow from the same donor (days 35 and 391). The donor had chromosomal abnormalities similar to those found in the patient and an abnormal growth of colony-forming unit in vitro. It is possible that the donor had latent FA and that the poorly functioning graft was the result of a defect in the donor's marrow cells. All patients had severe mucositis and six developed hemorrhagic cystitis. Four patients are still surviving 647-3435 days after grafting, of whom two are well and two have chronic GVHD that is improving. Overall, the literature reports a total of 21 patients with FA conditioned with high-dose cyclophosphamide. Of these 38% were long-term survivors, of whom 71% had acute GVHD. This result should be compared with that obtained with the modified conditioning regimen which includes very low doses of cyclophosphamide or none at all. Besides our own results, Auerbach showed that cells from patients with FA were no more sensitive than normal cells to procarbazine-induced chromosomal breakage (Auerbach et al. 1983). According to these results, a conditioning using 12.5 mg/kg procarbazine per day administered in three doses over 6 days, alternating with three doses of antithymocyte globulin (15 mg/kg per day) and followed by low-dose fractionated total body irradiation (7 Gy), was used in three patients. This regimen was well tolerated with mild mucositis. One patient died prematurely of cerebral hemorrhage, two patients are alive but follow-up was short at the time of publication.

Discussion

Current results of BMT for non-Fanconi aplastic anemia have, like those of FA, recently been improving: a 70% long-term survival rate has been obtained in different centers (Gluckman et al 1984b; Hows et al. 1981; Storb et al. 1982; Ramsay et al. 1983). Advances made in the last decade explain these results. These include better indications, improvement of gnotobiotic techniques and transfusion support, and utilization of new conditioning regimens and immunosuppressive agents such as CYA. A better knowledge of the nature of the underlying diseases for which BMT is performed will hopefully improve these results. FA is a good example of this: it was first shown by in vitro studies that patients experienced an unusual toxicity to the conditioning regimen. Subsequently, a decrease in the dose or omission of cyclophosphamide from the conditioning regimen improved the long-term survival rate from 38% to 70%. Therefore, accurate diagnosis of the disease is mandatory. FA is quite different from the other constitutional aplastic anemias: dyskeratosis congenita (DC) has been clearly distinguished by its later onset, the occurrence of nail dystrophy and leukoplasia of mucosal surfaces, and the high frequency of malignant epithelial tumors. Chromosomal findings were normal in most cases reported, but some authors described an increased number of chromosomal breaks. Our own experience shows that these two diseases can be clearly separated. We had the opportunity to perform transplants in two patients with DC complicated by severe aplastic anemia (SAA), neither of whom had chromosomal abnormalities. They were both conditioned with our SAA protocol including 150 mg/kg cyclophosphamide and 6 Gy TAI. There was no sign of intolerance to cyclophosphamide and the immediate outcome after transplantation was uneventful. Both developed (2 and 7 years after transplantation) signs of endothelial activation with diffuse vasculitis. The first patient died of cerebral hemorrhage due to hypertension, and a renal biopsy showed severe vascular damage. The second patient developed hypertension and veno-occlusive disease of the liver confirmed by biopsy 7 years after BMT. These observations suggest that endothelial cells of patients with DC may be abnormally sensitive to the agents used for conditioning.

Accurate diagnosis when familial history is negative for FA or when malformations are not observed is critical. It seems that, in the BMT setting, it is mandatory to test all juvenile patients suffering from aplastic anemia, not only for spontaneous chromosomal breaks but also for increased frequency of breaks after incubation with appropriate drugs. The standardization of techniques of this sort would be very useful for the detection of such cases. In our series of 183 patients who received transplants for SAA, the diagnosis of FA was usually easy. Nevertheless, mistakes were made in two cases. One patient developed aplastic anemia at the age of ten. He had no malformations suggestive of FA and there was no family history of the disease. Several cytogenetic studies were performed: some were normal, one showed 4% chromosomal breakage with an increase to 16% after incubation with nitrogen mustard. This abnormality was felt to be insufficient to confirm the diagnosis of FA. The patient was given a transplant at the age of 16 with 150 mg/kg cyclophosphamide and 6 Gy TAI. Shortly after transplantation, he developed hemorrhagic cystitis, gastrointestinal hemorrhages, and a skin rash, all symptoms similar to those in our first five patients with FA, who had received transplants after conditioning with high-dose cyclophosphamide. He died on day 40 of acute pulmonary edema and was classified as having had FA according to the clinical course of the disease.

The other patient was diagnosed at the age of 3 months as having Blackfan-Diamond erythroblastopenia. She had several malformations including microphthalmia, thumb and skeleton abnormalities, and cardiac malformations similar to those observed in FA. When she was 2 years old, in addition to anemia, she developed agranulocytosis with repeated severe infectious complications. Her platelet counts remained normal. Repeated cytogenetic analyses were discordant: one showed an increase in chromosomal breaks in peripheral blood lymphocytes, two other analyses were normal. The sensitivity to alkylating agents was not tested. A study of bone marrow cells showed an increase in chromosomal breaks; skin tests for radiosensitivity were abnormal. She was given the same conditioning treatment as patients with FA; she had a good take, but 6 months after transplantation the graft was rejected with a reappearance of erythroblastopenia and agranulocytosis.

In conclusion, FA seems to be a potentially curable disease. Secondary prevention could be performed by prenatal diagnosis if there is a family history of FA (Auerbach et al. 1981). BMT offers a good chance of cure providing that there is an HLA-identical healthy donor. The chances of finding a donor within the family for a patients with FA are slightly higher than for patients with other forms of SAA because the parents are frequently consanguinous. For those who have no HLA-identical donor, studies are in progress on the use of HLA-matched, unrelated donors or for the use of partially mismatched, related donors.

References

Auerbach AD, Wolman SR (1976) Susceptibility of Fanconi's anaemia fibroblasts to chromosome damage by carcinogens. Nature 261: 494-496

Auerbach AD, Wolman SR (1978) Carcinogen-induced chromosome breakage in Fanconi anemia heterozygous cells. Nature 271: 69-71

Auerbach AD, Adler B, Chaganti RSK (1981) Prenatal and postnatal diagnosis and carrier detection of Fanconi's anaemia by a cytogenetic method. Pediatrics 67: 128-135

Auerbach AD, Adler B, O'Reilly RJ et al. (1983) Effect of procarbazine and cyclophosphamide on chromosome breakage in Fanconi anemia cells - relevance to bone marrow transplantation. Cancer Genet Cytogenet 9: 25-36

Beard MEJ (1976) Fanconi anemia. In: Congenital disorders of erythropoiesis. Ciba Found Symp 103-114

Berger R, Bernheim A, Gluckman E et al. (1980a) In vitro effect of cyclophosphamide metabolites on chromosomes of Fanconi anaemia patients. Br J Haematol 45: 565-568

Berger R, Bernheim A, Le Coniat M et al. (1980b) Nitrogen mustard induced chromosome breakage: a tool for Fanconi anemia diagnosis. Cancer Genetics and Cytogenetics 2: 269-274

Berger R, Bernheim A, Leconiat M et al. (1980c) Bone marrow graft of Fanconi's anemia patient: cytogenetic study. Cancer Genet Cytogenet 2: 127-130

Deeg HJ, Storb R, Thomas ED et al. (1983) Fanconi's anemia treated by allogeneic bone marrow transplantation. Blood 61: 954-959

Dutreix J, Wambersie A, Bounik C (1973) Cellular recovery in human skin reactions - application to dose fraction number overall time relationship in radiotherapy. Eur J Cancer 9: 159-167

Fanconi G (1967) Familial constitutional panmyelocytopathy Fanconi's anemia. Clinical aspects. Semin Hematol 4: 233-240

Gluckman E, Devergie A, Schaison G et al. (1980) Bone marrow transplantation in Fanconi anaemia. Br J Haematol 45: 557-564

Gluckman E, Devergie A, Dutreix J (1983) Radiosensitivity in Fanconi anaemia: application to the conditioning regimen for bone marrow transplantation. Br J Haematol 54: 431-440

Gluckman E, Devergie A, Benbunan M et al. (1984a) Bone marrow transplantation in severe aplastic anemia using cyclophosphamide and thoraco-abdominal irradiation. In: Aplastic anemia - stem cell biology and advances in treatment. Liss, New York, pp325-333

Gluckman E, Devergie A, Poirier O et al. (1984b) Use of cyclosporine A as prophylaxis of graft versus host disease after human allogeneic bone marrow transplantation. Report of 38 patients. Transplant Proc 15: 2628-2633

Higurashi M, Conen PE (1971) In vitro chromosomal radiosensitivity in Fanconi's anemia. Blood 38: 336-342

Hows J, Harris R, Palmer S et al. (1981) Immunosuppression with cyclosporin A in allogeneic bone marrow transplantation for severe aplastic anemia: preliminary results. Br J Haematol 48: 227-236

Prindull G, Jentsch E, Hansmann L (1979) Fanconi's anaemia developing erythroleukaemia. Scand J Haematol 23: 59-63

Ramsay NKC, Kim TH, McGlave PB et al. (1983) Bone marrow transplantation for severe aplastic anemia using the conditioning regimen of cyclophosphamide and total lymphoid irradiation. Exp Hematol 10: 139-142

Storb R, Doney KC, Thomas ED et al. (1982) Marrow transplantation with or without donor buffy coat cells for 65 transfused aplastic anemia patients. Blood 59: 236-246

Swift MR (1976) Fanconi's anemia: cellular abnormalities and clinical predisposition to malignant disease. In: Congenital disorders of erythropoiesis. Ciba Found Symp 11-115

Part II

Spontaneous and Induced Chromosomal Breakage for Diagnosis of Patients with Fanconi Anemia and Their Relatives

Diepoxybutane Test for Prenatal and Postnatal Diagnosis of Fanconi Anemia*

A. D. Auerbach, R. Ghosh, P. C. Pollio, and M. Zhang

Introduction

Patients with Fanconi anemia (FA) show considerable heterogeneity in the age of onset, phenotypic expression, and clinical course of the disease, making diagnosis of the disorder on the basis of clinical manifestations alone both difficult and unreliable. The basis for this heterogeneity is unknown, as is the molecular basis for the syndrome. Complementation analysis has demonstrated the existence of at least two complementation groups (Duckworth-Rysiecki et al. 1985; Auerbach et al. 1986a; Moustacchi et al. 1986), but this genetic heterogeneity has not yet been correlated with the clinical heterogeneity seen in affected individuals. Since FA patients who lack congenital malformations, previously described as having the Estren-Dameshek syndrome (Estren and Dameshek 1947; Dallapiccola et al. 1980), are found in the same sibships as "classical" FA, with multiple congenital abnormalities (Glanz and Fraser 1982), this phenotypic diversity cannot be accounted for by genetic heterogeneity alone. The diagnosis of FA is also made difficult by the occurrence of other disorders, both genetic and nongenetic, which are characterized by many of the clinical features seen in FA. For these reasons, the development of a laboratory test which aids in the identification of FA individuals would be useful.

Schroeder et al. (1964, 1976) first suggested the use of spontaneous chromosomal breakage as a cellular marker for FA; however, longitudinal studies of chromosome instability in FA patients have shown a wide variation in the frequency of baseline breakage within the same individual, ranging from no baseline breakage to high levels (Schroeder et al. 1976; McIntosh et al. 1979). An abnormal sensitivity to a variety of DNA cross-linking agents has been demonstrated both in FA patients (Gluckman et al. 1980, 1984; Auerbach et al. 1982, 1983) and in cells from these patients (Sasaki and Tonomura 1973; Auerbach and Wolman 1976; Weksberg et al. 1979). We have suggested elsewhere that the hypersensitivity of cells from FA patients to the clastogenic effect of the DNA cross-linking agent diepoxy-

* This work was supported in part by Basil O'Connor Starter Research Grant No. 5-446 from the March of Dimes Birth Defects Foundation, by PHS Grant No. HL32987 from the National Institutes of Health, by a General Clinical Research Center Grant RR00102 from the National Institutes of Health to The Rockefeller University Hospital, and by support from the Pew Memorial Trust to the Laboratory for Investigative Dermatology.

T. M. Schroeder-Kurth A. D. Auerbach G. Obe (Eds.)
Fanconi Anemia, Clinical, Cytogenetic and Experimental Aspects

butane (DEB) can be used as a unique cellular marker for the syndrome, facilitating both prenatal and postnatal diagnosis (Auerbach et al. 1981, 1985, 1986b, 1989). Tests based on demonstrating an increased frequency of induced chromosomal breakage after exposure of cultured cells to a variety of DNA cross-linking agents such as mitomycin C (MMC) or nitrogen mustard are in use in some laboratories (Berger et al. 1980; Cervenka et al. 1981), as are tests based on the differential inhibition of cell growth when FA and normal lymphocytes are cultured in a medium containing MMC (German et al. 1987; Arwert and Kwee, this volume). In our experience, the use of DEB for diagnosis of FA appears to be more reliable than the use of MMC, as the latter can lead to false-positive diagnoses due to the wide range of sensitivity to MMC found in normal individuals. We are also concerned that FA patients with two populations of lymphocytes, in whom a majority of cells appear to be cross-link resistant (Auerbach et al., this volume), would be diagnosed as unaffected in cocultivation tests. In this chapter we present a detailed description of our methods for prenatal and postnatal testing using DEB, as well as an updated summary of our results using these methods.

Methods

Peripheral Blood Lymphocytes

The culture unit consisted of 0.4 ml of heparinized blood added to 10 ml of RPMI 1640 medium (Gibco) supplemented with 15% fetal bovine serum, 1-glutamine, penicillin-streptomycin, and phytohemagglutinin (PHA); this was incubated for 72 or 96 h at 37 °C in a 5% CO_2 atmosphere at high humidity. The culture vessel was either a washed and sterilized 2 oz glass medicine bottle or a 25 cm^2 disposable tissue culture flask. Cultures were set up in triplicate for DEB studies, and a replicate set of cultures was established, to serve as untreated controls. DEB, at a final concentration in the medium of 0.1 μg/ml, was added to the treated cultures 24 h after their initiation, thus exposing cells to the chemical for 48–72 h. This concentration was chosen because it induces multiple chromosomal breaks and gaps in cells from FA patients while having little clastogenic effect on normal cells. The mitotic index is usually not affected by this concentration. Dilutions were prepared just prior to the addition of DEB to cell cultures. In diluting the DEB, which is a liquid at room temperature, a density of 1.0 g/ml was used for calculation purposes. The first of three serial dilutions in phosphate-buffered saline (PBS) was prepared by adding 10 μl DEB to 10 ml PBS, resulting in a DEB concentration of 1 mg/ml. The half-life of DEB, a highly reactive DNA cross-linking agent, is approximately 4 days in aqueous solution. Cultures were harvested after 72–96 h, and chromosome preparations were made following standard methods.

As DEB is thought to be carcinogen, with unknown risk, all possible precautions were taken. Cultures with DEB were handled using latex gloves, and all work was carried out in a vertical laminar flow hood or a chemical fume hood (for the first part of the harvest procedure). Since DEB is rapidly inactivated by concentrated (50%) HCl, all disposable culture bottles and pipettes were rinsed with

HCl before being discarded. HCl was added to spent medium before disposal, and was used in case of spillage.

From each DEB-treated preparation, 50-100 Giemsa-stained metaphases were analyzed (25 metaphases in the case of very high breakage). If the frequency of DEB-induced chromosomal breakage was found to be above the normal range, 50 Giemsa-stained metaphases from the untreated preparation were also analyzed. To avoid bias in cell selection, consecutive metaphases which appeared unbroken with sufficiently well-defined chromosome morphology were selected for study. Each cell was scored for chromosome number and for the numbers and types of structural abnormalities. Achromatic areas less than a chromatid in width were scored as gaps, while exchange configurations, translocations, and dicentric and ring chromosomes were scored as rearrangements. Gaps were excluded from the calculations of the frequency of chromosomal breakage, and rearrangements were scored as two breaks.

Amniocentesis

Amniotic fluid samples (30 ml each) were obtained, and delivered to the laboratory in syringes or sterile nontoxic tubes. The amniotic fluid was centrifuged at 800 rpm for 10 min. The cell pellet was resuspended in a small volume of the patient's own amniotic fluid, the final concentration of which was at least 10% (vol/vol). For example, if the cells from 5 ml of amniotic fluid were plated in a 25 cm^2 tissue culture flask, the cell pellet was resuspended in at least 0.5 ml of the patient's own amniotic fluid and added to a flask containing 4.5 ml of medium. The preferred medium was complete Chang medium (Hana Media Inc., USA), which facilitates the growth of cells, especially after subculture. Increased chromosomal breakage, reported to be associated with this medium (Casey et al. 1983), does not interfere with the discrimination of affected fetuses. Six flasks were set up from 30 ml of amniotic fluid, cultures were incubated at 37 °C in an atmosphere of 5% CO_2, and the flasks were not disturbed for 4-5 days, allowing time for cell attachment. The culture medium was then aspirated, and 5 ml of fresh medium was added to each flask. Cultures were fed every 3-4 days thereafter and carefully monitored microscopically. When macroscopically visible colonies of 2-4 mm diameter were present, chromosome preparations for banding analysis were made from primary cultures. Metaphase spreads were examined for the presence of numerical or structural chromosome abnormalities. The best results were obtained when cultures were fed the day before chromosome preparations were made.

Two of the primary cultures were reserved for chromosomal breakage studies to determine whether the fetus was affected with FA. When the colonies reached a sufficient size, the cells were trypsinized and subcultured at a 1:2 or 1:3 split ratio in order to provide flasks for DEB-treated and untreated cultures. The growth medium in two or three flasks was replaced 24 h after subculture with fresh medium containing a nontoxic concentration (0.01 µg/ml) of DEB. This concentration is ten-fold lower than that used for blood cultures since DEB has a greater cytotoxic effect on cultured cells which grow attached to plastic than on lymphocyte cultures. Cells were allowed to grow in this medium for an additional 72 h, by which time the cultures were nearly confluent. To collect sufficient mitotic cells for cytogenic studies, cells were trypsinized and subcultured, at a 1:2 or 1:3 split ratio, into fresh medium without DEB. One of the flasks previously treated with DEB was kept in reserve, and refed with medium containing freshly diluted DEB. At the first mitotic wave after subculture, 24-48 h later, cells from the trypsinized DEB-treated cultures and from several of the untreated cultures were harvested, and chromosome preparations made according to standard procedures. Chromosomal breakage analysis was performed on 50-100 Giemsa-stained metaphases from each preparation, as described for peripheral blood cultures.

Chorionic Villus Sampling

Chorionic villi were obtained using a Portex catheter guided by high-resolution, real-time ultrasound scanning (Old et al. 1982; Brambati et al. 1985). Chorionic villi were differentiated from maternal tissue in the aspirate by direct examination under a dissecting microscope. They were washed in two changes of sterile saline and were then added to two 15 ml centrifuge tubes containing 5 ml of sterile saline for transport on ice from the obstetrical unit to the tissue culture laboratory. Tube 1 contained 5 mg of villus for direct preparation for routine cytogenetic study according to the method of Simoni et al. (1983). Tube 2 contained the rest of the sample, which was then prepared for tissue culture.

The villi were allowed to settle by gravity, and the supernatant saline was aspirated and discarded. A dissociation mix, consisting of 5 ml RPMI 1640 medium with 5% fetal bovine serum, hyaluronidase (10 mg, Type 1-S, Sigma, St. Louis, USA), collagenase (5 mg, Type 1 A, Sigma), and deoxyribonuclease II (10 mg, Type V, Sigma) was added to the tissue in the tube. The tube was then placed on a rocking platform at room temperature for 1 h, after which undissociated villi were allowed to settle by gravity. The supernatant was aspirated, and the cells pelleted by centrifugation. The supernatant dissociation mix was returned to the undissociated villi and the tube put back on the rocking platform for another hour. The pelleted cells were resuspended in 12 ml of complete Chang medium, added to three 25 cm^2 tissue-culture flasks, and incubated at 37 °C in an atmosphere of 5% CO_2.

The dissociation procedure was repeated hourly until the villi were completely dissociated (3 h was usually sufficient). Primary cultures were subcultured once or twice at a 1:3 split ratio. The growth medium in at least two flasks was replaced 24 h after subculture with fresh medium containing a nontoxic concentration (0.01 μg/ml) of DEB. Remaining flasks served as untreated controls for baseline chromosomal breakage studies. The cells were allowed to grow in this medium for an additional 72 h, after which time the cultures were nearly confluent. The cells were then subcultured at a 1:3 split ratio into fresh medium without DEB, and harvested 24-48 h later, at the first mitotic wave after subculture. Chromosome preparations were made according to standard procedures. In each group 50-100 metaphases were studied. The methods used to select and score metaphases for chromosomal breakage analysis were the same as described for selecting and scoring peripheral blood lymphocytes.

In order to rule out maternal cell contamination (a potential problem in long-term trophoblast cultures), maternal and paternal blood samples were cultured and harvested for cytogenetic studies. Slides from these samples and from the fetal culture were stained with quinacrine (Caspersson et al. 1970), and a comparative study of fluorescent polymorphism was carried out. The presence of paternal markers in cells from CVS ruled out overgrowth of cultures by maternal cells. HLA typing can also be used for this purpose (Callaway et al. 1986).

Results

Peripheral Blood Lymphocyte Studies

Patients were referred for DEB testing because they manifested some of the clinical features of FA. Some patients exhibited congenital abnormalities known to be associated with FA, others had hematologic manifestations such as aplastic anemia or leukemia, while still others had both aplastic anemia and malformations. In cases where the patient was unable to travel to The Rockefeller University Hospital for examination and blood sampling, heparinized blood was shipped to us by an express carrier with an overnight delivery service. A total of 222 patients have had DEB tests in our laboratory; baseline chromosomal breakage was studied in 124 of these. The results of the baseline chromosomal breakage studies are shown in Table 1. It is important to note that the mean chromosomal breaks per cell for 92 patients diagnosed as affected by FA ranged from 0.02 to 0.85 breaks per cell, while the range of baseline chromosomal breakage for the 32 patients with some FA-like phenotypic characteristics, but diagnosed as not affected on the basis of DEB studies, was 0 to 0.12 breaks per cell. The range of baseline breakage in peripheral blood lymphocytes cultured from the controls was 0 to 0.05 breaks per cell (Auerbach et al. 1981). Thus the baseline breakage rate in some FA patients did not differ from that in the controls, or from that in non-FA patients, and some FA patients would have been misdiagnosed if baseline breakage studies only had been considered. Similar results were found when the percentage of cells with aberrations was analyzed for each group.

The results of studies of DEB-induced chromosomal breakage are shown in Table 2. The breakage frequency for the FA group ranged from 1.06 to 23.9 mean breaks per cell, while the frequency for the non-FA group ranged from 0 to 0.36

Table 1. Baseline chromosomal breakage in FA and non-FA cases

Tissue	Diagnosis	Patients (*n*)	Mean breaks/cell ($\bar{x} \pm SE$)	Range of breaks/cell	Mean aberrant cells (%) ($\bar{x} \pm SE$)	Range of aberrant cells (%)
Peripheral blood	FA	92	0.25 ± 0.02	0.02–0.85	17.1 ± 0.93	2–40
	Non-FA	32	0.03 ± 0.01	0–0.12	2.8 ± 0.53	0–12
Amniotic fluid cells	FA	7	0.27 ± 0.04	0.18–0.45	24 ± 0.01	12–58
	Non-FA	34	0.04 ± 0.01	0–0.13	4.0 ± 0.59	0–12
Chorionic villus cells	FA	3	0.42 ± 0.06	0.30–0.50	29 ± 3.6	24–36
	Non-FA	11	0.07 ± 0.02	0–0.19	5.9 ± 1.4	0–16

Table 2. DEB-Induced chromosomal breakage in FA and non-FA cases[a]

Tissue	Diagnosis	Patients (n)	Mean breaks/cell ($\bar{x} \pm SE$)	Range of breaks/cell	Mean aberrant cells (%) ($\bar{x} \pm SE$)	Range of aberrant cells (%)
Peripheral blood	FA	98	8.7 ±0.46 (10.0 ±0.42)[b]	1.1 -23.9 (3.62-23.9)[c]	84.9±2.1	18-100
	Non-FA	124	0.06±0.1	0-0.36	5.0±0.39	0-22
Amniotic fluid cells	FA	7	0.83±0.04	0.70-0.96	50.0±3.1	38-58
	Non-FA	36	0.05±0.01	0-0.14	4.8±0.56	0-13
Chorionic villus cells	FA	3	1.6 ±0.41	1.0 -2.39	59.7±2.8	54-63
	Non-FA	12	0.10±0.02	0.02-0.19	7.7±1.3	2-17

[a] DEB concentration in peripheral blood cultures was 0.1 μg/ml.
DEB concentration in amniotic fluid cell cultures was 0.01 μg/ml.
DEB concentration in chorionic villus cell cultures was 0.01 μg/ml.

[b] Mean breaks per aberrant cell.

[c] Range of breaks per aberrant cell.

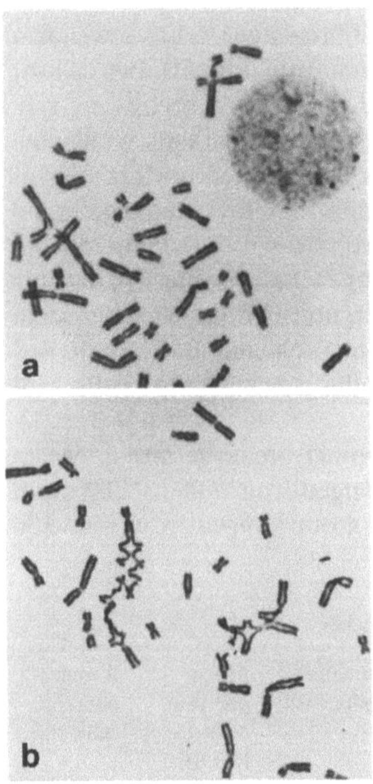

Fig. 1 a, b Part of a metaphase spread of an FA lymphocyte **a** showing spontaneous chromatid aberrations; **b** after exposure to 0.1 μg/ml DEB. The multiple complex chromatid exchange figures seen at this concentration of DEB are unique to FA cells. (Reproduced with permission from Auerbach et al. 1981.)

mean breaks per cell. The range for DEB-induced chromosomal breakage in the controls was 0-0.10 mean breaks per cell (Auerbach et al. 1981). There is thus no overlap in the range for the FA group compared with the non-FA and control groups. The ability to differentiate FA patients from other individuals on the basis of DEB studies is seen even more clearly if one analyzes the frequency of breaks

Table 3. Mean DEB-induced chromosomal breakage (breaks/cell) in subgroups of FA and non-FA patients

Aplastic anemia	Malformations			
	FA Patients		Non-FA patients	
	No	Yes	No	Yes
No	7.9[a]	11.1	0.04[b]	0.03
Yes	8.9	8.7	0.03	0.11

[a] Siblings of FA probands.
[b] Control subjects.
Analysis of variance: FA subgroups, $p > 0.2$; non-FA subgroups, $p < 0.001$

per aberrant cell for the FA patients. While most FA patients exhibited typical chromosomal breaks and exchanges in most or all cells analyzed after DEB exposure, some patients appeared to have two populations of cells (see Table 1, Auerbach, Rogatko and Schroeder-Kurth, this volume, pp. 3-17). In these individuals, there appeared to be no chromosomal breakage in the majority of DEB-treated cells, while the remainder of DEB-treated cells in each case exhibited the high number of breaks and exchanges typical of FA patients (see Fig. 1 for an example of such a cell). We have never observed even one DEB-treated cell with multiple chromatid exchanges in studies of non-FA patients. The mean frequency of breaks per aberrant cell for the 98 FA cases analyzed in our laboratory ranged from 3.62 to 23.9. Thus the induction of this type of breakage by DEB seems to be a unique marker for FA.

FA and non-FA patients were further classified into subgroups based on whether or not they exhibited birth defects and/or hematologic manifestations at the time of diagnosis (see Auerbach, Rogatko, and Schroeder-Kurth, this volume). Table 3 shows the mean frequency of DEB-induced chromosomal breakage for each of the subgroups. A one-way analysis of variance for the FA subgroups showed no significant differences in the breakage frequencies ($p > 0.2$). Thus, there is no correlation between the severity of the clinical manifestations and the frequency of DEB-induced chromosomal breakage. A similar analysis of the non-FA subgroups showed a significant difference among the groups ($p < 0.001$). Looking at the means for the non-FA subgroups, it was obvious which group was the different one, but to verify this, the data were subjected to several multiple comparison tests. Each confirmed the finding of a significant difference between the group with both birth defects and hematologic abnormalities and the other groups ($p < 0.001$). Since it is likely that the non-FA group is highly heterogeneous, comprising a variety of genetic and nongenetic entities, these results are not surprising.

Amniotic Fluid Cell Studies

Studies of amniotic fluid cells for prenatal diagnosis of FA have been performed in 42 patients with pregnancies at risk, including one twin pregnancy. These diagnostic studies were only performed in cases in which cross-link sensitivity had been demonstrated in the proband. The frequency of baseline chromosomal breakage in the seven cases diagnosed prenatally as affected by FA ranged from 0.18 to 0.45 mean breaks per cell, while the frequency in the cases diagnosed as unaffected on the basis of DEB studies ranged from 0 to 0.13 mean breaks per cell (see Table 1). The frequency of baseline chromosomal breakage in control studies was 0–0.12 mean breaks per cell (see Auerbach et al. 1985). DEB-induced breakage ranged from 0.7 to 0.96, 0 to 0.14, and 0 to 0.06 mean breaks per cell in affected fetuses, nonaffected fetuses at risk, and control fetuses respectively (see Table 2). Fetuses diagnosed as affected with FA thus exhibited at least a five-fold increase in DEB-induced chromosomal breakage when compared with fetuses diagnosed as nonaffected.

Two of the affected pregnancies were carried to term, whereas the other five were terminated. One newborn and two abortuses, diagnosed prenatally as affected, had congenital malformations including abnormalities of the thumb and radius. The other affected newborn had severe growth retardation from birth, and hematologic manifestations by the age of 18 months. No FA-associated malformations were found in any of the other fetuses or newborns studied. In all cases in which tissue was available for study, diagnoses were confirmed by chromosomal breakage studies in newborns or abortuses (Auerbach et al. 1985). Thus, analysis of baseline and DEB-induced chromosomal breakage in cultured amniotic fluid cells from fetuses at risk for FA can provide a reliable marker for prenatal diagnosis of the syndrome. Sonography can also be used to identify affected fetuses with malformations such as radial ray defects. However, this method should only be used in conjunction with chromosomal breakage studies in fetal cells since the absence of physical abnormalities does not rule out a diagnosis of FA. We have also observed that amniotic fluid cell cultures from affected fetuses grow slowly compared with cultures from nonaffected fetuses at risk, or from cultures studied because of advanced maternal age. Thus, poor growth of amniocytes from a fetus at risk for FA may be a useful indicator of an affected fetus, but should again be used in conjunction with cytogenetic studies, as slow growth of cells may be due to a number of nonspecific causes.

Chorionic Villus Studies

We have successfully monitored 15 pregnancies at risk for FA by studying cultured trophoblast cells obtained by chorionic villus sampling (CVS). In the three fetuses diagnosed as affected on the basis of DEB-induced chromosomal breakage, baseline chromosomal breakage in cultured cells was highly elevated (see Table 1). The frequency of baseline breakage in cells from fetuses diagnosed prenatally as nonaffected was similar to that found in simultaneously studied control cultures obtained by CVS performed in cases of advanced maternal age (see Auerbach et al. 1986b). DEB-induced chromosomal breakage in affected fetuses ranged from 1 to 2.39 mean breaks per cell compared with 0.02–0.19 and 0.02–0.14 mean breaks per cell in nonaffected fetuses at risk and normal controls respectively (see Table 2).

In the affected cases, the parents elected to terminate the pregnancy on the basis of these results. No obvious malformations were detectable in the abortuses. Results were confirmed by findings of markedly elevated chromosomal breakage rates in tissues obtained on termination of the pregnancy. The 12 pregnancies diagnosed as normal after CVS have reached term with no evidence of FA-associated malformations in the newborns. Most of these pregnancies diagnosed as normal were also monitored by amniocentesis, with confirmatory results. In most cases we were able to obtain peripheral blood samples from newborns; baseline and DEB-induced chromosomal breakage were within normal limits.

In addition to these 15 pregnancies at risk for FA, we have monitored a twin pregnancy at risk by the study of cells obtained by CVS. In twin A, a male, we found a frequency of baseline chromosomal breakage similar to that seen in affected fetuses, but no increase in the frequency of breakage after the cells were exposed to DEB. In twin B, a female, we found normal frequencies of both baseline and DEB-induced chromosomal breakage. HLA studies were performed on trophoblast cells from both twins; twin A was HLA identical to one of the affected children in this family, and twin B was HLA identical to their other affected child. A confirmatory amniocentesis from each of the twins was requested, but successful amniocyte cultures were only obtained from twin A by the laboratory referring the case. Results of baseline and DEB-induced chromosomal breakage in these cultures was similar to that seen in cultured cells obtained by CVS. Twin A died in utero soon after the amniocentesis was performed. Twin B showed marked intrauterine growth retardation at this time, but the pregnancy was continued. In the 38th week, twin B was delivered by Cesarean section. The baby, a 2551 g female, was observed at birth to be phenotypically normal. The placenta and cord insertion were also normal. Results of chromosomal breakage studies of cord blood and peripheral blood from the newborn showed markedly elevated baseline and DEB-induced chromosomal breakage, with frequencies similar to those found in FA patients. Results of studies of progenitor cells [colony-forming unit granulocyte-macrophage (CFU-GM), colony-forming unit granulocyte-erythroid-monocyte-megakaryocyte (CFU-GEMM) and burst-forming unit erythroid (BFU-E)] in cord blood indicated a deficiency of these cells compared with findings in cord blood from normal newborns (H. Broxmeyer, personal communication). The results of a complete blood cell count on this infant, obtained at 6 weeks of age, were normal. We interpret these findings as indicating a false-negative prenatal diagnosis in this case. The HLA studies indicate that there is no reason to suggest maternal contamination of either sample, as twin A expressed a single maternal haplotype and twin B expressed the other maternal haplotype. A single paternal haplotype was found in both twins. Since no amniocentesis was obtained from twin B, we cannot determine whether, in this family, chromosome instability is not expressed prenatally, or only not expressed during the first trimester at the time that CVS was performed. The baby will be followed closely for signs of hematologic manifestations of FA. We suggest that amniocentesis be performed in all cases in which the CVS study is negative and the pregnancy is continued.

Discussion

Despite the absence of knowledge of the specific molecular defect in FA, hypersensitivity of FA cells to the clastogenic effect of DNA cross-linking agents provides a unique marker for the syndrome. We have found that analysis of DEB-induced chromosomal breakage can be used to facilitate prenatal and postnatal diagnosis of FA. Data from the International Fanconi Anemia Registry (IFAR) show that at least 25% of FA patients have no congenital malformations (Auerbach, Rogatko, and Schroeder-Kurth, this volume). We therefore suggest that all young patients with aplastic anemia of unknown etiology should be tested for sensitivity to DEB in order to rule out a diagnosis of FA. Since treatment protocols for FA differ from those used for other forms of aplastic anemia, it is important to establish a conclusive diagnosis in these patients. Antithymocyte globulin (ATG) or cyclosporin are apparently ineffective drugs for the treatment of aplastic anemia in FA patients, while anabolic steroids are often useful. With the increasing reliance on bone narrow transplantation in the treatment of aplastic anemia, patients must be tested for sensitivity to DNA cross-linking agents, and hypersensitive patients subjected to a modified cytoreduction protocol, calling for a reduction in the dose of cyclophosphamide compared with that in general use in marrow transplant patients (Gluckman et al. 1980; Auerbach et al. 1983). In addition, the genotype of siblings being considered as marrow donors must be established, in order to avoid the transplantation of marrow from another affected individual. A diagnosis of FA must be also ruled out in cases of acute nonlymphocytic leukemia (ANLL) in children, since these patients will be hypersensitive to the chemotherapeutic agents used in standard treatment protocols, necessitating drastic dose reductions (Auerbach et al. 1982).

Once a diagnosis of FA has been established in a child, parents usually request prenatal monitoring of subsequent pregnancies. First trimester diagnosis by means of CVS, providing greatly reduced emotional and medical complications in cases where parents elect to terminate a pregnancy after diagnosis of an affected fetus, is of great benefit to families at risk for FA. In spite of our having experienced a case of false-negative diagnosis in cells cultured from chorionic villi, we still recommend this method. We suggest that all negative diagnostic studies be confirmed by amniocentesis. In ambiguous cases, or in cases which come to the attention of the physician too late to perform an amniocentesis, diagnosis of FA can be made in a few days by the study of lymphocytes from a fetal blood sample, using methods similar to those described for peripheral blood.

In our experience, FA families are often especially eager to have additional normal children in the hope of providing an HLA-identical healthy bone marrow donor for their affected child. While bone marrow transplantation offers a good chance of cure in these cases, a successful transplant using partially mismatched related donors or matched unrelated donors has not yet been reported in FA. Several families have requested HLA typing of cells obtained by CVS, which can now be accomplished (Callaway et al. 1986).

Conclusion

Our studies of DNA cross-link sensitivity in FA patients have led to the development of methods for prenatal and postnatal diagnosis of the disorder. These methods are indirect, relying on expression of a cellular marker. The ultimate goal of research in FA is to identify the biochemical and molecular defect. Conclusive identification of specific abnormal enzymes in FA cells has not yet been accomplished. The isolation of a DNA probe that would provide a direct assay for mutation at the FA locus may be achieved in the future. Until this can be accomplished, the diagnosis of FA using the methodology described in this chapter will be of great benefit to FA patients and their families.

Acknowledgement. We thank William Hamister for assistance with data management and statistical analysis.

References

Auerbach AD, Wolman SR (1976) Susceptibility of Fanconi's anaemia fibroblasts to chromosome damage by carcinogens. Nature 261: 494-496

Auerbach AD, Adler B, Chaganti RSK (1981) Prenatal and postnatal diagnosis and carrier detection of Fanconi anemia by a cytogenetic method. Pediatrics 67: 128-135

Auerbach AD, Weiner MA, Warburton D, Yeboa K, Lu L, Broxmeyer HE (1982) Acute myeloid leukemia as the first hematologic manifestation of Fanconi anemia. Am J Hematol 12: 289-300

Auerbach AD, Adler B, O'Reilly RJ, Kirkpatrick D, Chaganti RSK (1983) Effect of procarbazine and cyclophosphamide on chromosome breakage in Fanconi anemia cells: relevance to bone marrow transplantation. Cancer Genet Cytogenet 9: 25-36

Auerbach AD, Sagi M, Adler B (1985) Fanconi anemia: prenatal diagnosis in 30 fetuses at risk. Pediatrics 76: 794-800

Auerbach AD, Koorse RE, Ghosh R, Chiorazzi N (1986a) Mutagen sensitivity of Fanconi anemia (FA) homozygous, heterozygous and hybrid cell lines. Am J Hum Genet (Suppl) 39: A24

Auerbach AD, Zhang M, Ghosh R, Pergament E, Verlinsky Y, Nicholas H, Boué J (1986b) Clastogen-induced chromosomal breakage as a marker for first trimester prenatal diagnosis of Fanconi anemia. Hum Genet 73: 86-88

Auerbach AD, Rogatko A, Schroeder-Kurth TM (1989) International Fanconi Anemia Registry: relation of clinical symptoms to diepoxybutane sensitivity. Blood 73: 391-396

Berger R, Bernheim A, Le Conait M, Vecchione D, Schaison G (1980) Nitrogen mustard induced chromosome breakage: a tool for Fanconi's anemia diagnosis. Cancer Genet Cytogenet 2: 269-274

Brambati B, Simoni G, Danesino C, Oldrini A, Ferrazzi E, Romitti L, Terzoli G, Rossella F, Ferrari M, Fraccaro M (1985) First trimester fetal diagnosis of genetic disorders: clinical evaluation of 250 cases. J Med Genet 22: 92-99

Callaway C, Falcon C, Grant G, Maurer D, Auerbach AD, Rosenwaks Z, Pollack MS (1986) HLA typing used with cultured amniotic and chorionic villus cells for early prenatal diagnosis or parentage testing without one parent's availability. Hum Immunol 16: 200-204

Casey J, Ketterer D, Giles H (1983) Increased non-random chromosome breakage using Chang media. Am J Hum Genet 35: 128A

Caspersson T, Zech L, Johansson C, Modest EJ (1970) Identification of human chromosomes by DNA-binding fluorescing agents. Chromosoma 30: 215-227

Cervenka J, Arthur D, Yasis C (1981) Mitomycin C test for diagnostic differentiation of idiopathic aplastic anemia and Fanconi anemia. Pediatrics 67: 119-127

Dallapiccola B, Alimena G, Brinchi V, Isacchi G, Gandini E (1980) Absence of chromosome heterogeneity between classical Fanconi's anemia and the Estren-Dameshek type. Cancer Genet Cytogenet 2: 349-360

Duckworth-Rysiecki G, Cornish K, Clarke CA, Buchwald M (1985) Identification of two complementation groups in Fanconi's anemia. Somatic Cell Mol Genet 11: 35-43

Estren S, Dameshek W (1947) Familial hypoplastic anemia of childhood. Report of eight cases in two families with beneficial effect of splenectomy in one case. Am J Dis Child 73: 671-687

German J, Schonberg S, Caskie S, Warburton D, Falk C, Ray JH (1987) A test for Fanconi's anemia. Blood 69: 1637-1641

Glanz A, Fraser FC (1982) Spectrum of anomalies in Fanconi anaemia. J Med Genet 19: 412-416
Gluckman E, Devergie A, Schaison G, Bussel A, Berger R, Sohier J, Bernard J (1980) Bone marrow transplantation in Fanconi anaemia. Br J Haematol 45: 557-564
Gluckman E, Berger R, Dutreix J (1984) Bone marrow transplantation in Fanconi anemia. Semin Hematol 20: 20-26
McIntosh S, Breg WR, Lubiniecki AS (1979) Fanconi's anemia. The preanemic phase. Am J Pediatr Hematol Oncol 1: 107-110
Moustacchi E, Papadopoulo D, Diatloff-Zito C, Buchwald M (1986) Two complementation groups of Fanconi's anemia differ in their phenotypic response to a DNA cross-linking treatment. Hum Genet 75: 45-47
Old JM, Ward RTH, Petrou M, Karagozlu F, Modell B, Weatherall DJ (1982) First-trimester fetal diagnosis for haemoglobinopathies: three cases. Lancet II: 1413-1416
Sasaki MS, Tonomura A (1973) A high susceptibility of Fanconi's anemia to chromosome breakage by DNA cross linking agents. Cancer Res 33: 1829-1836
Schroeder TM, Anschütz F, Knopp A (1964) Spontane Chromosomenaberrationen bei familiärer Panmyelopathie. Humangenetik 1: 194-196
Schroeder TM, Tilgen D, Krüger J, Vogel F (1976) Formal genetics of Fanconi's anemia. Hum Genet 32: 257-288
Simoni G, Brambati B, Danesino C, Rossella F, Terzoli GL, Ferrari M, Fraccaro M (1983) Efficient direct chromosome analyses and enzyme determinations from chorionic villi samples in the first trimester of pregnancy. Hum Genet 63: 349-357
Weksberg R, Buchwald B, Sargent P, Thompson MW, Siminovitch (1979) Specific cellular defects in patients with Fanconi anemia. J Cell Physiol 101: 311-324

Chromosomal Breakage in Response to Cross-linking Agents in the Diagnosis of Fanconi Anemia

F. Arwert and M. L. Kwee

Symptoms Leading to the Diagnosis of Fanconi Anemia

The Fanconi anemia (FA) syndrome was originally described by Guido Fanconi in 1927. In his report he described three brothers with a condition resembling pernicious anemia. Evidently the anemia was the main symptom of the disease. Subsequently, other clinical symptoms (e.g., thumb aplasia and other skeletal abnormalities, café au lait spots, and growth retardation) frequently observed in FA have been described (Nilsson 1960; Fanconi 1967).

A cytogenetic symptom helpful for the differential diagnosis of FA was described by Schroeder et al. (1964). The authors showed that an increased level of spontaneous chromosomal damage was found in metaphases of cultured lymphocytes obtained from patients with FA. Not only could this feature be used to confirm the diagnosis of FA, but it was found to be present even in the premorbid stage of the disease.

However, inter- and intra-individual variation is often observed in the level of spontaneous chromosomal aberrations, the damage ranging from normal to high levels (Schroeder et al. 1976; McIntosh et al. 1979). This makes the absence of increased endogeneous damage an unreliable marker for the rejection of a diagnosis of FA.

Almost all FA cells show a specific susceptibility to the induction of chromosomal aberrations by cross-linking agents (Sasaki and Tonomura 1973). This sensitivity is well documented and reported for mitomycin C (MMC), nitrogen mustard, diepoxybutane (DEB), 8-methoxypsoralen plus near-UV light, cyclophosphamide, and *cis*-diamminedichloroplatinum II (*cis*-PtII) (Sasaki and Toramura 1973; Latt et al. 1975; Auerbach and Wolman 1976; Berger et al. 1980; Poll et al. 1982). Cytogenetic investigations in families with an FA proband have revealed that there may be clinically asymptomatic sibs without congenital FA-type malformations who show chromosomal sensitivity to cross-linking agents. These individuals invariably later develop anemia and must be diagnosed as FA "patients."

There are only a few reports where no difference was found between control cells and cells from FA patients in the induction of chromosomal damage after treatment with MMC or DEB (Sasaki 1978; Novotná et al. 1979; Cohen et al. 1982). The nonresponding cases reported by Sasaki (1978) were patients who were mistakenly diagnosed as having FA (M. S. Sasaki, personal communication). The unusual responses described by Novotná and by Cohen remain to be explained.

T. M. Schroeder-Kurth A. D. Auerbach G. Obe (Eds.)
Fanconi Anemia, Clinical, Cytogenetic and Experimental Aspects

However, two cases described below indicate that some patients with FA may exhibit virtually no chromosomal sensitivity to cross-linking agents following treatment of their peripheral blood lymphocytes.

Apart from these special cases, most authors agree that cross-link sensitivity is specific and essential for the diagnosis of FA. This feature seems to be the main symptom, is present before the onset of any sign of anemia, and is probably most closely related to the basic defect. Prenatal diagnosis of FA, as described by Auerbach et al. (1981), relies exclusively on the increased sensitivity of cells from FA patients to cross-linking agents.

Cocultivation Assay: A Cytogenetic Method for Rapid Diagnosis of FA Using Blood Lymphocytes

Sensitivity of FA lymphocytes to cross-linking agents is commonly measured as the number of breaks observed in, e.g., 100 metaphases. This figure is compared to that observed in control lymphocytes. Generally we screen 100 metaphases of an untreated and an MMC-treated blood sample of a patient in parallel with a treated and an untreated sample from a control. The procedure is reliable but time consuming, since hundreds of metaphases have to be analyzed carefully to determine the number of breaks present.

We have developed a more rapid test for the diagnosis of FA, using peripheral blood lymphocytes. The test is based on the fact that proliferation of FA cells is specifically inhibited by cross-linking agents (German et al. 1978; Ishida and Buchwald 1982). We used MMC as a cross-linking mutagen. When normal and FA lymphocytes from individuals of opposite sexes are mixed and cultured both in the presence and the absence of MMC, a difference in sensitivity to MMC becomes evident from a change in the sex ratio of metaphases in 60-h-cultures.

Figure 1 shows the MMC-dependent changes in the sex ratio observed in ten mixed cultures from control donors. It is evident that in nine combinations the sex ratio of control pairs is not significantly influenced by 0.01 μg/ml MMC. In one combination (no. 8) the sex ratio seems to be influenced by MMC. We calculated the significance of this change using the two-sample χ^2 test: $\chi^2 = \sum(O-E)^2/E$, where O represents the observed number of metaphases and E is the expected number. This calculation results in a p value of 0.083. Such a p value suggests that the change in the sex ratio may have occurred by chance, assuming that statistically significant differences show p values smaller than 0.05. As illustrated in Fig. 2, a significant MMC-dependent increase in the control-patient sex ratio was observed in six patients with FA (nos. 1-7), whereas no statistically significant changes in the sex ratio were observed in mixed cultures from controls with idiopathic aplastic anemia (nos. 11-13) or pure red cell aplasia (no. 10). As may be expected, neither a successfully transplanted FA patient (no. 9) nor an FA-heterozygous individual (no. 8) showed any significant change in the sex ratio.

The data presented in Figs. 1 and 2 indicate that the cocultivation assay is a reliable test to distinguish patients with FA from patients with other types of

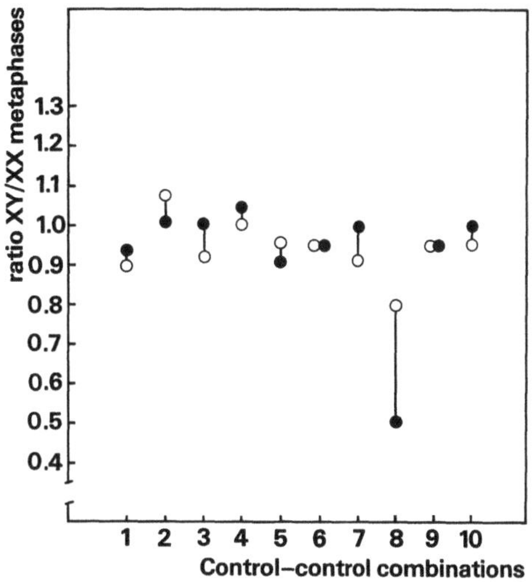

Fig. 1. MMC-dependent changes in the sex ratio observed in ten mixed cultures from controls. Whole blood cultures (0.25 ml male blood + 0.25 ml female blood) plus 6 ml Ham's F10 medium containing 15% fetal calf serum, 0.15 ml phytohemaglutinin, and the antibiotics penicillin and streptomycin were grown for 60 h at 37 °C. One culture contained MMC (0.01 μg/ml) *(filled circles)*, the other was grown without MMC *(empty circles)*. Chromosome preparations were made according to an established procedure (Moorhead et al. 1960), and stained with quinacrine. The presence or absence of a fluorescent Y chromosome was recorded in about 100 well-spread metaphases, using a Leitz fluorescence microscope with epiillumination

aplastic anemia. Since the assay is less time consuming than the chromosomal breakage test, the cocultivation assay may be preferred when large numbers of blood samples are to be investigated for differential diagnosis in cases of aplastic anemia.

No false-positive results were observed when cases positive in the cocultivation assay were studied using the chromosomal breakage test (MMC stress). False-positive cases might be expected when lymphocytes from xeroderma pigmentosum-group A (XP-A) patients are used in the cocultivation assay, since XP-A cells are reported to be sensitive to MMC (Hartley-Asp 1978; Fujiwara et al. 1977). Confusion over a diagnosis of FA or of xeroderma pigmentosum is unlikely to occur when this is based on clinical symptoms.

Maraschio et al. (1986) described a patient who was suffering from a possibly new chromosomal instability disorder. In this patient, the increase of chromosomal breakage in comparison with that in controls was evident after cells from the patient were cultured in the presence of low concentrations of MMC. Such a case, we think, would appear FA-positive in the cocultivation assay. However, without further knowledge about the sensitivity of the patient's cells to other cross-linking agents, it is difficult to conclude whether this patient represents a new chromosomal disorder, a variant of ataxia-telangiectasia (which two possibilities were discussed by Maraschio et al.), or possibly a variant of FA.

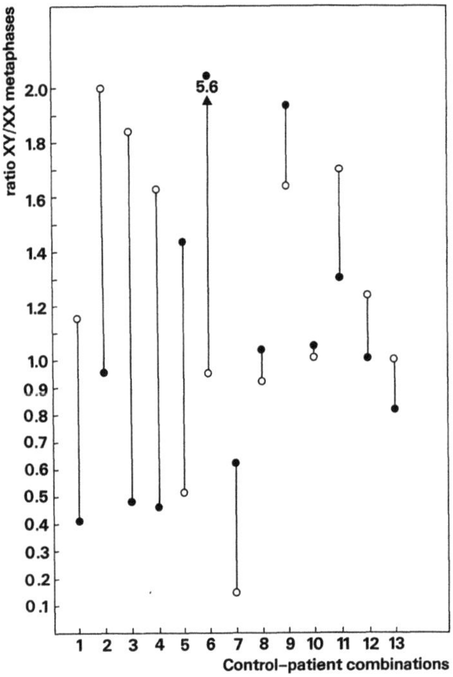

Fig. 2. MMC dependent changes in the sex ratio observed in 12 mixed cultures from patients with aplastic anemia and one from a FA heterozygous person. Experimental procedure and symbols are as in Fig. 1. Control/patient combinations are: nos. 1 and 2, a male patient with FA, tested on two occasions. This patient was described by Kwee et al. (1983). Nos. 3 and 4, male patients with FA described previously by Joenje et al. (1981). No. 5, a female FA patient, is case JV in Kwee et al. (1983). No. 6, a female patient with FA, is case WK 8013 in Poll et al. (1984). No. 7, a female patient with FA, GW, has not previously been described. No. 8 is an FA-heterozygous female, no. 9 a female with FA after bone marrow transplantation, no. 10 a female with pure red cell aplasia, no. 11 a male and nos. 12 and 13 female patients with idiopathic aplastic anemia. In all cases where a significant change in the sex ratio was observed (cases 1-7), the diagnosis FA was made and confirmed by the hypersensitivity of lymphocyte cultures to chromosomal breakage by MMC. Similarly the diagnosis FA was excluded for cases 10, 11, 12 and 13 by absence of hypersensitivity of lymphocyte cultures to chromosomal breakage by MMC. In the combination with FA patients the MMC-dependent change in the sex ratio was statistically significant ($p<0.05$). In the other cases (nos. 8-13), p values greater than 0.05 were obtained with the two-sample χ^2 test, suggesting an arbitrary change in the sex ratio

Auerbach et al. (1981) published a report on the case of a 9-year-old girl whose lymphocyte cultures showed only 20% DEB-responsive cells. With such a proportion (80%) of cells showing a normal response, it is doubtful whether a statistically significant change in the sex ratio would be found in the cocultivation assay. Therefore, the cocultivation assay seems suitable for the rapid differentiation of cases of FA from other aplastic anemias, but in cases with a negative result in the cocultivation assay a chromosomal breakage test has to be performed because of known mosaicism in the blood cells of some FA patients. (Auerbach et al. 1981; Kwee et al. 1983). The screening of 100-200 metaphases for the presence of highly cross-link-sensitive cells is recommended for accurate diagnosis. The cocultivation assay seems more generally applicable to demonstrate sensitivity to specific drugs. The use of bleomycin or neocarzinostatin is likely to allow identification of ataxia-telangiectasia patients (Taylor et al. 1979; Cohen and Simpson 1983). When an automated procedure is used to prepare chromosome slides from blood cultures, in combination with computer-aided metaphase identification, the cocultivation assay may allow in population screening the identification of individuals with an increased sensitivity to any other drug.

Cross-link Sensitivity in Special Cases of FA

Case JdW

In 1983 we published a report on a case of FA with an unusual response to bifunctional cross-linking agents (Kwee et al. 1983). Case JdW was exceptional because only 40% of his cultured blood cells showed an "FA-like," cross-link-dependent chromosomal breakage, while 60% of his lymphocytes responded like those from a normal individual. As can be seen from Fig. 2, pair nos. 1 and 2, a proportion of only 40% sensitive cells was sufficient, using the cocultivation assay, to identify JdW as having FA. During follow-up studies of JdW we reinvestigated the fraction of MMC-resistant cells, using the procedure as published. This time, 2½ years later, the fraction of nonresponsive cells was 53%, a value close to the 60% originally observed. So there had been little change in the proportion of these cells over a period of 2 years. One might expect MMC-resistant cells to have a growth advantage over sensitive cells. This would result in a gradual increase in the proportion of resistant cells. In case JdW, however, this phenomenon was not observed.

Fibroblast cultures were initiated from a skin biopsy from JdW in order to investigate whether other tissues also contain MMC-resistant cells. The results of this study (Fig. 3) suggest that no unresponsive fraction was present in fibroblast cultures from patient JdW.

At present, JdW is 28 years old and few patients with FA who have not received a transplant reach this age. One may surmise that the presence of resistant cells in the blood is beneficial to JdW, preventing a hematological crisis. Such a hypothesis suggests that a resistant fraction may be found in elderly patients with FA. We investigated two of JdW's sibs who had FA, JD (a married female, aged 30) and FD (sister, aged 18), but their blood cells were found to be extremely MMC-sensitive and no resistant function was observed (Fig. 4). The data from JD and FD suggest that no general correlation exists between the age of FA patients and the presence of resistant blood cells.

Case ST

ST is a girl, born in 1966. Her younger brother PT, born in 1969, was diagnosed as having FA, based on the finding of café-au-lait spots, hypospadia, aplastic anemia, and an increased chromosomal breakage rate. In the search for an HLA-compatible donor a family investigation was made and ST was diagnosed as suffering

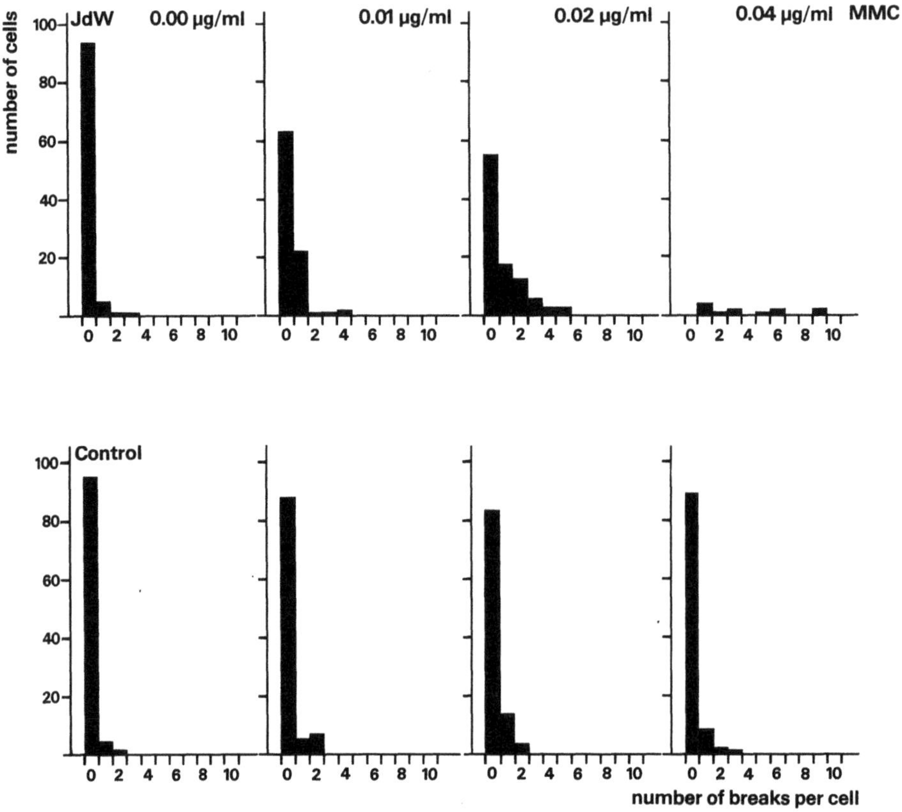

Fig. 3. Chromosomal breakage in cells from patients with FA and controls. Skin fibroblast cultures from JdW were grown in Ham's F10 medium with 15% fetal calf serum. When the cells reached confluency, the cultures were split 1:3. After 24 h MMC was added and 48 h later, colchicine. Cultures were harvested after 2 h of treatment with colchicine and chromosome preparations were made as described for lymphocyte cultures. At all concentrations the chromosomal damage in 100 metaphases was scored, except in the case of JdW at the highest concentration of MMC (0.04 µg/ml), where only 15 metaphases were found

from FA because she had a "typical FA habitus." PT died at the age of six from incurable aplastic anemia. Every year, ST is asked to go for an examination by the hospital hematology department, but she usually refuses because she feels well and has no complaints. When ST was 15 years old, we investigated a blood sample for spontaneous chromosomal damage and found two breaks in 100 metaphases. This is within the range of the number of breaks found in controls, but, as mentioned before, it does not rule out a diagnosis of FA. A cocultivation test was done using the cells of a male control. The results are given in Table 1. A significant ($p<0.001$, two-sample χ^2 test) MMC-dependent change in the sex ratio was observed confirming the earlier clinical diagnosis.

A blood sample was obtained from ST when she was 19 years old and investigated for the possible presence of MMC-unresponsive (resistant) cells. At that time ST felt healthy, as she feels today. As illustrated in Table 2, ST's lymphocytes

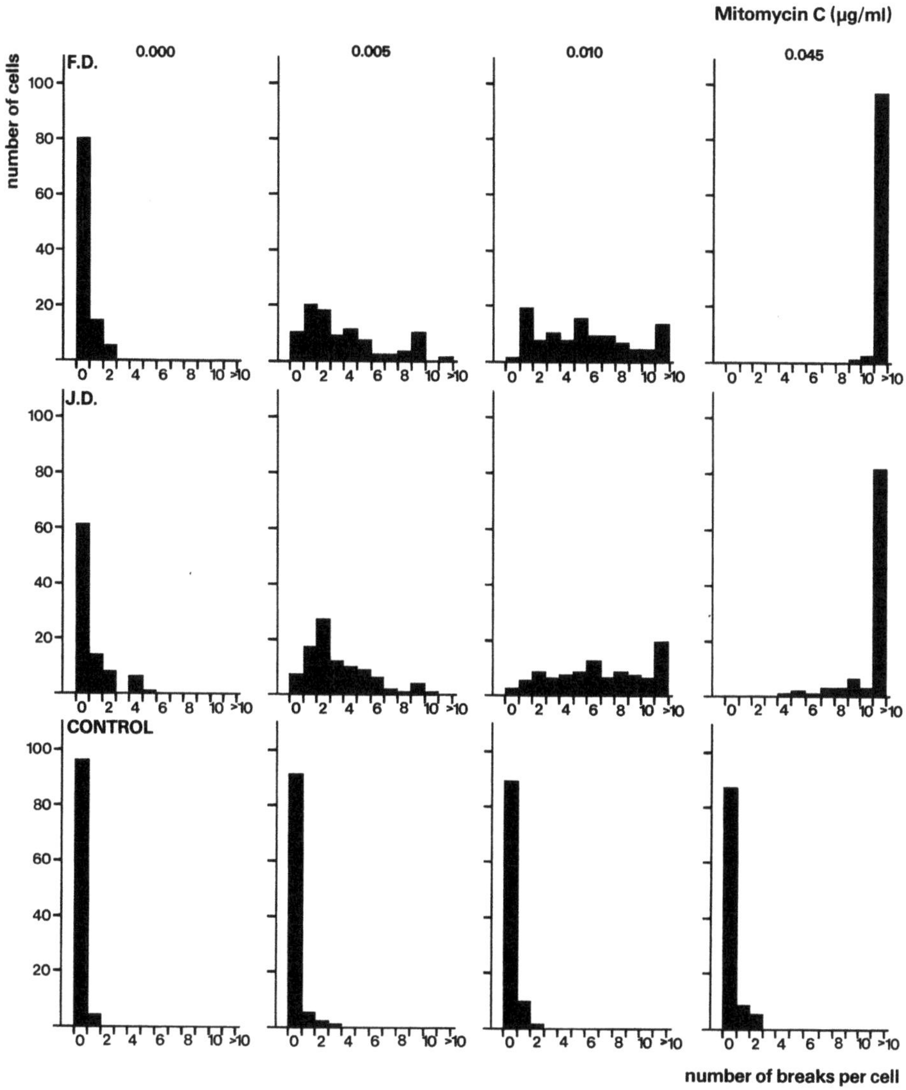

Fig. 4. Chromosomal breakage induced by various concentrations of MMC in lymphocytes in cultures from a healthy individual and two FA patients, FD and JD. At each concentration the number of cells damaged in 100 well-spread metaphases was recorded

Table 1. Effect of mitomycin C on mitotic activity in mixed lymphocyte cultures from case ST (female) and a normal male

MMC	Number of metaphases analyzed		Male to female ratio of karyotypes
	Male karyotype	Female karyotype	
–	32	78	0.41
+(0.01 µg/ml)	52	48	1.08

Table 2. Spontaneous and MMC-induced chromosomal damage in lymphocyte cultures from two normal controls and from case ST

MMC (μg/ml)	Breaks[a] (*n*)	Damaged metaphases (%)
Control 1		
0	2	2
0.005	7	7
0.015	14	9
0.045	36	23
Control 2		
0	8	8
0.005	3	3
0.015	3	3
0.045	22	21
Case ST		
0	0	0
0.005	5	5
0.015	11	11
0.045	18	16

[a] At each concentration the number of breaks in 100 metaphases was scored.

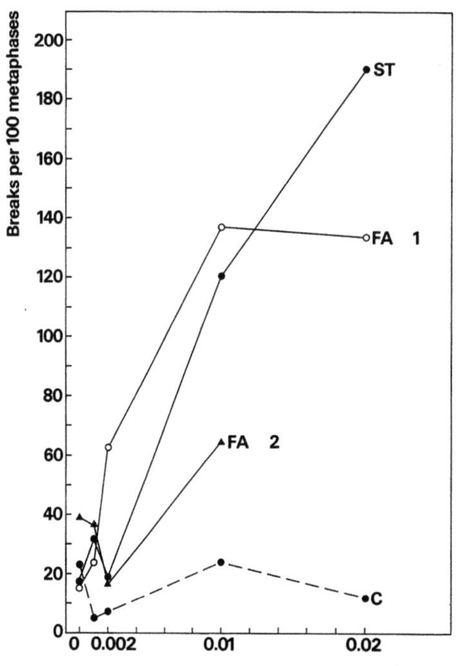

Fig. 5. Chromosomal breakage induced by treatment with MMC in fibroblast cultures from control, *C* (●- - -●), case ST (●——●), and two (○——○ and ▲——▲) patients with FA, *FA 1* and *FA 2*. *FA 1* is case JaVo, described by Poll et al. (1984); *FA 2* is case GM 2053 (obtained from the Camden Cell Bank)

were completely resistant to MMC, and responded similarly to those of two controls, which were grown in parallel.

This result raised the question whether the diagnosis of FA in the case of ST was indeed correct. Fortunately, a fibroblast cell line from ST was available and these fibroblasts were clearly hypersensitive to MMC (Fig. 5). ST is therefore certainly affected by FA, and the unusual response of her lymphocytes to MMC suggests an apparently complete replacement of MMC-sensitive cells by MMC-resistant ones.

The interesting point in the case of ST is that without her having been investigated through the case of her brother, PT, and without the cocultivation test performed when she was still asymptomatic, the diagnosis made when she was 19 years old, based on the response of the lymphocyte cultures to MMC, would, mistakenly, have been "not FA." Case ST illustrates that the diagnosis of FA cannot always be ruled out with certainty by a cross-link sensitivity test of peripheral blood cells. A correct diagnosis was made from the results of fibroblast cultures, but fibroblast cell lines are not always available from patients with an unknown aplastic anemia. From case ST, we believe that in FA families, sibs should be investigated as early as possible, and using not only blood cell cultures, but preferably also fibroblast cell lines.

Acknowledgements. We are grateful to Miss A. B. Oostra, Mrs D. Boden and Miss A. H. Wanamarta for their expert technical assistance, and to Miss C. de Lint for preparing the manuscript.

References

Auerbach AD, Wolman SR (1976) Susceptibility of Fanconi's anaemia fibroblasts to chromosome damage by carcinogens. Nature 261: 494-496

Auerbach AD, Adler B, Chaganti RSK (1981) Prenatal and postnatal diagnosis and carrier detection of Fanconi's anaemia by a cytogenetic method. Pediatrics 67: 128-135

Berger R, Bernheim A, Le Coniat M, Vecchione D, Schaison G (1980) Nitrogen mustard-induced chromosome breakage: a tool for Fanconi's anemia diagnosis. Cancer Genet Cytogenet 2: 269-274

Cohen MM, Simpson SJ (1983) Increased clastogenicity and decreased inhibition of DNA synthesis by neocarzinostatin and tallysomycin in ataxia telangiectasia lymphoid cells. Mutat Res 112: 119-128

Cohen MM, Simpson SJ, Hongi GR, Maurer HS, Nicklas JW, Martin AO (1982) The identification of Fanconi anemia genotypes by clastogenic stress. Am J Hum Genet 34: 794-810

Fanconi G (1927) Familiäre infantile perniziosaartige Anämie (perniziöses Blutbild und Konstitution). Jahrb Kinderheilkd 117: 257-280

Fanconi G (1967) Familial constitutional panmyelopathy, Fanconi's anemia (FA). Semin Hematol 4: 233-240

Fujiwara Y, Tatsumi M, Sasaki MS (1977) Cross link repair in human cells and its possible defect in Fanconi's anemia cells. J Mol Biol 113: 635-649

German J, Caskie S, Schonberg S (1978) A simple cytogenetic test for increased mutagen-sensitivity. J Supramol Struct (Suppl) 2: 89

Hartley-Asp B (1978) The influence of caffeine on the mitomycin C-induced chromosome aberration frequency in normal human and xeroderma pigmentosum cells. Mutat Res 49: 117-126

Ishida R, Buchwald M (1982) Susceptibility of Fanconi's anemia lymphoblasts to DNA crosslinking and alkylating agents. Cancer Res 42: 4000-4006

Joenje H, Arwert F, Eriksson AW, De Koning H, Oostra AB (1981) Oxygen-dependence of chromosomal aberrations in Fanconi's anaemia. Nature 290: 142-143
Kwee ML, Poll EHA, Van de Kamp JJP, De Koning H, Eriksson AW, Joenje H (1983) Unusual response to bifunctional alkylating agents in a case of Fanconi anaemia. Hum Genet 64: 384-387
Latt SA, Stetten G, Juergens LA, Buchanan GR, Gerald PS (1975) Induction by alkylating agents of sister chromatid exchanges and chromatid breaks in Fanconi's anemia. Proc Natl Acad Sci USA 72: 4066-4070
Maraschio P, Peretti D, Lambiase S, Lo Curto F, Caufin D, Gargantini L, Minoli L, Zuffardi O (1986) A new chromosome instability disorder. Clin Genet 30: 353-365
McIntosh S, Breg WR, Lubiniecki AS (1979) Fanconi's anemia. The preanemic phase. Am J Pediatr Hematol Oncol 1: 107
Moorhead PS, Nowell PW, Mellman WJ, Batips DM, Hungerford DA (1960) Chromosome preparations of leukocytes cultured from peripheral blood. Exp Cell Res 20: 613-617
Nilsson LR (1960) Chronic pancytopenia with multiple congenital abnormalities (Fanconi's anemia). Acta Paediatr 49: 518-529
Novotná B, Goetz P, Surkova NI (1979) Effects of alkylating agents on lymphocytes from controls and from patients with Fanconi's anemia. Hum Genet 49: 41-50
Poll EHA, Arwert F, Joenje H, Eriksson AW (1982) Cytogenetic toxicity of antitumor platinum compounds in Fanconi's anemia. Hum Genet 61: 228-230
Poll EHA, Arwert F, Kortbeek HT, Eriksson AW (1984) Fanconi anaemia cells are not uniformly deficient in unhooking of DNA interstrand crosslinks, induced by mitomycin C or 8-methoxypsoralen plus UVA. Hum Genet 68: 228-234
Sasaki MS (1978) Fanconi's anemia condition possibly associated with a defective DNA repair. In: Hanawalt PC, Friedberg EC, Cox CF (eds) DNA repair mechanisms. ICN-UCLA symposia on molecular and cellular biology, vol IX. Academic Press, New York San Francisco London, pp 675
Sasaki MS, Tonomura A (1973) A high susceptibility of Fanconi's anemia to chromosome breakage by DNA-crosslinking agents. Cancer Res 33: 1829-1836
Schroeder TM, Anschütz F, Knopp A (1964) Spontane Chromosomenaberrationen bei familiärer Panmyelopathie. Humangenetik 1: 194-196
Schroeder TM, Drings P, Beilner P, Buchinger G (1976) Clinical and cytogenetic observations during a six-year period in an adult with Fanconi's anaemia. Blut 34: 119-132
Taylor AMR, Rosney CM, Campbell JB (1979) Unusual sensitivity of ataxia telangiectasia cells to bleomycin. Cancer Res 39: 1046-1050

Cytogenetic Studies in Fanconi Anemia: Induced Chromosomal Breakage and Cytogenetics of Leukemia

R. Berger and M. Le Coniat

Introduction

Fanconi anemia (FA) has belonged to the group of chromosomal breakage or chromosome instability syndromes since the first description, by Schroeder et al. (1964), of chromosomal breakage in the cultured peripheral lymphocytes of patients with FA. The rate of chromatid and chromosomal breakage varies from one patient to another as well as in the same patient over time (review in Polani 1976; Berger et al. 1975, 1977; Schroeder et al. 1976b; Berrebi et al. 1979). Consequently, for diagnostic purposes, a cytogenetic test more reliable than the simple quantitative estimation of chromosomal breakage in cultured cells became necessary.

The high sensitivity of FA cells to alkylating agents and carcinogens was ascertained by several authors (Schuler et al. 1969; Sasaki and Tonomura 1973; Auerbach and Wolman 1976). The high sensitivity of patients with FA to the conditioning regimens used for bone marrow transplantation (BMT), which include treatment with cyclophosphamide and X-rays is a common observation (Gluckman et al. 1980). We therefore investigated the possible relationship between this clinical observation and the hypersensitivity of FA cells seen by cytogenetic studies. These studies led us to establish a diagnostic test for FA using an alkylating agent introduced into the culture medium (Berger et al. 1980a). In this chapter we report on our experience with this test.

FA is considered a preleukemic condition since a number of patients eventually develop acute leukemia. We report our data on the cytogenetic analysis of acute leukemia in FA patients; data of this type are still relatively rare.

Chromosomal Breakage as a Tool for Diagnosis of FA

The first series of experiments were performed using the serum of a patient treated with cyclophosphamide. A significant increase of chromosomal breakage was found when this serum was added to a culture medium of stimulated lymphocytes from patients with FA (Berger et al. 1980b). Because of difficulties in the handling of cyclophosphamide and the uncertainties concerning the dose of cyclophosphamide metabolites, we decided to use the bifunctional alkylating nitrogen mustard, mechlormethamine hydrochloride ($C_5H_{12}Cl_3N$; trade name, Caryolysin, Delagrange Laboratories) which has a short half-life in vitro and in vivo (Berger et al.

T. M. Schroeder-Kurth A. D. Auerbach G. Obe (Eds.)
Fanconi Anemia, Clinical, Cytogenetic and Experimental Aspects

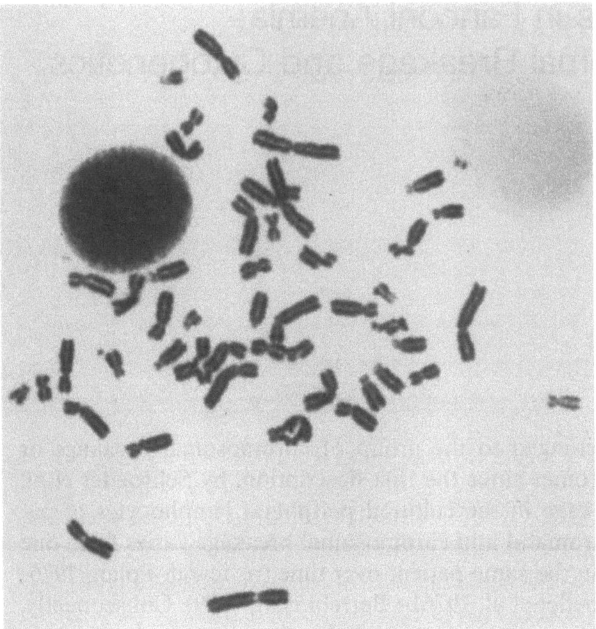

Fig. 1. Example of chromosomal breakage induced by nitrogen mustard

1980a). Chromosome preparations of 72-h phytohemagglutinin (PHA)-stimulated whole blood cultures were made using routine methods (culture medium RPMI 1640 supplemented with 17% fetal calf serum and antibiotics; hypotonic solution, 0.075 *M* KCl; fixative, methanol-acetic acid 3:1; air drying; Giemsa staining). Nitrogen mustard was added to the cultures at a concentration of 0.05 μg/ml, 24 h after their initiation (Berger et al. 1982a). The drug solution was prepared immediately before use. For each blood sample one culture remained untreated, thus allowing a direct comparison of the untreated and treated cultures.

Chromosome abnormalities were scored according to the recommendations of the International System for Human Cytogenetic Nomenclature (ISCN 1978); chromatid gaps were not scored. The number of breaks per cell was recorded as follows: chromatid and chromosomal breaks, fragments, and deletions were recorded as one break, translocations, dicentrics, rings, triradials, and quadriradials as two breaks (Fig. 1). The diagnosis was ascertained by familiar clinical and hematological data in FA patients as well as in other forms of bone marrow hypoplasia or aplasia.

Up to now, 46 FA patients have been investigated using this method (Table 1). As expected, both the spontaneous and the induced chromosomal breakage rates varied from patient to patient. The spontaneous breakage rate varied from 0.04 to 0.92 breaks per cell and the induced rate varied from 0.22 to 11.9 breaks per cell. Treatment of lymphocytes with the alkylating agent resulted in a clear-cut increase in chromosomal breakage in every patient with FA studied, irrespective of considerable quantitative variations. There was an uneven distribution of the induced breaks among the cells, suggesting different sensitivities of subpopulations of lymphocytes. Three FA patients had a low spontaneous chromosomal breakage rate;

Table 1. Chromosomal breakage in patients with Fanconi anemia, parents and sibs of patients with Fanconi anemia, patients with aplastic anemia, and patients with dyskeratosis congenita

Patients/ relatives studied	Cases (*n*)	Nitrogen mustard concentration (μg/ml)	Mean breaks per cell (*n*)	Standard error	Range (breaks per cell)
FA	46	0	0.24	0.15	0.04- 0.92
		0.05	2.92	2.35	0.17-11.9
P	8	0	0.015	0.028	0 - 0.08
		0.05	0.035	0.055	0 - 0.06
S	10	0	0.002	0.006	0 - 0.02
		0.05	0.016	0.018	0 - 0.04
AA	27	0	0.02	0.07	0 - 0.34
		0.05	0.01	0.02	0 - 0.06
DC	3	0	0.03		0 - 1
	2	0.05	0.04		0 - 1

FA, Fanconi anemia; P, parents; S, sibs; AA, aplastic anemia; DC dyskeratosis congenita

in one of them the increase in the frequency of breaks with nitrogen mustard was relatively low, suggesting that this patient might have a special form of FA. However, the increase in chromosomal breakage induced by nitrogen mustard was high in the other two patients.

Interestingly, no increase in the chromosomal breakage rate was observed in patients with the Zinsser-Engmann-Cole syndrome (dyskeratosis congenita). Chromosomal breakage was not increased in eight obligate heterozygous parents of patients with FA, in 10 sibs of patients with FA, in seven supposed normal homozygous controls (Berger et al. 1980a, 1982), or in 27 patients investigated because of non-FA bone marrow aplasia or hypoplasia with various causes (Table 1). One non-FA patient with bone marrow aplasia of unknown origin was of interest because he had a relatively high spontaneous breakage rate. The absence of elevated frequencies of chromosomal breakage with nitrogen mustard was in accordance with the diagnosis of non-FA bone marrow aplasia.

Finally, the test was applied to patients with FA and surviving after BMT. One of them (Berger et al. 1980c, case PR 1952) did not exhibit chromosomal breakage 45 and 52 months after BMT, neither did patient CG 2728. These results showed that the engrafted cells behave like normal cells in spite of their introduction into an FA host, indicating that there is no diffusible breaking factor from the host. These results are in accordance with experiments indicating a correction or suppression of chromosomal breakage by cocultivation with normal cells, assuming that most of the chromosomal breaks arise during in vitro culture (Nordensen et al. 1980). In conclusion, the use of nitrogen mustard provides a useful diagnostic tool for FA. It may be more reliable than tests using mitomycin C (Cohen et al. 1982; Cervenka and Hirsch 1983). The method does not allow the recognition of heterozygotes, as was supposed by Auerbach and Wolman (1978) to be possible with diepoxybutane (DEB). As far as clinical and hematological data are concerned, FA is thought to be a heterogeneous disease (Schroeder et al. 1976b; Duckworth-Rysiecki et al. 1984; see Digweed et al., this volume). Recently, two complementation groups have been recognized using somatic cell hybrids (Duckworth-Rysiecki et al. 1985), and the sensitivity of FA cells from different complementation groups may vary (Weksberg et al. 1979; Moustacchi and Diatloff-Zito 1985). The mechanism(s) of the hypersensitivity of FA cells to chromosomal breakage remains controversial and will not be discussed here.

Our test showed that the rate of induced chromosomal breakage varied from one patient to another without a clear correlation with the rate of spontaneous breakage. This was taken into account when the protocol for a pre-BMT regimen was discussed; the reduction of the cyclophophamide dose administered improved the result of BMT in patients with FA, who are so fragile (Gluckman et al. 1984; see also Gluckman et al., this volume).

Cytogenetics of Acute Leukemia and Preleukemia in Patients with FA

The occurrence of cancer and leukemia in patients with FA was recognized relatively late (German 1983, for review). Acute nonlymphoblastic leukemia (ANLL) is now known to be often associated with FA and this led some authors to classify FA as a preleukemic syndrome. In a few patients the occurrence of ANLL or a preleukemia led to the diagnosis of FA (Auerbach et al. 1982; our case CG 2358). The evolution towards ANLL has been estimated to occur in 5%-10% of cases of FA (Alter and Potter 1983) and occurred in up to 30% (including preleukemia) in a series of 44 FA patients analyzed in the same hospital between 1962 and 1976 (Schaison et al. 1983). The cytological types of ANLL are variable (German 1983).

In a few cases chromosome studies were performed in FA patients with ANLL. Various chromosomal changes were found, as expected from the diversity of ANLL studied, but the involvement of chromosomes 1 and 7 has been reported several times (Table 2). However, three points deserve special attention.

First, the finding of clonal chromosomal abnormalities does not mean that the cells are malignant, since they may be associated without any sign of leukemia or preleukemia (Liskér and Cobo de Gutiérrez 1974; Berger et al. 1975, 1980d; Schroeder et al. 1976a; Huret et al. 1986). However, a clonal chromosomal change may occur several months before a frank leukemia with a long preleukemia phase (Berger et al. 1977).

Second, partial duplications are unusually frequent in our experience (Berger et al. 1977, 1980d, our case CG 2575, unpublished) and other cases of partial duplications have been reported (for review see Huret et al. 1986). The spontaneous occurrence of partial duplication of the long arm of chromosome 5 in a culture of FA fibroblasts has also been reported (Auerbach et al. 1980). The question therefore arises: are these duplications related to abnormalities of DNA replication in relation to chromosome instability?

Third, a homozygosity of chromosomal segments has been reported in the preleukemic and leukemic phases of a patient with FA (Berger et al. 1977). This homozygosity was thought to be related to the observation of mitotic missegregations which could be explained as being due to mitotic irregularities as observed by Schroeder (1966). Whatever the mechanisms may be, it seems important to search for homozygosity in FA-leukemic cells in the future.

Table 2. Clonal chromosomal abnormalities in leukemia and preleukemia occuring in patients with Fanconi anemia

Disease	Chromosomal abnormalities	References
Acute myelomonocytic l	46, XY, t (5; 18) (q.q)	Bourgeois and Hill (1977)
Preleukemia	46, XX, dup (3) (q12q27), 12q+	Berger et al. (1977)
Acute myeloblastic l	46, XX, 1p+, dup (3) (q12q27), 7p+, 12q+	
Erythroleukemia	46, XY, dup (1) (p32p34), trip (3) (q12q27), del (7) (p11)	Berger et al. (1980d)
Preleukemia	46, XX, dup (2) (q24q36)/47, XX, dup (2) (q24q36), +?4p	Berger et al. (1980d)
Acute l	46, XY, der (6) t (1; 6) (q32; p25)/46, XY, der (6) t (1; 6) (q25; p23), der (11) t (11; ?) (q25, ?)	Obeid et al. (1980)
Acute l	der (6) t (1; 6) (q22 or q23; pter)/der (6) t (1; 6) (q22 or q23; pter), 5q−	Tanzer et al. (1980)
Acute myeloblastic l	der (14) t (1; 14) (q12 or q21; q23), 4q−, 6q+, 7q−, 13q+, 20q−	Tanzer et al. (1980)
Acute myeloblastic l	46, XX, −7, −8, +mar 1, +mar 2/complex −7, mar/complex mar, without −7	Auerbach et al. (1982)
Erythroleukemia	1p+, t (13; 15)	Rotzak et al. (1982)
Acute myeloblastic l	45, XY, −7	Stivrins et al. (1984)
Preleukemia	46, XX, −17, t (10,?) (q26; ?), del (12) (p11), der (17) t (1; 17) (q21; p13)	Nowell et al. (1984)
Acute myeloblastic l	46, XX, 7q−, 9q−	Woods et al. (1985)
Acute myeloblastic l	47, XY, +20, −22, dup (1) (q22q34), +del (22) (q11)	(R. Berger et al. unpublished material)

l, leukemia

References

Alter BP, Potter NU (1983) Long-term outcome in Fanconi's anemia: description of 26 cases and review of the literature. In: German J (ed) Chromosome mutation and neoplasia. Liss, New York, pp 43-62

Auerbach AD, Wolman SR (1976) Susceptibility of Fanconi's anemia fibroblasts to chromosome damage by carcinogens. Nature 261: 494-496

Auerbach AD, Wolman SR (1978) Carcinogen-induced chromosome breakage in Fanconi's anemia heterozygous cells. Nature 271: 69-71

Auerbach AD, Wolman SR, Chaganti RSK (1980) A spontaneous clone of Fanconi anemia fibroblasts with chromosome abnormalities and increased growth potential. Cytogenet Cell Genet 28: 265-270

Auerbach AD, Weiner MA, Warburton D, Yeboa K, Lu L, Broxmeyer HE (1982) Acute myeloid leukemia as the first manifestation of Fanconi anemia. Am J Hematol 12: 289-300

Berger R, Bussel A, Schenmetzler C (1975) Anomalies chromosomiques et anémie de Fanconi. Étude de 4 cas. Nouv Rev Fr Hematol 15: 539-550

Berger R, Bussel A, Schenmetzler C (1977) Somatic segregation and Fanconi anemia. Clin Genet 11: 409-415
Berger R, Bernheim A, Le Coniat M, Vecchione D, Schaison G (1980a) Nitrogen mustard-induced chromosome breakage: a tool for Fanconi's anemia diagnosis. Cancer Genet Cytogenet 2: 269-274
Berger R, Bernheim A, Gluckman E, Gisselbrecht C (1980b) In vitro effect of cyclophosphamide metabolites on chromosomes of Fanconi anemia patients. Br J Haematol 45: 565-568
Berger R, Bernheim A, Le Coniat M, Vecchione D, Devergie A, Gluckman E (1980c) Bone marrow graft of Fanconi's anemia patient. Cytogenetic study. Cancer Genet Cytogenet 2: 127-130
Berger R, Bernheim A, Le Coniat M, Vecchione D, Schaison G (1980d) Chromosomal studies of leukemic and preleukemic Fanconi's anemia patients. Examples of acquired chromosomal amplification. Hum Genet 56: 59-62
Berger R, Bernheim A, Le Coniat M, Vecchione D, Schaison G (1982) Anémie de Fanconi et chromosomes. In: Actualités Hématologiques, 15èmme Série. Masson, Paris, pp 217-225
Berrebi A, Chemke J, Rappaport S, Barak Y (1979) 14 years follow-up in a patient with Fanconi anemia. Clinical, hematological and cytogenetic study. Haematologica 64: 472-478
Bourgeois CA, Hill FGH (1977) Fanconi anemia leading to acute myelomonocytic leukemia. Cytogenet Studies. Cancer 39: 1163-1167
Cervenka J, Hirsch BA (1983) Cytogenetic differentiation of Fanconi anemia, idiopathic aplastic anemia and Fanconi anemia heterozygotes. Am J Genet 15: 211-223.
Cohen MM, Simpson SJ, Honig GR, Maurer HS, Nicklas JW, Martin AO (1982) The identification of Fanconi anemia genotypes by clastogenic stress. Am J Hum Genet 34: 794-810
Duckworth-Rysiecki G, Hultén M, Mann J, Taylor MR (1984) Clinical and cytogenetic diversity in Fanconi's anemia. J Med Genet 21: 197-203
Duckworth-Rysiecki G, Cornish K, Clarke CA, Buchwald M (1985) Identification of two complementation groups in Fanconi anemia. Somatic Cell Mol Genet 11: 35-41
German J (1983) Patterns of neoplasia associated with the chromosome-breakage syndromes. In: German J (ed) Chromosome mutation and neoplasia. Liss, New York, pp 97-134
Gluckman E, Devergie A, Schaison G, Bussel A, Berger R, Sohier J, Bernard J (1980) Bone marrow transplantation in Fanconi anemia. Br J Haematol 45: 557-564
Gluckman E, Berger R, Dutreix J (1984) Bone marrow transplantation for Fanconi anemia. Semin Hematol 21: 20-26
Huret JL, Benz E, Guilhot F, Brizard A, Tanzer J (1986) Fluctuation of a clone 46, XX, i (7q) in bone marrow in a Fanconi anemia. Hum Genet 74: 98-100
ISCN (1978) In: International system for human cytogenetics nomenclature. Cytogenet Cell Genet 21: 309-404
Liskér R, Cobo de Gutiérez A (1974) Cytogenetic studies in Fanconi's anemia. Description of a case with bone marrow clonal evolution. Clin Genet 5: 72-76
Moustacchi E, Diatloff-Zito C (1985) DNA semi-conservative synthesis in normal and Fanconi anemia fibroblasts following treatment with 8-methoxypsoralen and near ultraviolet light or with X-rays. Hum Genet 70: 236-242
Nordenson I, Björksten B, Lundh B (1980) Prevention of chromosomal breakage in Fanconi's anemia by co-cultivation with normal cells. Hum Genet 56: 169-171
Nowell PC, Bergman G, Besa E, Wilmoth D, Emanuel B (1984) Progressive preleukemia with a chromosomally abnormal clone in a kindred with the Estren-Dameshek variant of Fanconi's anemia. Blood 64: 1135-1138
Obeid DA, Hill FGH, Harnden D, Mann J, Wood BSB (1980) Fanconi anemia. Oxymetholone hepatic tumors, and chromosome aberrations associated with leukemia transition. Cancer 46: 1401-1404
Polani PE (1976) Cytogenetics of Fanconi anemia and related chromosome disorders. In: Congenital disorders of erythropoiesis. Ciba Found Symp (new series) 37: 261-302
Rotzak R, Kaplinsky N, Chaki R, Blei F, Berkowitz M, Goldman B, Frakl O (1982) Giant marker chromosome in Fanconi's anemia transforming into erythroleukemia in an adult. Acta Haematol 67: 214-216
Sasaki MS, Tonomura A (1973) A high susceptibility of Fanconi's anemia to chromosome breakage by DNA cross-linking agents. Cancer Res 33: 1829-1836

Schaison G, Leverger G, Yildiz C, Berger R, Bernheim A, Gluckman E (1983) L'anémie de Fanconi. Fréquence de l'évolution vers la leucémie. Presse Med 12: 1269-1274
Schroeder TM (1966) Cytogenetische und cytologische Befunde bei enzymopenischen Panmyelopathien und Pancytopenien. Humangenetik 2: 287-316
Schroeder TM, Anschütz F, Knopp A (1964) Spontane Chromosomenaberrationen bei familiärer Panmyelopathie. Humangenetik 1: 194-196
Schroeder TM, Drings P, Beilner P, Buchinger G (1976a) Clinical and cytogenetic observations during a six-year period in an adult with Fanconi's anemia. Blut 34: 119-132
Schroeder TM, Tilgen D, Krüger J, Vogel F (1976b) Formal genetics of Fanconi's anemia. Hum Genet 32: 257-288
Schuler D, Kiss A, Fabian F (1969) Chromosomal peculiarities and in vitro examinations in Fanconi's anemia. Humangenetik 7: 314-322
Stivrins TJ, Davis RB, Sanger W, Fritz J, Purtilo DT (1984) Transformation of Fanconi's anemia to acute nonlymphocytic leukemia associated with emergence of monosomy 7. Blood 64: 173-176
Tanzer J, Frocrain C, Desmaret MC (1980) Anomalies du chromosome 1 dans 3 cas de leucémie compliquant une aplasie de Fanconi (FA) (Abstract). Nouv Rev Fr Hematol 22 (Suppl XCIII)
Weksberg R, Buchwald M, Sargent P, Thompson MW, Siminovitch L (1979) Specific defects in patients with Fanconi anemia. J Cell Physiol 101: 311-324
Woods WC, Nesbit ME, Buckley J, Lampkin BC, McCreadie S, Kim TH, Pionelli S, Kersey JH, Feig S, Bernstein I, Hammond D, for the Children's Cancer Study Group (1985) Correlation of chromosome abnormalities with patient characteristics, histologic subtype, and induction succes in children with acute nonlymphocytic leukemia. J Clin Oncol 3: 3-11

Aplastic Anemia and Fanconi Anemia: Response of Lymphocytes to X-Rays and Mitomycin C*

A. T. Natarajan, J. M. J. J. Vossen, and M. H. van Weel-Sipman

Introduction

Aplastic anemia (AA) und Fanconi anemia (FA) are characterized by peripheral blood pancytopenia. While FA is an inherited autosomal recessive disorder, AA may be congenital or acquired. Patients with FA often manifest various congenital abnormalities, whereas such abnormalities are rare in AA patients. Cells derived from patients with FA generally exhibit an increased frequency of baseline chromosomal aberrations and respond with increased sensitivity to DNA cross-linking agents such as mitomycin C (MMC) and diepoxybutane (Sasaki and Tonomura, 1973). These patients' response to X-rays has been reported to be variable (Natarajan et al. 1984). It has been shown that the lymphocytes of some patients with AA respond with increased sensitivity to bleomycin, as measured by the uptake of tritiated thymidine (Morely et al. 1978). We previously reported an increased sensitivity to X-rays and not to mitomycin C of lymphocytes in some patients with AA (Natarajan et al. 1984). Since then we have screened several patients with AA and with FA for the response of their lymphocytes to X-rays and to MMC. The results obtained indicate that the majority of these two types of patients can be distinguished by their differential response to X-rays and MMC.

Materials and Methods

The group of patients studied were children exhibiting symptoms of prolonged bleeding and/or anemia.

Venous blood was drawn in lithium heparin tubes and whole blood cultures were set up in Ham's F10 medium supplemented with 15% fetal calf serum, penicillin, streptomycin, and phytohemoglutinin (Wellcome). The cultures were incubated at 37 °C in a 5% CO_2 atmosphere. Colcemid was added to the cultures 3 h before harvest. The cells were centrifuged, washed in Hanks balanced salt solution, subjected to hypotonic shock (0.75 m*M* KCl for 15 min at 37 °C) and fixed in acetic methanol (1:3). Routine air dried preparations were made and stained with 5% aqueous Giemsa solution for 10 min.

---

* These studies were partly supported by an IAEA grant and an Euratom contract with the University of Leiden.

T. M. Schroeder-Kurth A. D. Auerbach G. Obe (Eds.)
Fanconi Anemia, Clinical, Cytogenetic and Experimental Aspects

To determine the frequencies of baseline aberrations, the cells were harvested 48 h after initiation of the culture. At this time most of the lymphocytes are expected to be in their first mitotic division.

Cultures grown for 69 h were X-irradiated using an ENRAF apparatus at 150 kV, 6 mA at a dose rate of 1 Gy/min. Colcemid was immediately added to the culture and the lymphocytes harvested and fixed after 3 h. The mitotic cells accumulated represented G_2 cells at the time of irradiation.

To treat with MMC, the drug (Kyoga, Japan) was added to 48-h cultures to give the desired concentrations (0.01-0.06 μg/ml) and the cultures were incubated for an additional 24 h. The cultures were harvested and fixed as above. Mitotic cells accumulated using this protocol should contain mostly cells which have been treated at the most sensitive stage of the cell cycle, namely the S phase.

The cells were scored for the presence of chromosomal aberrations, namely, chromatid gaps, chromatid breaks, chromosome breaks (isochromatid breaks), chromatid exchanges, and chromosome exchanges (dicentrics and rings). For each condition, 100 cells were scored. All types of aberrations were pooled and are presented in Tables 1-4.

Results and Discussion

Normal Individuals

The frequency of spontaneously occurring aberrations in normal individuals varies from 0 to 10 aberrations per 100 cells. Many confounding factors have been found for this variation (for a review see Carrano and Natarajan 1988). The types of aberrations encountered are usually gaps and chromatid breaks, the exchange type of aberrations being rare - about 1 in 1000 cells. The frequency of X-ray-induced aberrations in adults has been found to be between 18 and 127 per 100 cells following a G_2 irradiation with 1 Gy (Natarajan et al. 1982). Parallel data in children (of the age group 1-15) are lacking. The concentrations of MMC chosen in our study induced up to 50 chromosomal aberrations per 100 cells in normal individuals.

Table 1. The frequency of chromosomal aberrations induced by X-rays (1 Gy) or mitomycin C in lymphocytes of patients with FA

Patient	Aberrations per 100 cells		
	Baseline	X-rays	MMC (μg/ml)
FA1	17.0	271	172 (0.03)
FA2	30.0	210	154 (0.01)
FA3	47.0	nd	152 (0.01)
FA4	57.0	nd	147 (0.02)
FA5	45.0	208	383 (0.03)
FA6	31.0	105	97 (0.03)
FA7	22.5	434	89 (0.03)

nd, no data

Fanconi Anemia

The results obtained from the patients with FA are presented in Table 1. All the patients exhibited an increased frequency of baseline chromosomal aberrations. This characteristic of FA patients has been widely recognized for a long time (Schroeder et al. 1964). The aberrations observed were mostly of the chromatid type. The frequency of aberrations varied between patients, ranging from 17 to 57 per 100 cells. Since the aberrations found were of the chromatid type, one may speculate that these arise due to some defect associated with DNA replication. However, unlike Bloom's syndrome cells which are defective in some stages of DNA replication (e.g. retarded chain elongation and deficiency in DNA ligase 1) and exhibit increased frequencies of sister chromatid exchanges (SCEs), cells in patients with FA do not exhibit an increased frequency of baseline SCEs.

The frequency of X-ray-induced aberrations in G_2 cells also varies among patients with FA, a situation similar to the one found among normal individuals (Natarajan et al. 1982). The basis for this interindividual variability is not clear; it could be due either to differential radiosensitivity or to a differential rate of progression of irradiated G_2 cells to mitosis. Among the patients with FA studied, one (FA7) responded with a very high frequency of aberrations following 1 Gy of X-rays. The others responded like normal individuals, though the values were in the upper limits of the range encountered in normal individuals.

The response to MMC is also presented in Table 1. Though several concentrations were studied, for comparative purposes, only data from treatment with 0.03 μg/ml or below are presented. The low concentration of MMC we chose induces low frequencies of aberrations in normal cells (a maximum of about 50 aberrations per 100 cells), making it easy to detect patients with FA who respond unequivocally with a higher frequency of aberrations. There was also interindividual variation in the response to MMC among patients with FA (Table 1). Using the response to MMC as an indicator, we tried to study the obligate heterozygotes (parents) of two of the FA patients. In both cases, the parents responded like normal individuals (Table 2), indicating that we cannot rely on response to MMC for the detection of heterozygotes. Though response to diepoxybutane has been claimed to be a good marker for FA heterozygosity in fibroblasts (Auerbach and Wolman 1978), this approach did not work with MMC or DEB in lympho-

Table 2. Frequency of chromosomal aberrations induced by X-rays (1 Gy) or mitomycin C (0.03 μg/ml) in two patients with FA and their parents

	Aberrations per 100 cells		
	Baseline	X-rays	MMC
FA5	45	208	383
Father	1	226	48
Mother	1	132	28
FA6	31	105	97
Father	7	66	26
Mother	8	88	16

cytes. In one patient (FA4), we studied the frequencies of baseline and MMC-induced chromosomal aberrations prior to and after bone marrow transplantation. The results are presented in Table 3. The frequency of baseline aberrations as well as MMC-induced aberrations was very high prior to transplantation. The response to MMC became normal following bone marrow transplantation.

Aplastic Anemia

The data pertaining to patients with AA are presented in Table 4. Unlike patients with FA, the lymphocytes of AA patients have a very low frequency of baseline chromosomal aberrations (1-11 per 100 cells). This frequency is similar to the frequency in controls and is much lower than that observed in patients with FA. The response to MMC in patients with AA is also very similar to that observed in normal individuals indicating, unlike in FA, no hypersensitivity to this cross-linking agent. On the other hand, the lymphocytes of some AA patients responded with a much higher frequency of chromosomal aberrations following G_2 X-irradiation. The observation that the lymphocytes of some of the patients with AA were hypersensitive to bleomycin (Morley et al. 1978), an agent which induces DNA strand

Table 3. Frequency of chromosomal aberrations induced by MMC in lymphocytes of a patient with FA (FA4) before and after bone marrow transplantation

Status	MMC (μg/ml)	Aberrations per 100 cells			
		Gaps	Breaks	Exchanges	Total
Before transplantation (frozen lymphocytes)	0.00	8	44	5	57
	0.01	6	54	13	73
	0.02	9	134	5	148
After transplantation	0.00	2	0	0	2
	0.01	8	10	0	18
	0.02	9	4	0	13
	0.03	9	29	11	49

Table 4. Frequency of chromosomal aberrations induced by X-rays (1 Gy) or mitomycin C (0.03 μg/ml) in lymphocytes of patients with AA

Patient	Aberrations per 100 cells		
	Control	X-rays	MMC
AA1	4.0	1266	9.0
AA2	5.5	237	8.0
AA3	7.5	666	32.0
AA4	5.5	464	19.0
AA5	3.0	417	14.5
AA6	6.5	880	32.0
AA7	4.0	498	13.0
AA8	2.0	404	27.0
AA9	1.0	273	10.0
AA10	1.5	438	14.0

breaks, like X-rays, indicates that these cells may be defective in correctly repairing DNA strand breaks. The basic defect in the radiation-defective syndromes, including ataxia-telangiectasia, is not clear. Biochemical studies with cells from patients with AA may throw some light on whether there is a defect or defects associated with this condition.

Conclusion

Patients with AA and those with FA can be distinguished from each other by the response of their lymphocytes to X-rays and DNA cross-linking agents. FA cells are hypersensitive to MMC and their sensitivity to X-rays is variable. On the other hand, most patients with AA demonstrate a hypersensitive response to X-rays, while their response to MMC is similar to that in normal individuals.

Acknowledgement. The expert technical assistance of Jaap van Rijn is gratefully acknowledged.

References

Auerbach AD, Wolman SR (1978) Carcinogen induced chromosome breakage in Fanconi's anemia heterozygous cells. Nature 271: 69-71

Carrano AV, Natarajan AT (1988) Considerations for population monitoring using cytogenetic techniques - ICPEMC document. Mutat Res 204: 379-406

Morley A, Seshadri R, Trainor K, Sorrell J (1978) Is aplastic anaemia due to abnormality of D. N. A.? Lancet ii 9-11

Natarajan AT, Meijers M, van Rijn JLS (1982) Individual variability of human cells in induction of chromosomal alterations by mutagens. In: Sorsa M, Vainio H (eds) Mutagens in our environment. Liss, New York, 75-88

Natarajan AT, Vossen JMJJ, van Rijn JLS (1984) Cytogenetic response of Fanconi's anaemia to mitomycin C, X-rays and DNA repair inhibitors. Clin Genet 25: 210

Sasaki MS, Tonomura A (1973) A high susceptibility of Fanconi's anemia to chromosme breakage by DNA cross linking agents. Cancer Res 33: 1829-1836

Schroeder TM, Anschütz F, Knopp A (1964) Spontane Chromosomenaberrationen bei familiärer Panmyelopathie. Humangenetik 1: 194-196

Variation in Cellular Sensitivities Among Fanconi Anemia Patients, Non-Fanconi Anemia Patients, Their Parents and Siblings, and Control Probands*

T. M. Schroeder-Kurth, T. H. Zhu, Y. Hong, and I. Westphal

Introduction

The well-documented spontaneous chromosomal breakage in Fanconi anemia (FA) patients varies considerably from patient to patient, but also within the individual during the course of the disease, and is not correlated with the state of health or with the treatment (Schroeder et al. 1976; Schroeder 1982).

Some observations in newborns and young children have shown that the characteristic chromosomal breakage in FA homozygotes may develop within a few months (Schroeder 1982; Gebhart et al. 1985). From family investigations and chromosome analyses in cases tentatively diagnosed as FA, it appears that significant spontaneous breakage can be observed later in life years before the onset of the anemic stage of the disease (Schroeder et al. 1964, 1976; Schroeder and Kurth 1971; Gebhart et al. 1985). Other FA patients, however, may escape detection simply because their endogenous breakage frequency is not significantly higher than that in controls, and, in addition, the types of the few aberrations found, such as gaps and breaks, are nonspecific. Healthy persons also exhibit low frequencies of chromosomal breakage in their lymphocytes, for unknown reasons.

The problems involved in the differential diagnosis of FA, such as the wide range of clinical symptoms, the identification of patients, and prognosis, are described by Auerbach, Rogatko and Schroeder-Kurth (this volume, pp. 3-17).

In the absence of clinical features of typical FA (i.e., aplastic anemia and/or malformations), in sporadic cases or in prenatal chromosome analysis, marginal or significantly increased nonspecific chromosomal abnormalities must arouse suspicion of FA. Without further efforts to clarify the diagnosis such cases should at present, however, not be classified as FA. Conclusions based on biochemical investigations alone may prove incorrect in these cases (Klocker et al. 1983).

Since the observations of Schuler et al. in 1969, cytogeneticists have repeatedly shown that lymphocytes and fibroblasts from cases of FA are particularly sensitive to alkylating agents, which cause adducts and cross-links in chromosomal DNA. This leads to a drastic increase of chromatid and chromosomal aberrations and to reduced clonal cell survival (for review see Schroeder 1982; Ray and German 1981; Wunder and Fleischer 1983). In 1976 and 1978, Auerbach and Wolman re-

* This study is supported by the Deutsche Forschungsgemeinschaft. T. H. Zhu and Y. Hong were in receipt of grants from the People's Republic of China.

T. M. Schroeder-Kurth A. D. Auerbach G. Obe (Eds.)
Fanconi Anemia, Clinical, Cytogenetic and Experimental Aspects

ported a high specificity of diepoxybutane (DEB) for cytogenetic differential diagnosis of FA and other aplastic anemias, or for diagnosis in nonanemic children with skeletal and skin abnormalities similar to those in patients with FA (Auerbach and Wolman 1976, 1978; Auerbach et al. 1981).

The specific DEB sensitivity of FA cells led to the definition of FA for the International FA Registry (IFAR), whose aim is to evaluate basic questions concerning clinical pictures and prognoses of the patients, to carry out familial observations, offer genetic counseling, and identify relevant problems for further biochemical or genetic investigation (see Auerbach et al., this volume, pp. 3-17).

With respect to cytogenetic diagnoses there are still inherent difficulties and uncertainties even in those cases registered in the IFAR. In this paper, we report on the variations in spontaneous and induced chromosomal instabilities in patients with FA and their family members. The aim is to demonstrate the limits of cytogenetic parameters, and to discuss the evaluation of the cytogenetic finding of increased chromosomal instability.

Patients with FA, their parents, and siblings were tested cytogenetically for spontaneous and induced chromosomal instability by treatment of lymphocytes in vitro with DEB, mitomycin C (MMC), and isonicotinic acid hydrazide (INH). Some persons were investigated repeatedly and this allows description of the individual pattern of sensitivity of such patients and to observe an individual or interfamilial variation. From our own observations and from the few data in the literature (Gebhart et al. 1985) we would expect families to have distinct patterns of sensitivity, that individuals with FA have constant sensitivity patterns, and that a genetic heterogeneity could be recognized by such cytogenetic analyses.

In addition to DEB, we chose MMC and INH in order to test for variable sensitivity. MMC is widely used for the diagnosis of FA, since handling it is less dangerous compared to DEB; the hypersensitivity to INH was reported by us (Schroeder and Stahl-Maugé 1979). Using these substances for tests enabled us to compare our results with those from other laboratories. Parallel experiments were performed with patients with suspected FA, their relatives, and control probands as laboratory standard.

Cytosine arabinoside (ara-C) was applied to the lymphocyte cultures of four patients with FA and of controls. The bone marrow transplantation center at the Children's Hospital of the University of Ulm was planning to introduce this substance for conditioning before bone marrow transplantation (Ebell et al., this volume; Friedrich et al. 1987). The experiments with ara-C are included in this paper because the results allow comparison with those of biochemical investigations with cell strains from FA patients of complementation groups A and B (Duckworth-Rysiecki 1985; Moustacchi and Diatloff-Zito 1985 et al., 1987; see also chapters by Buchwald et al. and Moustacchi et al., this volume).

Material and Methods

Patients and Probands

In our laboratory, the European Center for the IFAR, 32 families with a total of 34 patients, 30 parents, 14 siblings, and 7 further relatives were studied from 1982 to October 1986. We investigated 41 patients suspected of having FA, along with family members (21 parents, 9 siblings). Not all of these families are included in the statistical analysis of the IFAR done by Auerbach et al. (this volume, pp. 3-17).

A number of control subjects were included in this program, which is still going on. Pediatricians and physicians in other specialties referred their patients for cytogenetic differential diagnosis, sending a 5- to 8-ml blood sample and a registry form containing information about the patient, the course of the disease, and treatment.

Lymphocyte Cultures and Experiments

Lymphocyte cultures were set up in quadruplicate in Chromosome Medium B (Biochrom KG, FRG). Each culture contained 0.4 ml buffy coat in plasma, 7.6 ml medium, and 2 ml interleukin-2 (Lymphocult-T, Biotest-Institut, FRG), which stimulates the mitotic activity of the lymphocytes (Gillis et al. 1982). DEB (Aldridge, Chicago) and MMC (Serva, Heidelberg) were added in final concentrations of 0.1 μg/ml, 48 and 24 h before harvest, respectively; the final concentration of INH (Serva, Heidelberg) was 14 m*M*. The doses were chosen in accordance with the literature (DEB: Auerbach et al. 1981; MMC: Sasaki 1975, Sasaki and Tonomura 1973; INH: Schroeder and Stahl-Maugé 1979). Ara-C (Mack) was tested in final concentrations of 10^{-8}-10^{-6} *M* in lymphocyte cultures of four patients with FA, three parents, and 20 controls.

Chromosome preparations were made following standard techniques. For karyotyping, the chromosomes were G-banded, using a modification of the method of Wang and Federoff (1972). The slides for chromosomal breakage studies were stained in 2% Giemsa (Gurr) phosphate buffer solution at pH 7.2.

Evaluation

Karyotypes. These were checked according to standard methods. The only abnormality found was a 47, XYY constitution in a healthy brother of one of the patients in the group with forms of aplastic anemia who were diagnosed as having non-FA anemia. All other patients and probands had normal karyotypes.

Breakage Studies. Whenever possible, 100 metaphases were analyzed in each experiment. Since lymphocytes of FA patients tend to grow poorly, this was not always possible. Experiments which gave less than 25 cells were excluded from the study. Even after stimulation with interleukin-2, 29.5% of the lymphocyte cultures of all probands could not be evaluated.

Chromatid and chromosomal aberrations were scored and photographed according to Schroeder and Kurth (1971) and to the ISCN (1985). The number of metaphases evaluated, the number of aberrant cells, the number of breaks, the number of breaks per cell and breaks per aberrant cell, and the multiples of spontaneous breakage rates obtained after treatment with mutagens were recorded. The value for the breaks per cell was chosen for comparison with other authors' data, although much information was lost by considering only this measurement. Borderline sensitivity, in particular, has to be discussed when looking at an individual case or at a familial pattern of sensitivity. The number of aberrant cells, the degree of damage in the aberrant cell, and the various types of aberrations found have to be considered for final judgement.

Table 1. Synopsis of clinical and cytogenetic data of 34 patients with FA

Case	IFAR no.	Age at first examination (years)	Clinical data		Breakage rate (breaks/cell)			
			Malformations	Anemia	Spontaneous	After treatment with		
						INH	MMC	DEB
FA 1	1043/1	11	+/−	+	0.18	0.16	2.03	3.54
FA 2	1025/1	15	+/−	+	0.13	0.18	2.84	>10.0
FA 3	1015/1	17	+/−	+	0.14	0.44	1.28	2.02
FA 4	1052/1	8	0	+	0.18	0.09	1.50	>10.0
FA 5	1052/2	10	0	+	0.06	0.12	1.76	>10.0
FA 6	1011/1	4	+/−	+	0.30	0.23	4.82	4.30
FA 7	1046/1	6 months	++	0	0.07	0.16	0.82	>10.0
FA 8	1058/1	4	+/−	+	0.05	0.20	0.60	1.98
FA 9	1038/1	8	++	+	0.35	0.51	1.16	3.80
FA 10	1017/1	18	++	+	0.74	0.50	n	9.32
FA 11	1050/1	6	0	+	0.59	0.70	2.76	>10.0
FA 12	1001/1	11	0	+	0.23	0.18	1.45	>10.0
FA 13	1030/1	9	+/−	+	0.47	0.65	2.36	>10.0
FA 14	1047/1	4	+	+	0.12	n	n	4.82
FA 15	1062/1	2	++	0	0.24	0.20	1.36	0.88
FA 16	1029/1	11	+/−	+	0.15	0.15	n	1.80
FA 17	1031/1	5	++	+	0.09	0.34	1.72	>10.0
FA 18	1022/1	10	+	+	0.23	0.20	>10.0	>10.0
FA 19	1022/2	5	0	0	0.27	0.16	>10.0	>10.0
FA 20	1019/1	16	+	+	0.37	0.26	1.46	8.05
FA 21	1049/1	20	+/−	+	0.37	0.51	2.10	2.92
FA 22	1040/1	4	++	+	0.13	0.35	2.68	>10.0
FA 23	3002/1	3	++	+	0.19	n	n	>10.0
FA 24	3001/1	13	+/−	+	0.06	n	2.57	>10.0
FA 25	1004/1	13	++	+	0.88	0.96	1.86	3.48
FA 26	1083/1	2	++	+	0.20	0.06	1.50	9.40
FA 27	1124/1	6	+	+	0.36	0.43	0.66	3.34
FA 28	1124/2	11	+	+	0.13	0.06	2.36	3.02
FA 29	1014/1	10 months	++	0	2.40	3.63	n	n
FA 30	1055/1	6	+	+	0.18	0.14	0.86	1.98
FA 31	1073/1	4	++	+	0.50	0.20	1.60	4.00
FA 32	1013/1	6	++	+	0.19	0.32	n	n
FA 33	1086/1	6	++	+	0.22	0.20	1.96	2.30
FA 34	1089/1	8	++	+	0.15	0.08	0.63	1.10

++, Typical malformation pattern in FA; +, single but typical malformation, or anemia present; +/−, unspecific anomaly; 0, absent; n, not done, no result
Dosages: INH, 14 m*M;* MMC and DEB, o.i. μg/ml

Identification of Lymphocyte Cultures

Each FA family is or will be recorded in the IFAR. For this study, Table 1 lists the patients with FA by number in the first column (FA 1, FA 2, etc.) and refers in the second column to the IFAR number which is allocated to each FA family. Siblings with FA have consecutive numbers added to the family IFAR registration number (e.g., 1052/1, 1052/2, etc.), while healthy members have a letter added indicating their relationship to the patient (FA-F, father; FA-M, mother; FA-B, brother; FA-S, sister; for other labels see footnote to Table 9).

Probands who were investigated because they were suspected of having FA are also registered in the IFAR with a family number (Table 2), but they are listed in subsequent tables as group P. Their parents and siblings have the same IFAR number with the suffixes F, M, S, and B as described above. Control persons are listed as C1 to C26. No complete family studies were available in this group.

Results

The description of our results concerning variations in sensitivities of cells when treated with INH, MMC, and DEB is predetermined by the definition of FA: FA cells are highly sensitive to the induction of chromosomal aberrations by DEB (Auerbach et al., this volume, pp. 3-17). Thus the patients primarily suspected of having FA are classified in the FA group of 34 patients, their obligate heterozygous parents, and siblings. Forty-one DEB-nonsensitive patients are classified as non-FA patients and their relatives (P group). Since this is a study which concentrates on individual sensitivity patterns, the description of the results will include interpretations and critical remarks on the criteria used.

Sensitivity Patterns

FA Homozygous Patients

Table 1 gives information on 34 patients with FA including the IFAR numbers for identification, their age at the time of the first cytogenetic investigation, and some information about the clinical picture, i.e., their age at the time of the first investigation, the presence or absence of anemic symptoms, and other patterns of abnormalities typical for FA: thumb and/or radial defects, microcephaly and kidney anomalies (++), one single symptom (+), unspecific anomalies (+/−), or no such anomalies (0).

The cytogenetic results are given as breaks per cell; in some cases, single experiments were unsuccessful (n). Treatment particularly with DEB, but also with MMC, led to breakage rates of more than 10 per cell, which means that each metaphase contained more than 10, sometimes innumerable breaks.

Lymphocytes from four out of 34 patients with FA did not show an increase in spontaneous chromosomal instability (FA 5, FA 7, FA 8, and FA 24). Three of these were clearly identified as suffering from FA by their abnormal sensitivity to INH, MMC, and/or DEB. FA 8, however, deserves special attention, because the cells had a relatively low sensitivity in addition to the absence of a spontaneously

Table 2. Synopsis of clinical and cytogenetic data of the probands P1-P41 (non-FA patients)

Case	IFAR no	Age at examination (years)	Clinical data		Chromosomal breakage rates in lymphocytes			
			Malformations	Anemia	Spontaneous	Treatment with		
						INH	MMC	DEB
P 1	1023/1	1	+	0	0.02	0.04 (2.0)[a]	0.52 (26.0)	0.13 (6.5)
P 2	1078/1	3	0	+	0.08	n	n	n
P 3	1032/1	1 month	+	0	0.01	0.01 (1.0)	n	0.05 (5.0)
P 4	1020/1	1	0	+	0.12	0.18 (1.5)	0.58 (4.8)	0.41 (3.4)
P 5	1063/1	9	0	+	0.01	0.03 (3.0)	0.11 (11.0)	0.06 (6.0)
P 6	1028/1	8	0	+	0.06	0	0.14 (2.3)	0.04 (0.7)
P 7	1039/1	14	0	+	0.10	0.04 (0.4)	0.31 (3.1)	0.11 (1.1)
P 8	1074/1	10	AT		0.13	0.38 (2.9)	n	6.00 (46.2)
P 9	1059/1	14	0	+	0.02	0.05 (2.5)	0.12 (6.0)	0.02 (1.0)
P 10	1027/1	6 months	+	0	0[b]	0	0.23 (23.0)	0.05 (5.0)
P 11	1034/1	1 month	+	0	0[b]	0	0	0
P 12	1061/1	6	0	+	0.10	0.10 (1.0)	0.26 (2.6)	0.22 (2.2)
P 13	1060/1	1	+	0	0.03	0.05 (1.7)	0.46 (15.3)	0.30 (10.0)
P 14	1021/1	2	+	0	0.03	0.02 (0.7)	0.24 (8.0)	0.02 (0.7)
P 15	1036/1	13	0	+	0[b]	0	0.07 (7.0)	0.03 (3.0)
P 16	1075/1	34	+	0	0.01	0	0.14 (14.0)	0
P 17	1068/1	3 months	+	+	0.06	0.02 (0.3)	0.10 (1.6)	0.04 (0.7)
P 18	1077/1	6	+	0	0[b]	0	0.03 (3.0)	0.007 (0.7)
P 19	1125/1	14	0	+	0.05	n	n	0.01 (0.2)
P 20	1065/1	3 months	+	0	0.02	0	0.03 (1.5)	0.01 (0.5)
P 21	1069/1	10	0	+	0[b]	0.02 (2.0)	0.22 (11.0)	0
P 22	1111/1	8	0	+	0[b]	n	n	0.44 (44.0)
P 23	1080/1	1 month	+	0	0[b]	n	n	0.06 (6.0)
P 24	1057/1	23	+/−	0	0.05	0.02 (0.4)	0.21 (4.2)	0.15 (3.0)
P 25	1044/1	3	0	+	0.06	0.04 (0.7)	0.52 (8.6)	0.06 (0)
P 26	1085/1	5	0	+	0.06	0.02 (0.3)	0.02 (0.3)	0.04 (0.7)
P 27	1082/1	9	+/−	+	0.18	0.20 (1.1)	0.80 (4.4)	0.19 (1.1)
P 28	1090/1	13	0	+	0.10	0.02 (0.5)	0.26 (2.6)	0.14 (1.4)
P 29	1054/1	2	0	+	0[b]	0.02 (2.0)	0.20 (20.0)	0.01 (1.0)
P 30	1095/1	14	+/−	+	0.07	0 (7.0)	0.19 (2.7)	0.01 (0.1)
P 31	1100/1	2	+/−	+	0[b]	n	0.03 (3.0)	0.04 (4.0)
P 32	1071/1	6 months	+	0	0[b]	n	0.07 (7.0)	0.01 (1.0)
P 33	1092/1	11	+	+	0.15	0.19 (1.3)	n	n
P 34	1097/1	10 months	0	+	0[b]	n	n	0.01 (1.0)
P 35	1053/1	9	0	+/−	0.17	0.02 (0.1)	0.55 (3.2)	0.03 (1.2)
P 36	1106/1	16	0	+	n	n	0.37	0.30 -
P 37	1106/2	12	0	+/−	0.20	n	0.74 (3.7)	0.21 (1.0)
P 38	1114/1	10	0	+	0.32	0.12 (0.4)	1.75 (5.5)	0.59 (1.8)
P 39	1103/1	8	+/−	+	0.02	n	0.05 (2.5)	0.02 (1.0)
P 40	1093/1	7	0	+	0.04	n	n	0 (0)
P 41	1093/2	7	0	+/−	0.06	0.04 (0.6)	0.10 (1.6)	0.02 (0.3)

Cases mentioned in text; + +, typical malformation pattern in FA; +, single but typical malformation, or anemia present; +/−, unspecific anomaly; 0, absent; n, not done, no result
Dosages: INH, 14 m*M;* MMC and DEB, 0.1 μg/ml

[a] The values in ( ) indicate the multiple of the spontaneous breakage rate

[b] The sensitivity of the probands' lymphocytes is expressed in these cases as a multiple of a spontaneous breakage rate of 0.01

Table 3a. Breakage rates, means, and ranges by groups of probands

Designation	Probands (*n*)	Breakage			
		Spontaneous	Induced		
			INH (14 m*M*)	MMC (o.i. μg/ml)	DEB (o.i. μg/ml)
FA patients	34	0.44 (0.05-2.40)	0.40 (0.06-3.63)	2.38 (0.60-10.0)	6.29 (0.88-10.0)
Parents of FA patients	30	0.05 (0-0.28)	0.05 (0-0.30)	0.39 (0.01-1.88)	0.16 (0-1.08)
Siblings of FA patients	14	0.03 (0-0.06)	0.03 (0-0.06)	0.16 (0.02-1.00)	0.08 (0.08-0.16)
Non-FA patients	41	0.06 (0-0.32)	0.04 (00.20)	0.29 (0-1.75)	0.11 (00.59)
Parents of non-FA patients	21	0.07 (00.34)	0.23 (03.00)	0.36 (0-2.85)	0.34 (0-1.69)
Siblings of non-FA patients	9	0.03 (0-0.10)	0.13 (0-0.30)	0.35 (0-0.99)	0.07 (0-0.22)
Ataxia-telangiectasia	1	0.13	0.38	-	6.00
Control persons I	22	0.02 (0-0.08)	0.03 (0-0.10)	0.33 (0-0.59)	0.05 (0-0.22)
Control persons II	5	0.11 (0.01-0.68)	0.09 (0.03-0.26)	0.63 (0.32-1.08)	0.21 (0-0.42)

Table 3b. Breaks per aberrant cell, means, and ranges in patients with FA, non-FA probands, and control persons

Subjects	*n*	Breaks			
		Spontaneous	Induced		
			INH (14 m*M*)	MMC (0.1 μg/ml)	DEB (0.1 μg/ml)
FA patients	34	1.48 (1.00-2.00)	1.54 (1.20-2.44)	4.96 (1.66- > 10.0)	8.23 (2.22-12.19)
Non-FA probands	41	1.27 (1.00-2.00)	1.47 (1.00-2.00)	1.56 (1.00-1.87)	1.51 (1.00-2.00)
Control persons I	22	1.04 (1.00-1.50)	1.00 (1.00-1.50)	1.53 (1.00-3.71)	1.14 (1.00-2.50)
Control persons II	5	2.09 (1.00-3.37)	1.73 (1.00-2.00)	2.78 (1.95-3.50)	1.66 (1.34-2.10)

elevated breakage rate. This case was diagnosed as one of FA because DEB induced an aberration rate of 0.98, higher than that in any non-FA individual (Table 3 a, b). While only 48% of the cells exhibited breakage, some cells had multiple breaks typical of FA. Considering cytogenetic results only, it is clear from this case that with statistically significant aberration rates alone, setting the limits for

Table 4. Individual sensitivity of FA lymphocytes to DEB

Case no.	Multiples of baseline breakage-rates	Aberrant cells		Breaks per aberrant cell	
		n	%	Untreated	After treatment
FA 5	166.7	6	100	1.00	> 10.00
FA 24	166.7	6	100	1.00	> 10.00
FA 7	142.9	4	100	1.75	> 10.00
FA 17	111.1	7	100	1.28	> 10.00
FA 22	76.9	15	100	1.11	> 10.00
FA 2	76.9	10	84	1.30	11.90
FA 4	55.6	13	100	1.64	> 10.00
FA 23	52.6	12	82	1.58	12.19
FA 26	47.0	10	100	2.00	9.40
FA 12	43.5	17	98	1.35	10.20
FA 18	43.5	14	100	1.64	> 10.00
FA 14	40.2	10	90	1.20	5.35
FA 8	39.6	4	48	1.25	4.12←
FA 19	37.0	18	97	1.50	10.30
FA 28	23.2	10	88	1.30	3.43
FA 20	21.8	20	100	1.47	8.05
FA 13	21.3	29	100	1.62	> 10.00
Mean (17 cases)	68.6	12.4	93.4	1.41	9.11
FA 1	19.7	9	90	2.00	1.96
FA 11	16.9	36	100	1.63	10.00
FA 3	14.4	12	62	1.16	3.25
FA 6	14.3	16	98	1.87	4.38
FA 10	12.6	46	100	1.60	9.32
FA 16	12.0	11	64	1.34	2.62
FA 30	11.0	14	66	1.28	3.00
FA 9	10.9	26	71	1.35	5.35
FA 33	10.6	17	68	1.29	2.99
Mean (9 cases)	13.8	20.8	79.9	1.50	4.76
FA 27	9.3	21	86	1.75	3.88
FA 31	8.0	26	82	1.92	4.87
FA 21	7.9	21	82	1.76	3.56
FA 34	7.3	12	52	1.11	2.09←
FA 25	4.0	52	96	1.69	3.62←
FA 15	3.7	18	40	1.33	2.20←
Mean (6 cases)	6.7	25.0	73.0	1.59	3.37

Three arbitary groups of patients with FA were formed according to higher or lower sensitivity to DEB: > 20-fold (17 cases), > tenfold (9 cases), and < tenfold the baseline breakage rate (6 cases). ←, Cases mentioned in text.

differential diagnosis remains a problem. A complete evaluation of the breakage analysis, including the types of aberrations, could be decisive. In case FA 8, even in the untreated lymphocytes, one of the four aberrations found was a nonhomologous chromatid translocation, and in the experimental cultures a low but significant increase in these typical aberrations was found. Thus, the classification of this

Table 5. Individual sensitivity to MMC of FA lymphocytes

Case no.	Multiples of baseline breakage rates	Aberrant cells		Breaks per aberrant cell	
		n	%	Untreated	After treatment
FA 18	43.5	14	100	1.58	> 10.00
FA 24	42.8	6	52	100	4.94
FA 19	37.0	18	98	1.50	> 10.00
FA 5	29.3	6	50	1.00	3.52
FA 17	22.2	7	56	1.28	3.07
FA 2	21.8	10	70	1.30	4.05
FA 22	20.6	15	65	1.11	4.12
FA 28	18.2	10	74	1.30	3.18
FA 6	16.1	16	71	1.87	6.78
FA 8	12.0	4	36	1.25	1.66 ←
FA 7	11.7	4	31	1.75	2.64 ←
FA 1	11.3	9	47	2.00	4.31
Mean (12 cases)	23.9	10	63	1.41	4.86
FA 3	9.1	12	46	1.16	2.78
FA 33	8.9	17	19	1.29	2.03
FA 4	8.3	13	40	1.38	3.78
FA 26	7.5	10	36	2.00	4.16
FA 12	6.3	17	32	1.35	4.53
FA 15	5.7	18	42	1.33	3.23
FA 21	5.7	21	54	1.76	3.88
FA 13	5.0	29	47	1.62	5.02
FA 30	4,8	14	34	1.28	2.52
FA 11	4.7	36	78	1.63	3.53
FA 34	4.2	12	27	1.11	2.03
FA 20	3.9	26	57	1.47	2.56
FA 9	3.3	26	41	1.35	2.82
FA 31	3.2	26	42	1.92	3.80
FA 25	2.1	52	92	1.62	2.02 ←
FA 27	1.9	21	66	1.71	2.27
Mean (16 cases)	5.3	22	47	1.50	3.19

Patients with FA were split into two groups about an arbitrary level of increase in the breakage rates: the "highly sensitive" (12 out of 28), with an increase > tenfold, the rest the "less sensitive," with an increase < tenfold.
←, Cases mentioned in text

patient as having FA was certainly correct. The girl had no severe physical abnormalities, but aplastic anemia started in infancy and she died of a fatal graft-versus-host reaction after a bone marrow transplant at age of 4 years.

In Tables 4, 5, and 6 we have tried to specify the sensitivity of patients with FA to DEB, MMC, and INH, as expressed in multiples of the individual baseline breakage. In addition, the tables contain, for comparison, two independent values: the percentage of aberrant cells and breaks per aberrant cell in the untreated as well as in the treated cells. Only 12 out of 34 cases of FA had 100% damaged cells when treated with DEB. After MMC or INH treatment only one case from each treatment had 100% aberrant cells. Experimental conditions as well as back muta-

Table 6. Individual sensitivity of FA lymphocytes to INH

Case no.	Multiple baseline breakage rates	Aberrant cells		Breaks per aberrant cell	
		n	%	Untreated	After treatment
FA 8	4.0	4	15	1.25	1.33
FA 17	3.8	7	22	1.28	1.54
FA 3	3.1	12	18	1.16	2.44
FA 22	2.7	15	25	1.11	1.40
FA 7	2.3	4	12	1.75	1.33
FA 5	2.0	6	8	1.00	2.00
FA 32	1.7	15	25	1.13	1.21
FA 29	1.5	62	100	3.87	4.39←
FA 9	1.5	26	30	1.35	1.70
Mean (9 cases)	2.5	17	28	1.54	1.91
FA 2	1.4	10	13	1.30	1.38
FA 13	1.4	29	46	1.62	1.41←
FA 21	1.4	21	31	1.76	1.64
FA 11	1.2	36	42	1.63	1.66
FA 27	1.2	21	27	1.71	1.59
FA 25	1.1	52	40	1.69	2.40←
FA 16	1.0	36	42	1.34	1.25←
FA 1	0.9	9	10	2.00	1.60
FA 18	0.9	14	16	1.64	1.25
FA 33	0.9	17	14	1.29	1.42
FA 6	0.8	16	15	1.87	1.53
FA 12	0.8	17	14	1.35	1.28
FA 15	0.8	18	16	1.33	1.24
FA 30	0.8	14	10	1.28	1.40
FA 10	0.7	46	26	1.60	1.92
FA 20	0.7	26	18	1.47	1.44
FA 19	0.6	18	11	1.50	1.45
FA 34	0.5	12	3	1.11	2.40←
FA 4	0.5	13	8	1.38	1.20
FA 28	0.5	10	12	1.30	1.00
FA 31	0.4	26	12	1.92	1.66
FA 26	0.3	10	12	2.00	1.00
Mean (22 cases)	0.9	21	20	1.55	1.51

Differing reactions to INH divided patients with FA into two groups: one had low sensitivity with multiples of baseline breakage >1.5-fold, a slight increase in the number of aberrant cells and aberrations per aberrant cell. The other group was considered nonsensitive to INH on the basis of an individual multiple of baseline breakage <1.5-fold; as a group the other parameters were unchanged when compared to reactions in untreated conditions. There are again exceptions (←) in both groups, where ranking would have been different if another parameter, like increase of aberrant cells or increase of breaks per aberrant cell, had been taken.

←, Cases mentioned in text

tions could account for undamaged cells. Thus, the number of breaks per aberrant cell can serve as an additional parameter in defining whether or not cells are sensitive to a clastogen. Again, for comparison, breaks per aberrant cell in the untreated and in the treated cultures are listed. Taking the multiples of baseline breakage rates after treatment with DEB (Table 4), MMC (Table 5), and INH (Table 6), the cases of FA were ranked in an order which differed between the clastogens. For each treatment, the attempt was made to group the patients with FA, according to higher or lower sensitivity in order to test for simple rules which might be useful for cytogenetic diagnosis.

DEB Sensitivity. Patients with FA were divided according to their individual DEB sensitivity into three arbitrarily decided groups: in 17 patients, a more than 20-fold, in nine more than tenfold, and in six a less than tenfold increase of baseline breakage rates was found. The group with the highest sensitivity was characterized by a relatively low percentage of aberrant cells in untreated cultures (mean 12.4%) with a relatively low index of breaks per aberrant cell (mean 1.41). After treatment with DEB the proportion of aberrant cells increased drastically (mean 93.4%) and the index of breaks per aberrant cell reached values between 3.43 and more than 10 (mean > 9.11). Case FA8 is noteworthy for its lack of the drastic increase of aberrant cells (only 48%). However, the other parameters confirm the ranking in this group. (See also Tables 3a, b).

In the middle group, with a 13.8-fold mean increase of baseline breakage rates, there were more damaged cells and less pronounced increases of aberrant cells (79.9%) and of the index of breaks per aberrant cell (4.76).

This tendency could also be seen in the low-sensitivity group after DEB treatment: in the untreated cultures, 25% of the cells showed chromosomal damage, a value which increased to 73% after treatment, while the index of breaks per aberrant cell was the highest among the three groups (1.59), with an increase to 3.37 after DEB treatment.

MMC Sensitivity. After MMC treatment the FA cases fell into two groups according to multiples of baseline breakage: higher than tenfold (12 patients) and less than tenfold (16 patients). Higher sensitivity to MMC can be attributed to cases of FA with a relatively low proportion of damaged cells (10%) and a relatively low index of breaks per aberrant cell in the untreated culture (1.41). After MMC treatment the percentage of aberrant cells increased to 63% in this group with an index of breaks per aberrant cell of 4.86. In the lower sensitivity group (a 5.3-fold increase in baseline breakage rates), 22% of the cells were found to be damaged in the untreated cultures, with an index of 1.5 breaks per aberrant cell. After MMC treatment, 47% of the cells showed chromosomal aberrations with an index of 3.19 breaks per aberrant cell (Table 5).

INH Sensitivity. INH treatment induced fewer chromosomal abnormalities in the cells of FA patients than MMC or DEB. Two groups of FA patients are listed in Table 6 according to their sensitivity to INH: nine cases were sensitive, the sensitivity increasing more than 1.5-fold, and with a mean individual baseline breakage which increased 2.5-fold. Of the untreated cells, 17% showed chromosomal abnormalities in this group, with an index of 1.54 breaks per aberrant cell. After treatment, 28% of the cells were damaged; the incidence of breaks per aberrant cell increased to 1.91. There were 22 patients who were considered not sensitive to INH, since the quotient of breaks per cell in the untreated culture divided by breaks per cell in the treated culture was less than 1.5. As a group, the other parameters were unchanged when compared with untreated conditions. The cases were ranked according to the multiples of baseline breakage. The ranking in each experiment would have been different if the other parameter demonstrated in the table had been considered. Thus, looking at single cases in the various groups, there are exceptions which do not follow the simple correlations drawn from the means of the groups. Some of the exceptions are indicated by arrows in Table 4. In addition to FA8, which has already been mentioned, the ranking would have been different if another parameter such as the increase in the number of aberrant cells, the increase of aberrations per aberrant cell, or the increase in the breakage rate were taken. In cases FA 15, FA 16, FA 30, and FA 34, treatment with MMC and DEB led to a significant increase in the breakage rate; however, there was a clear spontaneous chromosomal instability. Again, the aberration types were characteristic for FA (chromatid breaks, nonhomologous chromatid translocations, and fragments; Schroeder and German 1974) as were the clinical pictures. It should be stressed that in such cases, repeated cytogenetic investigations may be necessary to confirm the diagnosis of FA.

Cases FA 3 and FA 21 also demonstrated relatively low sensitivities, thus posing problems for differential diagnosis. FA 3, FA 16 and FA 21 suffer from a typical aplastic anemia; FA 15 was identified as a patient only because of a suspect malformation pattern. The number of breaks per cell over baseline in this case increased 5.7-fold with MMC and 3.7-fold with DEB (Tables 4 and 5); again, however, the types of aberrations found clearly support the diagnosis of FA. It is interesting that a similar increase in the breakage rates was observed in cases in which FA was suspected (Table 7, P 4, P 5, P 13, P 14), in obligate heterozygotes or

Table 7. Patterns of sensitivity to INH, MMC, and DEB, expressed in magnitudes of the increase of chromosomal breaks per cell over the individual baseline breakage rates

Group	INH	MMC	DEB	Case nos.
I	0	+ + +	+ + +	2, 18, 19
		+ +	+ +	1, 6
		+	+	15, 34, 31
II	0	+ +	+ + +	28
III	0	+	+ + +	13, 12, 20, 4, 26
			+ +	21, 16, 11, 27, 25, 30
IV	+	+ + +	+ + +	17, 23, 5, 22
		+ +		8, 7
V	+	+	+ +	3, 9

+ + +, >20-fold increase; + +, >10-fold increase; +, >1.5-fold increase; 0, <1.5-fold increase

siblings (Table 9, family 1058 FA-F, family 1050 FA-M, family 1022 FA-F and -M, FA-S) and in healthy unrelated persons (Table 8, C 13, C 15, C 24). Thus, even a statistically significant increase in the breakage rate may not be relevant for differential diagnosis, but it may be of diagnostic value when considered together with other factors, i. e., detailed cytogenetic results and clinical findings.

Patterns of sensitivity represent recurrent combinations of sensitivity to a battery of clastogens. We have established five basic groups of patients with FA on the basis of individual sensitivity to the three agents. These are shown in Table 7.

In a study of sensitivity to INH, the lymphocytes of 25 of 31 FA patients did not show a significant increase of chromosomal damage following INH treatment (Table 6). Some of these cases were sensitive to MMC and DEB to the same extent (FA 18 and FA 19, who are siblings); in others the sensitivity, expressed as multiples of the individual spontaneous breakage rates, was higher following treatment with DEB than following treatment with MMC (groups II and III). There were also some cases in group I, with low sensitivity, which reacted in a similar fashion to both DEB and MMC (FA 15, FA 31, and FA 34); however, in case FA15 MMC was more effective in break induction per aberrant cell. This effect was also apparent in cases FA 1 and FA 6. This may account for the slightly higher sensitivity to MMC in these cases, but also raises the question of borderline results, particularly since non-FA cases show similar patterns (Table 2).

Only six cases were, in addition to being highly sensitive to DEB and MMC, sensitive to INH (group IV); however, the induction of breaks after INH treatment was comparatively low. In FA 3 and FA 9, there was a similar sensitivity pattern, with a less pronounced increase in the breakage rate following DEB and MMC treatment, but relatively more breaks per aberrant cell as a result of break induction by INH.

Non-FA Proband (P Cases)

Table 2 gives a survey of clinical and cytogenetic findings on individuals with some clinical symptoms resembling FA, but in whom the diagnosis of FA was excluded on the basis of cytogenetic studies with DEB. Most cases (30) had normal spontaneous breakage rates (range 0–0.08); only 10 cases showed elevated levels (0.1–0.32). INH and DEB treatment led to a significant increase of aberrations in one case only. This case was investigated accidentally because the blood was sent erroneously. The clinical report arrived later and showed that this patient was suffering from ataxia-telangiectasia (AT). The cytogenetic investigation did not support the clinical diagnosis. There were no clonal t(7; 14) or other translocations, but, as shown in Table 2 (case P 8) the lymphocytes were surprisingly sensitive to DEB and to INH. The cultures treated with MMC did not give enough metaphases, indicating a severe toxic reaction.

Twenty-one out of 32 cases were sensitive to MMC, and six out of 38 to DEB, i. e., they had statistically significant increases in breakage rates after treatment as compared to the individual baseline breakage. The absolute values of the breakage rates however, did not exceed the values of 0.2 (INH), 1.75 (MMC) and 0.59 (DEB), with the exception of P 8, the patient with AT, who died before the investigation could be repeated. It should be pointed out that MMC-induced breakage rates in some of the group of patients with FA (FA 6; FA 7, FA 29, FA 30, and

FA 34) were similar to the values among some probands (P 1, P 4, P 13, P 27, P 37, and P 38), particularly when the multiples of the baseline breakage rates are considered (P 1, 26 × ; P 13, 15.3 × ; versus FA 7, 11.7 × ; FA 8, 12.0 × ; Tables 2 and 5). With respect to the types of aberrations induced by INH, MMC, or DEB, the increase in breaks and chromatid translocations, particularly with MMC, makes the classification of these individuals difficult. However, the sensitivity of these cases to DEB, measured as an absolute value of breaks per cell or breaks per aberrant cell (not shown), is low, in contrast to a significant increase in breakage rates. It has not been decided how many breaks per cell after DEB treatment are significant for the definition of FA: the findings in P 38 left considerable doubt about the nature of the anemia. The diagnosis in P 14 seemed to be more certain: although breakage induction by MMC and DEB was significant, the spontaneous breakage rate was normal. FA lymphocytes, however, sometimes show spontaneous breakage rates within the normal range.

The patterns of sensitivity found by comparing sensitivity to INH, MMC, and DEB were quite different from those of patients with FA: MMC induced more breaks in more cells than DEB (means 0.29 for MMC versus 0.11 for DEB). Breakage rates after treatment with INH varied, and were mostly within the normal range (except P 8).

Controls

In this group, 26 persons were investigated who had no clinical signs of FA and who were not related to the probands of the group of patients with FA or with the group of probands. Six children were between the ages of 1 month (C 22) and 9 years [C 2, C 13, C 17, C 18 (monozygotic twins), C 21]; five probands were 10-19 years old (C 11, C 15, C 16, C 19, and C 20); C 14 was 20 years old; C 12 was 25 years old; the other probands were older than 30. Thus, the control group was not age- and sex-matched. It is extremely difficult to get blood samples from healthy children for experimental purposes.

Table 8 has two parts, the results being divided into those for one group of probands who were investigated between 1983 and 1986 (C 1-C 22), and those from four individuals who were studied as laboratory controls in 1987 (C 23-C 26) on two occasions. The results were not pooled together in order to show the considerable variation among voluntary blood donors and between experimental conditions at different times. In the first group, the spontaneous breakage rates ranged from 0.0-0.08. Treatment with INH led to small but significant increases of aberration frequencies in two of the 16 cases, with less than 0.1 breaks per cell. MMC induces considerable breakage frequencies in normal cells. In nine out of 12 cases, we found a significant increase of aberrations, which, in some cases, were as frequent as in the probands or even in cases of FA (C 12, C 13, C 14, C 15, and C 16).

The sensitivity to DEB in this group was different from that to MMC, although there was considerable variation. The highest breakage rate was 0.22 in C 20, which is 3.1 times the baseline value. Treatment with both MMC and DEB led to a significant increase in the breakage frequencies in the control group. The types of aberrations were the same as in the P group, mostly chromatid breaks. In normal cells, treatment with MMC causes chromatid translocations of the same

Table 8. Chromosome instability of healthy control persons

	Case no.	Breakage rate (breaks per cell)			
		Spontaneous	After treatment with		
			INH	MMC	DEB
	C 1	0			
	C 2	0			
	C 3	0.05	0.02	0.12 (2.4)	0.02
	C 4	0.04	0.02	0.16 (4.0)	0.09
	C 5	0.02	n	n	0.09
	C 6	0	0.00	n	0.01
	C 7	0.02	0.015	1.20 (60.0)	0.02
	C 8	0.005	0.015	0.50 (100.0)	0.10 (20.0)
	C 9	0.03	0.01	0.33 (11.0)	0.015
	C 10	0.005	0.015	0.34 (68.0)	0.01
	C 11	0.02	n	0.09	n
	C 12	0.01	0.07	0.42 (42.0)	0.10 (10.0)
1982-1986	C 13	0	0.10 (10.0)	0.59 (59.0)	0.10 (10.0)
(I)	C 14	0	0.06 (6.0)	0.59 (59.0)	0.00
	C 15	0	0.05	0.43 (43.0)	0.10 (10.0)
	C 16	0.08	0.06	0.27 (3.4)	0.13
	C 17	0	0.02	0.02	0.00
	C 18	0	0.00	0.03	0.03
	C 19	0	0.01	0.17 (17.0)	0.10
	C 20	0.07	0.06	0.10	0.22 (3.0)
	C 21	0.01	0.09 (9.0)	0.16 (16.0)	0.04
	C 22	0	n	0.00	n
	Mean	0.02	0.04 (2.0)	0.31 (15.5)	0.07 (13.5)
	C 23	0.67	0.26 (0.55)	1.08 (2.30)	0.42 (0.89)
	C 24	0.01	0.04	0.70 (7.00)	0.00
1987	C 25	0.09	0.06	0.66 (7.33)	0.20 (2.2)
(II)	C 26	0.03	0.06 (2.0)	0.32 (11.0)	0.06 (2.0)
	C 27	0.05	0.03	0.39 (7.8)	0.35 (7.0)
	Mean	0.11	0.009 (0.7)	0.63 (4.8)	0.21 (1.6)

C 17 and C 18 are identical twins C 8 and C 19 are mother and son C 13 and C 16 are sisters
Dosages: INH, 14 m*M*; MMC and DEB, 0.1 μg/ml
( ), Multiples of spontaneous breakage rates; n, not done, no result

nonhomologous types as in FA cells. There are only quantitative differences between MMC's effect on normal cells and on FA cells, which are often not verified by those who do not perform breakage studies routinely.

The second group of five C individuals was characterized by relatively high sensitivity to MMC when the breakage rates were compared with those of the first group. The highest breakage rate was found in C 23, who also had an unusual and unexpected spontaneous breakage rate (0.47), while the other three were within the control range (C 1-C 22) in spontaneous as well as in INH- and MMC-induced breakage rates. However, C 23 was neither sensitive to INH nor to DEB. Since this case seemed to be exceptional, and since the group of four was investigated separately, they were not included in calculations of control means but appear separately in Tables 3a and b as "control persons II."

The sensitivity pattern in this group was dominated by the reaction to MMC in cases in which DEB caused low breakage rates similar to the patterns in P probands mentioned above (C 12, C 13, C 15, C 16, C 19, C 24, C 25, and C 26). Probands C 14, C 21, and C 24 were not sensitive to DEB at all, but they were sensitive to MMC. The lymphocytes of the identical twins C 17 and C 18 were insensitive to all three compounds, indicating the existence of a genetically controlled pattern.

Investigations of Relatives of Patients with FA

We tested 15 fathers, 15 mothers, 14 sisters and brothers, and six closely related family members of FA patients for their sensitivity pattern. The results are presented in Table 9; for better comparison the findings in the patients of each family are also listed.

In Table 9, it can be seen that, with the exception of family 1124 (see also section "Intrafamilial Constancy of Sensitivity Pattern"), the spontaneous and INH-induced chromosomal instability of parents of FA patients was within the range of control subjects. The cells of FA heterozygotes, however, were generally more sensitive to MMC (mean 0.35) and to DEB (mean 0.18) than controls (Table 3a). At the individual level, however, some family members showed no reaction to the clastogens (families 1017, 1030, 1031, 1058, 1055, 1083, and 1073). The cells of some parents were sensitive to INH (1058, father of FA 8), to MMC (1058, father; 1050, mother; 1022, both parents; 3001, father; 1083, father; 1124, both parents) or to DEB (1050, mother; 3002, mother). Some siblings and more distant relatives showed individually increased sensitivity (1124, paternal grandmother: to INH, MMC, and DEB; 1083, brother to MMC; 1022, sister to MMC). Family 1024 seemed to be exceptional in that parents and most of the other relatives demonstrated higher than normal spontaneous and induced chromosomal instability.

Table 9. Sensitivity patterns of FA family members

Family	Case no.	Breakage rate (breaks per cell)			
		Spontaneous	After treatment with		
			IHN	MMC	DEB
1014	FA 29	2.40	3.63	-	-
	FA-F	0	0.05	-	-
	FA-M	0.04	0.07	-	0.08
	FA-S	0.04	0.01	-	0.11
	FA-S	0.01	-	-	0.03
1017	FA 10	0.74	0.50	-	9.32
	FA-F	0	0.06	0.01	0.03
1030	FA 13	0.47	0.65	2.36	> 10.00
	FA-F	0.04	0	0.07	0.04
	FA-M	0	0.03	0.04	0.02

Table 9 (continued)

Family	Case no.	Breakage rate (breaks per cell)			
		Spontaneous	After treatment with		
			IHN	MMC	DEB
1031	FA 17	0.09	0.34	1.72	> 10.00
	FA-F	0.06	0.02	0.04	0.08
	FA-M	0.18	0	0.10	0.04
1038	FA 9	0.35	0.51	1.16	3.80
	FA-M	0.10	0.04	0.11	0.09
1047	FA 14	0.12	-	-	4.82
	FA-M	0.04	0.02	0.06	0
	FA-F	0.02	0.06	0.16	0.10
	FA-S	0.02	0	0.14	0
	FA-S	0	0.02	0.26	0.02
	FA-B	0.02	0.02	0.04	0
1050	FA 11	0.59	0.70	2.76	> 10.00
	FA-M	0.06	0.14	1.10	1.08
1055	FA 30	0.18	0.14	0.86	1.98
	FA-S	0.02	-	0.02	0.10
	FA-B	0.02	0.04	0.04	0
1058	FA 8	0.05	0.20	0.60	1.98
	FA-M	0	0	0.08	0.02
	FA-F	0.04	0.30	0.34	0.08
	FA-B	0.06	0.02	0.04	0.06
1083	FA 26	0.20	0.06	1.50	9.40
	FA-F	0.12	-	1.40	0.10
	FA-M	0.20	-	0.20	0
	FA-B	0.06	0.06	0.66	0.08
1073	FA 31	0.50	0.20	1.60	4.00
	FA-F	0	0.04	0.04	0.02
	FA-M	0	0	0.02	0
	FA-B	0.04	0.04	0.04	0.14
1086	FA 33	0.22	0.20	1.96	2.30
	FA-F	0			0.04
	FA-M	0		0.04	0.10
	FA-B	0.02	0.06	0.08	0.02
1089	FA 34	0.15	0.08	0.63	1.10
	FA-F	0.01	0.03	0.27	0
	FA-M	0.02	-	0.28	0
	FA-S	0.01	0.03	0.25	0
3001	FA 24	0.06	-	2.57	> 10.00
	FA-F	0.01	-	1.11	0.36
3002	FA 23	0.19	-	-	> 10.00
	FA-M	0.02	-	-	0.93
	FA-F	0.03	-	-	0.06

Table 9 (continued)

Family	Case no.	Breakage rate (breaks per cell)				
		Spontaneous	After treatment with			
			IHN	MMC	DEB	
	Families with two affected children					
1022	FA 18	0.23	0.20	< 10.00	> 10.00	same
	FA 19	0.27	0.16	> 10.00	> 10.00	
	FA-F	0.07	0.05	0.69	0.07	similar
	FA-M	0.06	0.02	0.64	0.16	
	FA-S	0.01	0	1.00	0.05	
1052	FA 4	0.26	0.15	0.72	> 10.00	same
	FA 5	0.08	0.12	0.80	> 10.00	
	FA-F	0	0	0.04	0.32	similar
	FA-M	0	0	0.08	0.26	
	FA-S	0.02	0	0.02	0.16	
1124	FA 27	0.36	0.43	0.66	3.34	different
	FA 28	0.13	0.06	2.36	3.02	
	FA-F	0.22	0.20	1.16	0.29	different
	FA-M	0.28	0.08	1.88	0.15	
	FA-GP-Fm	0.46	-	0.18	0.14	
	FA-GP-Mm	0.20	0.10	0.80	0.22	
	FA-U	0.28	-	0.12	0.14	
	FA-U	0.50	0.18	0.80	0.18	
	FA-GP-Mp	-	0.44	0.78	0.34	
	FA-A	0.10	0.04	0.36	0.06	

F, father; M, mother; B, brother; S, sister; GP-M, grandmother; GP-F, grandfather; m, maternal; p, paternal; U, uncle; A, aunt
Dosages: INH, 14 m*M;* MMC and DEB, 0.1 μg/ml

Pairs of parents whose cells showed similar reactions to the treatment were found in families 1030, 1031, 1073, 1086 and 1089; the parents of 1124 and 1022 were specifically sensitive to MMC. A comparison of the findings in patients and in both parents showed two patterns of sensitivity. In most families, the patient was the only sensitive one in the family (1058, 1047, 1030, 1031, 1086, 1073, 1052, 1059). In some other families there were significant breakage rates after treatment with one clastogen in the father (1083), in the mother (3002), or in both (1022 and 1124). This was also the case in incomplete families (father, 3001; in family 1050 the mother was also sensitive to MMC and DEB).

Healthy siblings of patients with FA showed normal values (means, Table 3a, b). The specific findings within single families like 1083 favored the interpretation that the brother is a possible heterozygote for the FA gene; this would explain the increased chromosomal instability which was apparent after MMC treatment, as in the father and in the patient.

The question whether there is a family-related pattern of breakage induced by various agents can only be answered when more than one patient in a family, together with both parents and more distant relatives, can be analyzed. This will be discussed in the section "Intrafamilial Constancy of Sensitivity Pattern."

Investigations of Parents and Siblings of P Cases (Non-FA)

In this group, 9 fathers, 12 mothers and 9 siblings were investigated. The results are presented in Table 10. For comparison of the familial pattern of sensitivity, the findings of the respective patients are included in the table.

Table 10. Sensitivity patterns of non-FA family members

Family	Case no.	Breakage rate (breaks per cell)			
		Spontaneous	After treatment with		
			INH	MMC	DEB
1020	P 4	0.12	0.18	0.58	0.41
	P-F	0.02	0.03	0.13	0.61
	P-M	0	0	0.02	0
1021	P 14	0.03	0.02	0.24	0.02
	P-F	0.24	–	0.26	0.77
	P-M	0.34	0.14	0.46	0.40
1028	P 6	0.06	0.00	0.14	0.04
	P-F	0.01	–	–	–
	P-M	0.02	–	–	–
	P-B	0.03	0.11	0.30	0.07
1036	P 15	0.00	0.00	0.07	0.03
	P-M	0.11	0.03	0.17	0.07
1039	P 7	0.10	0.04	0.31	0.11
	P-M	0.12	0.11	0.69	0.18
	P-S	0.02	0.28	0.26	0.10
1063	P 5	0.01	0.03	0.11	0.06
	P-S	0.07	0.03	0.99	0.09
1060	P 13	0.03	0.05	0.46	0.30
	P-F	0.02	–	0.16	0.22
	P-M	0.08	0.05	0.35	1.01
1065	P 20	0.02	0.00	0.03	0.01
	P-F	0.06	0.04	0.16	0.24
	P-M	0.00	0.00	0.02	0.12
	P-S	0.04	0.02	0.02	0.00
1077	P 18	0.00	0.00	0.03	0.007
	P-F	0.01	0.00	0.00	0.04
	P-M	0.03	0.00	0.07	0.19
1082	P 27	0.18	0.20	0.80	0.19
	P-M	0.14	0.06	0.19	0.13
1093	P 40	0.04	–	–	0.00
	P 41	0.06	0.04	0.10	0.02
	P-F	0.06	0.08	0.10	0.04
	P-M	0.08	0.00	0.12	0.02
	P-S	0.00	0.02	0.10	0.06

Table 10 (continued)

Family	Case no.	Breakage rate (breaks per cell)			
		Spontaneous	After treatment with		
			INH	MMC	DEB
1097	P 34	0.00	–	–	0.01
	P-F	0.07	–	–	0.16
	P-M	0.03	–	–	0.04
	P-B	0.01	–	–	0.10
1111	P 22	0.00	–	–	0.44
	P-B	0.00	0.08	0.00	0.00
	Families with two affected children				
1100	P31[a]	1. 0.00	–	0.03	0.04
		2. 0.82	0.06	0.62	0.40
	P-F	0.26	3.00	2.85	1.69
	P-M	0.08	0.36	0.64	0.46
	P-B	0.08	0.18	0.68	0.22
	P-S[a]	1. 0.10	0.30	0.50	0.06
		2. 0.12	–	0.79	0.40

Dosages: INH, 14 m*M;* MMC and DEB, 0.1 μg/ml
[a] P 31 and P-S examined together on two separate occasions

The spontaneous breakage rate was within the range of controls (0–0.08) or of the FA heterozygous parents (0–0.28), with only one exception in family 1021 M. INH-induced breakage was within the control range in most cases, elevated in some (1000 M, F, and B; 1028 B) and abundant in two probands (1039 M, increased 14-fold; 1100 F, increased 11.5-fold). Note the exceptionally high value of INH-induced breakage in these two cases, which compares only to FA 29! The highest MMC-induced (2.85) and DEB-induced (1.69) breakage rates in this group were also found in 1100 F, as were the most sensitive cells of all non-FA probands (P 8 excluded). His values increased the means (Table 3 a, b) considerably. There seemed to be no correlation between the breakage rate found in the members of family 1100 and the patient P 31, since his cells were not sensitive at all, and the tests were performed on the same day. In individual cases, significant breakage rates were observed, when compared with spontaneous levels after treatment with MMC and DEB (1020, 1021, 1039, 1060, 1065, 1077, 1082, 1097); the same holds for some siblings (1028, 1039, 1063), but not for others (1065, 1093, 1097, 1110, 1111). This was also expressed in the means of the experiments (Table 3 a, b), which were surprisingly high in this heterogeneous group of family members compared with those for members of families with a patient affected by FA or controls.

Intrafamilial Constancy of Sensitivity Pattern

In Table 9 the results from a study in three families with two affected siblings are shown. In these cases we wanted to analyze whether the sensitivity pattern in such families is influenced by the defect in the FA gene. If there is genetic heterogeneity, and if the sensitivity to induced and spontaneous cellular damage has something to do with the gene defects and with specific familial genetic backgrounds, one would expect constant cellular sensitivity in such cases. Since conclusions are drawn from values like breaks per cell before and after treatment with certain chemicals, we wanted to know how reliable such values are and how they are influenced by genetic parameters.

In the three families with two FA patients (1022, 1052, and 1124), the extent of spontaneous breakage in the affected children was independent of cytopenia. In family 1022, both children with FA had extremely high levels of cellular sensitivity to MMC and DEB, although the 5-year-old daughter was still clinically healthy. Cells of the parents and of one unaffected sister showed significant increased breakage frequencies after MMC, but not after DEB treatment.

In family 1052, the cells of the affected children were extremely sensitive to DEB, but not to MMC. Both girls were suffering from severe aplastic anemia. The cells of the parents and of the unaffected sister were not sensitive to MMC, but slightly sensitive to DEB. The analyses of the members of each family were made on the same day, which is important for the interpretation of such results.

In family 1124, the situation was different. The cells from the two affected children showed different levels of sensitivity to INH and to MMC, although the investigations were made on the same day. Their reactions to DEB were similar. Their parents had high spontaneous breakage rates. Both were extremely sensitive to MMC. The absolute values of both parents were higher than that of one affected child (FA 27). Their DEB sensitivity was not significantly higher than the baseline values. Other family members had high endogenous breakage rates and some of them were highly sensitive to MMC. The only difference between affected and unaffected family members was the high sensitivity to DEB in the patients with FA. The reason for the high spontaneous breakage rates in this family was unclear. In this family the two affected siblings were examined on the same day, while all the other family members were investigated together on another day, later than the patients.

One family with two P probands (1093, identical twins, suffering from unspecific aplastic anemia) was interesting in this context. None of the patients, parents, or sisters had sensitive cells. This adds information on the question of the influence of genes within a family. In this family, the genetic constitution did not lead to abnormal cellular sensitivity to INH, MMC, or DEB (data not shown).

Constancy of Individual Patterns of Sensitivity

It can be shown from the results of our study that variation in the spontaneous breakage rates is a constant feature of patients with FA. Table 11 presents all repeated investigations of FA patients, together with the repeated investigations of P individuals. The results show that the frequency of induced breaks can be constant or variable to a considerable extent in both patients with FA and P individuals. The following questions are raised:

1. Can sensitivity develop during the course of the disease?
2. Is specific sensitivity to INH, MMC, or DEB a constant feature of the cells?
3. To what extent can changes of sensitivity be attributed to laboratory effects?

The results of this study provide some preliminary answers to these questions.

Independently of spontaneous breakage rates, the sensitivity to INH remained high in FA 3, developed in time in FA 11 and in FA 17, and remained low in FA 4 and in FA 5 (sisters), FA 12, FA 18 and FA 19 (sisters), and in the P probands.

Sensitivity to MMC was constantly observed in several patients at a relatively low level [FA 4, FA 5, (sisters), FA 11 and P 14]. However, we also observed changes which might influence the interpretation of cytogenetic results in such patients: cells of FA 18 and FA 19 (sisters) had the highest breakage rates at the first

Table 11. Examination of intra-individual consistency of the 11 FA patients and two non-FA patients

Case no.	Age at test	Breakage rate (breaks per cell)			
		Spontaneous	After treatment with		
			INH	MMC	DEB
FA 3	13 yrs.	0.20	0.42	–	–
	17 yrs	0.14	0.44	1.28	2.02
FA 4	8 yrs. 6 mo.	0.11	0.18	0.72	4.62
	9 yrs.	0.18	0.09	1.50	10.0
FA 5	10 yrs.	0.28	0.12	0.80	5.36
	10 yrs. 6 mo.	0.06	0.12	1.76	10.0
FA 7	6 mo.	0.07	0.16	0.82	10.0
	1 yr. 6 mo.	0.02	–	–	3.60
FA 10	18 yrs.	0.80	0.54	–	9.56
	19 yrs.	0.28	–	–	–
FA 11	6 yrs. 5 mo.	0.22	0.16	1.92	1.60
	6 yrs. 7 mo.	0.59	0.70	2.76	10.0
FA 12	10 yrs.	0.31	0.15	–	5.40
	11 yrs.	0.22	0.18	1.47	10.0
FA 15	1 yr. 5 mo.	0.08	–	–	1.94
	1 yr. 10 mo.	0.24	0.20	1.36	0.86
FA 17	4 mo.	0.02	0.02	–	–
	1 yr.	0.14	0.11	–	–
	5 yrs.	0.09	0.34	1.72	10.0
FA 18	10 yrs.	0.23	0.20	10.0	10.0
	11 yrs.	0.27	0.16	0.90	10.0
FA 19	5 yrs.	0.27	0.16	10.0	10.0
	6 yrs.	0.29	0.32	0.48	7.36
P 13	6 mo.	0.025	0.05	0.46	0.30
	1 yr. 8 mo.	0	0	0.04	0.03
P 14	2 yrs. 5 mo.	0.032	0	0.16	-
	3 yrs. 6 mo.	0.03	0.02	0.24	0.02
P 31	2 yrs. 5 mo.	0	–	0.03	0.04
	2 yrs. 8 mo.	0.82	0.06	0.62	0.40
	3 yrs. 5 mo.	0	0	0.34	0.02

Dosages: INH, 14 m*M;* MMC and DEB, 0.1 μg/ml

investigation following treatment with MMC. One year later very low breakage rates were found; however, the spontaneous as well as the DEB-induced breakage rates remained constantly high.

The lymphocytes of the two pairs of sisters (FA 4 and FA 5, FA 18 and FA 19) were investigated on the same day, thus excluding the considerable influence of laboratory conditions. The main result was that the observed changes were similar in both pairs of sisters after their cells had been treated with MMC and DEB (FA 4 and FA 5), and that these changes could be extreme. The interpretation of high or low sensitivity to MMC as correlating to different genetic defects in the FA gene should be avoided. Even the sensitivity to DEB changed considerably, so that breakage rates alone cannot be indicative of special types of FA gene(s) [FA 4 and FA 5 (sisters), FA 7 and FA 11] or other genes involved in P cases (P 13). In addition, the activity of the MMC solution may not be consistent between different experiments. More experimental analyses have to be performed during the course of the disease of a greater number of patients for us to understand whether induced or spontaneous breakage rates can be used to identify complementation groups in FA.

Sensitivity of FA Lymphocytes to Cytosine Arabinoside

Ara-C was tested in patients with FA because this chemical might be helpful in conditioning for bone marrow transplantation (see Friedrich et al. 1987). The following results were obtained:

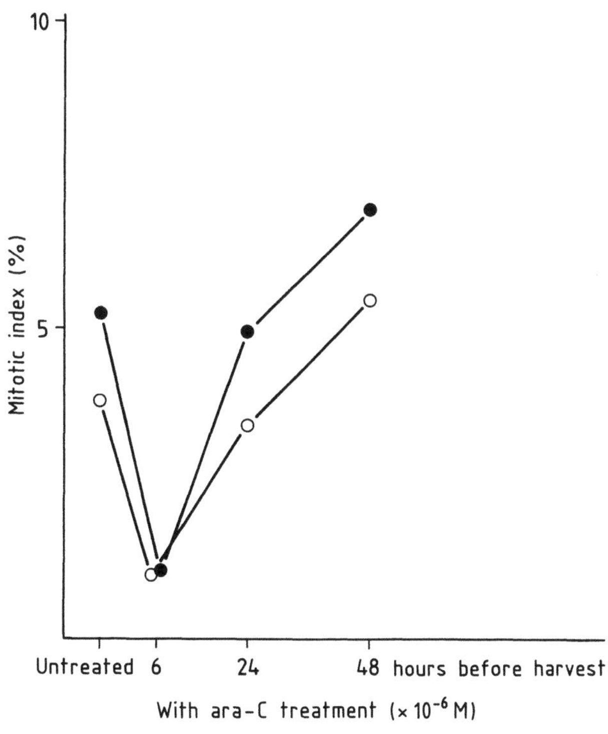

Fig. 1. Mitotic depression of control lymphocytes from two cell lines by ara-C (10^{-6} *M*) 6, 24 and 48 h before harvest

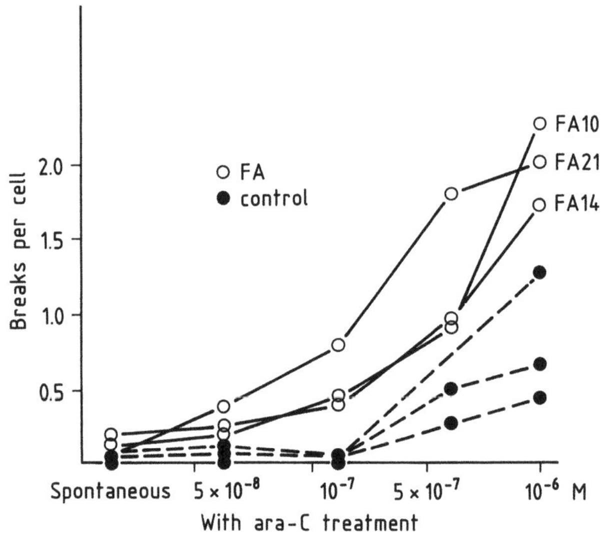

Fig. 2. Dose-effect curve for chromosomal aberrations induced by ara-C (final concentrations: 5×10^{-8} *M*–10^{-6} *M*, 6 h treatment) in FA and control lymphocytes

- Mitotic depression in control cells was maximal when the cultures had been treated with ara-C for 6 h immediately before fixation (Fig. 1).
- Dose-effect curves found in the cells of three patients with FA (FA 10, FA 21, and FA 14) and of three controls showed relatively low, but significantly elevated break frequencies in FA patients (Fig. 2).
- The types of aberrations induced by ara-C in FA cells were different from other chemically induced aberrations. Regardless of treatment time, only breaks were observed; no chromatid translocations were found. Obviously FA cells are not able to produce chromatid translocations following ara-C treatment. The control cells did not show chromatid translocations either; however, in a very small number of cases, two breaks were present in the aberrant cells.
- Lymphocytes of controls and of obligate heterozygous parents of patients with FA demonstrated an increase in the breakage rate when treated 6 h before harvesting, but not when treated for 24 h. This may be a result of repair of induced damage (Fig. 3). FA lymphocytes behaved differently as shown in Fig. 4: the lymphocytes of three patients with FA (FA 14, FA 21, and FA 22) showed the same levels of chromosomal breakage irrespective of whether they had been treated for 24 h or for 6 h.

The lymphocytes of one FA patient (FA 10) were obviously able to repair ara-C-induced damage when treated for 24 h, like normal and heterozygote cells, since breakage induction by ara-C when the lymphocytes were treated for 6 h was the same as in cases FA 14 and FA 21. Further studies will show whether recovery experiments of this type will make it possible to differentiate between the complementation groups A and B, as described by Buchwald et al. and Moustacchi et al. (this volume), using routine cytogenetic methods.

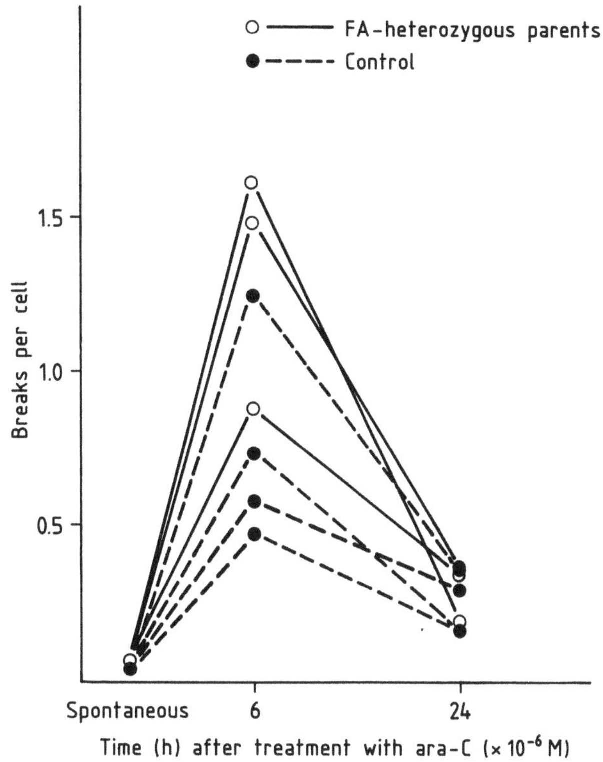

Fig. 3. "Recovery" of lymphocytes after treatment with ara-C

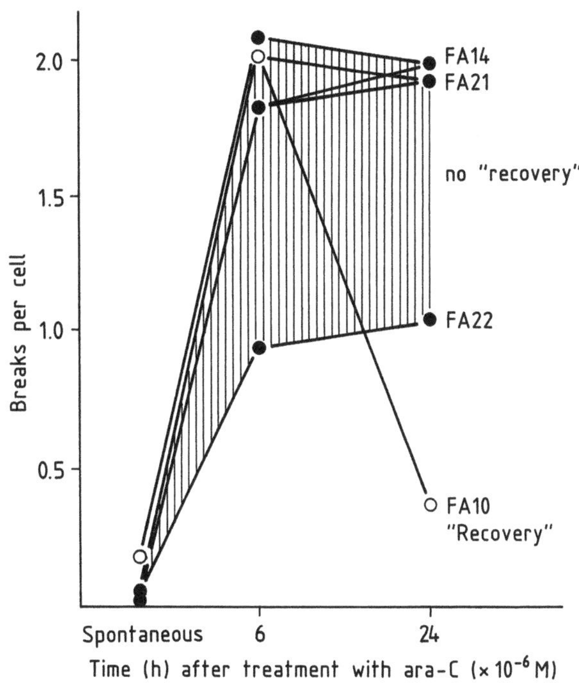

Fig. 4. "Recovery" and "nonrecovery" of FA lymphocytes after treatment with ara-C

Discussion and Conclusion

The aim of this study was to analyze the pattern of sensitivity in individual FA and non-FA patients and their family members to see whether there were groups of cases which reacted alike, thus indicating subtypes of the disease. A reproducible, abnormal increase in chromosomal aberrations after treatment with chemicals as compared with the baseline breakage rate of untreated cells of the same person describes the cellular sensitivity of the individual. Since baseline breakage in cases of FA can be marginal or even fall within the range of breakage frequencies of normal cells, and normal cells with a zero breakage baseline may react with a significant increase of breakage after treatment, the judgement on sensitivity is still subject to interpretation.

In order to define FA, a constant sensitivity of lymphocytes and fibroblasts to DEB would prove useful. The collection of cases in the IFAR as presented by Auerbach et al. (this volume, pp. 3-17) included patients sensitive to DEB, whether or not they were suffering from aplastic anemia or from associated malformations. This definition, solely dependent on sensitivity to DEB, must necessarily put other, nonsensitive cases formerly diagnosed as FA into another group of diseases. At the same time, patients with malformations indicative of FA would be excluded from the diagnosis of FA and its fatal prognosis. The question remains, for all those who are involved in classifying diseases or entities based on chemicals for cytogenetic studies or other laboratory tests, how to deal with these non-FA cases.

Sensitivity to DEB has been shown to be genetically determined and specifically related to the FA gene(s), irrespective of whether the patient belongs to complementation group A or B. (Auerbach and Wolman 1976, 1978; Auerbach et al. 1981, 1986; Gebhart et al. 1985; Marx et al. 1983; Zhu 1986). In FA families, therefore, it is possible to identify sibs in a premorbid stage of the disease by DEB testing. This has also led to the successful use of DEB testing for prenatal diagnosis (Auerbach et al. 1981, 1985, 1986).

The data from this study were interpreted against this background. If the sensitivity to DEB is genetically determined, then a sensitivity pattern formed by various sensitivities to different chemicals may also depend on genetic variation. We expected to find familial sensitivity patterns. From our results in three families with two FA patients in each, there is no doubt that there are family-specific patterns. Such patterns also exist in isolated cases, and can sometimes, but not always, be traced to parents and siblings.

An attempt was made to group FA patients into five general groups whose patterns of sensitivity were similar. Whether these patterns indicate specific classes or variants within the DEB-sensitive FA patients will be investigated. It could very well be that a particular sensitivity pattern, such as high sensitivity to DEB and MMC associated with low or zero sensitivity to INH, or high sensitivity to DEB and lower sensitivity to MMC and INH, will prove useful for classification of a complementation group (A or B as suggested by Digweed et al., this volume). The authors described the constancy of sensitivity to MMC in one cell line of a patient with a low breakage rate and thought that this would be indicative for complementation group B - the mild form of FA. Recently, Digweed et al. (1988) completed this study, showing that the case does belong indeed to complementation group B.

The results of our studies of FA families could suggest that in families 1022 and 1052, both parents have the same or a similar mutation in the FA gene which gives offspring with identical patterns of sensitivity. In family 1024, the parents demonstrated different patterns of sensitivity, which could suggest that they have different mutations in the FA gene. Further modifications, such as intragenic deletions, recombinations, or point mutations, must be postulated in one of the parents. The combination of two FA alleles with different mutations could also result in an unstable situation, which could induce additional modifications of the gene. One connecting link which may explain the specific effects of FA genes in cells, such as the exceptional increase in sister chromatid exchanges (SCE) in heterozygotes of the FA cluster around Bloemfontein in South Africa (Marx and Smith, this volume), is a particular ligase defect. Ligase deficiency was discovered by Hirsch-Kauffmann et al. (1978) in one case of FA, and a heterozygous state was interpreted from results in the cells of the patient's mother (reviewed by Digweed et al., this volume, Table 1).

Recently, at least two different ligase defects have been described in Bloom's syndrome cells, which are characterized by an increase in SCEs: one temperature-sensitive ligase and one ligase deficiency, which could also account for the slow growth rate of DNA replicates (Hand and German 1977; Willis and Lindahl 1987; Willis et al. 1987). Thus, it would not be surprising if a pronounced ligase deficiency could be demonstrated in the South African cases.

From our study of individual patterns of sensitivity it can be concluded that MMC treatment of lymphocytes from DEB-sensitive FA patients, their relatives, and unrelated probands leads to a wide range of breakage frequencies. To define a particular disease like FA, MMC alone is not reliable. The overlap of the breakage rates of DEB-positive cases of FA and non-FA probands with MMC is too wide, so that we cannot recommend MMC alone for differential diagnosis in a single case.

In DEB-positive cases of FA, less than half of the patients investigated were sensitive to INH. The induction of breakage was less pronounced with INH than with DEB or MMC. However, the reaction to INH was used for evaluation of sensitivity patterns because of the findings of our earlier study (Schroeder and Stahl-Maugé 1979).

DEB itself, although very specific for FA, does not induce a high frequency of breaks exclusively in FA lymphocytes. In our study, a patient with AT was investigated because his blood was sent for testing to the FA laboratory without further information. His lymphocytes had the same sensitivity to DEB and INH as FA cells, so a differentiation between FA and AT was not possible from our results. Lymphocytes of two other patients with AT whom we were able to investigate were not sensitive to DEB, MMC, or INH.

Earlier, Auerbach and Wolman (1979) reported sensitivity to DEB in the fibroblasts of two patients with AT. However, the amount of breakage after treatment with DEB was only twice the spontaneous breakage rate, while in our case (P8), DEB induced a 46.2-fold increase in chromosomal damage. Bleomycin was found to induce a two- to threefold increase in the breakage rate in 80 lymphocytes (Taylor et al. 1979), which we unfortunately did not test in our patients. Another parameter for variation in patterns of sensitivity within the group with AT seems to emerge if lymphocytes are exposed to X-rays: in contrast to Taylor et al. (1976), we found no increase in chromatid breakage after the irradiation of the lymphocytes of two sisters with AT (unpublished results).

In addition to our experience with FA patients and with P probands, these results reflect once more that specific individual patterns of sensitivity exist among patients affected with the same disease, most probably genetically determined. We therefore speculate that the patients with AT who were highly sensitive to DEB belonged to a different complementation group than the other unrelated patients with AT. We believe that chromosomal breakage studies, using a battery of clastogens, could help to differentiate subtypes within the AT group.

In our study, the sensitivity to DEB of the lymphocytes of FA heterozygotes and other family members, non-FA patients and their family members, as well as of unrelated healthy probands was occasionally significantly increased above the baseline breakage rate of the individual. This means that in our study the range of breakage frequency in these groups are wide compared to those of other studies (Auerbach et al. 1981, 1986; Marx et al. 1983). It is not possible to identify FA heterozygotes by testing with DEB, MMC, or INH alone, or with combinations of these.

Multiples of baseline breakage alone are not reliable for differential diagnosis of FA, non-FA, and other conditions. Setting limits for significant sensitivity, despite statistical significance, leaves problems in individual cases. Another parameter for differential diagnosis could be the appearance of cells, in cases of FA, which demonstrate more than ten aberrations after treatment with MMC or DEB. According to our own experience this phenomenon can be considered in addition to other factors. However, not in all cases of FA are there such cells, and we also have to state that these cells can be observed in experiments with lymphocytes from healthy persons, from P probands, and from family members of all patients. Thus they are not exclusively seen in cases of FA.

Ara-C was included in the study, because this substance might be useful for conditioning patients before bone marrow transplantation. We were able to test only four FA homozygotes, three obligate heterozygotes and 20 normal probands. The most interesting result was that the FA cell lines could be differentiated into two groups by a recovery experiment: three FA cell lines showed the same levels of chromosomal breakage when treated with ara-C for 24 or for 6 h. One FA cell line had a high level of breakage when treated for 6 h, but showed baseline breakage again when the cells were treated with ara-C for 24 h before harvesting. If this recovery experiment allowed identification of complementation group A or B, then treatment with ara-C and a chromosomal breakage study could serve on a broad scale to subtype DEB-positive cases of FA. This interpretation of our finding is of course speculative, but could serve as a working hypothesis (Hong and Schroeder-Kurth, 1986).

We feel that it is not surprising to see more differentiation when several clastogens are used for testing. Wunder and Fleischer (1983) reported a test system for the identification of FA homozygotes by inducing quantitatively controlled DNA damage in cloned lymphocytes and testing their survival after treatment. They used 8-methoxypsoralen (8-MOP) plus UVA light (PUVA) as a mutagen in various dosages and implanted the treated lymphocytes in capillaries on agar. After 7 days, the surviving colonies were counted. Numbers and sizes of the colonies are related to the sensitivity of the treated lymphocytes to 8-MOP (see also Wunder et al., this volume). Lymphocytes of pretested FA patients were extremely sensitive to this treatment. The majority of lymphocytes from their heterozygous parents were more sensitive than those of a group of nonrelated healthy probands. There is, however, an overlap between normal and obligate heterozygotes.

We have continued to test the survival capacity of lymphocytes of nearly all patients with FA, their relatives, and P patients, together with their family members. There are patients without anemia but with malformations resembling those in FA, who are sensitive to neither INH, MMC, nor DEB, but extremely sensitive to PUVA in the survival test.

A family described by Kantner et al. (1986) at the 7th International Congress of Human Genetics in Berlin is particularly interesting in the light of our results: a child with a unilateral radial aplasia was diagnosed as non-FA, but as having another disease associated with sensitivity to PUVA, like FA. Both parents of this child were investigated, and their lymphocytes showed partial sensitivity to PUVA, like those of many FA heterozygotes. The conclusion was that, in this family, sensitivity to PUVA was inherited in an autosomal recessive mode. During genetic counseling, the parents were informed that there is a 25% risk that any subsequent child would be sensitive to PUVA and possibly have abnormalities. Their second child was born, after an uneventful pregnancy, with unilateral radial aplasia. Ultrasonic investigation had been performed but failed to show the recurrence of a malformation. The lymphocytes of this child showed the same pattern of sensitivity: no spontaneous breaks, no increase of breaks after treatment with INH, MMC, or DEB, but extreme sensitivity to PUVA in a lymphocyte colony survival test.

We suggest that in this family, the sensitivity to PUVA alone identifies a genetically determined disease characterized by skeletal abnormalities, particularly of the upper extremities (radius and thumb), similar to those in patients with FA. It could very well be that many of the P probands, classified as non-FA because of the DEB-negative reactions of their lymphocytes, will fall into this group, if properly tested. The correlation between sensitivity to PUVA and malformations remains as unclear in these patients as in patients with FA.

In the selected group of patients we tested, we found two other patients with similar clinical pictures who were sporadic cases but possibly belonged to the same genetic group (Table 12, line 6). In addition, there were ten anemic children without malformations who had the same pattern of sensitivity as the four children described above, again indicating an overlap with other diseases. Another small group of patients showed sensitivity to MMC and to PUVA (line 5). They might have been misclassified as FA, had they not been tested with DEB. Two other patients were found to be insensitive in all tests (Table 11, line 7). On the other hand, there are a few DEB-sensitive patients with FA whose lymphocytes were not sensitive to PUVA. Counseling of the family with the nonanemic but malformed child (arrow, line 4) becomes extremely difficult in view of these test results.

Table 12. Results of multiple sensitivity testing including the results of sensitivity to 8-methoxypsoralene plus UVA in the lymphocyte-colony survival test in a group of FA patients and non-FA patients, indicating individual patterns of sensitivity

Disease		Sensitivity				Patients' condition			Patients (*n*)
		Chromosomal breakage			Lymph. surv. PUVA	Anemia only	Anemia + malform.	Malform. only	
		DEB	MMC	INH					
FA	1	+	+	+	+	10	1	1	18
	2	+	+	-	+	1	0	0	4
	3	+	+	+	-	0	1	1	2
→	4	+	+	-	-	0	0	1	1
Non-FA	5	-	+	-	+	3	0	2	5
	6	-	-	-	+	10	0	4	14
	7	-	-	-	-	2	0	0	2

Dosages: INH, 14 m*M;* MMC and DEB, 0.01 μg/ml; PUVA range 0.002–0.02 μg/ml
→, see text

We conclude that certain sensitivity patterns can help to identify genetically determined diseases or subgroups of clinically similar conditions. The investigation of specific sensitivities is essential for genetic counseling and prenatal diagnosis, in particular for those cases who undergo treatment. In patients with FA, it is life-saving to know the cellular response to the chemical compounds necessary for conditioning before bone marrow transplantation. For genetic research, the sensitivity pattern might prove useful for complementation experiments. We would speculate that once subgroups of DEB-sensitive cases of FA are diagnosed as belonging to a particular complementation group (A, B, or some other), it might be possible to identify these subgroups by simpler methods and routine chromosome studies.

Acknowledgements. Some of these results are presented in the thesis of T. H. Zhu, Tianjin (Faculty of Theoretical Medicine, University of Heidelberg, 1986). The study on the effects of ara-C was carried out by Y. Hong, Wuhan. We wish to thank R. Schwinger, U. Paschetto, and G. Fuchs for their assistance. We are very grateful to our colleagues and the families affected by FA for their continuing interest in and support of our study.

References

Auerbach AD, Wolman SR (1976) Susceptibility of Fanconi's anemia fibroblasts to chromosome damage by carcinogens. Nature 261: 494–496
Auerbach AD, Wolman SR (1978) Carcinogen-induced chromosomal breakage in Fanconi's anaemia heterozygous cell. Nature 271: 69–71
Auerbach AD, Wolman SR (1979) Carcinogen-induced chromosome breakage in chromosome instability syndromes. Cancer Genet Cytogenet 1: 21–28
Auerbach AD, Adler B, Chaganti RSK (1981) Prenatal and postnatal diagnosis and carrier detection of Fanconi anemia by a cytogenetic method. Pediatrics 67: 128–135

Auerbach AD, Sagi M, Adler B (1985) Fanconi anemia: prenatal diagnosis in 30 fetuses at risk. Pediatrics 76: 794-800

Auerbach AD, Zhang M, Ghosh R, Pergament E, Verlinsky Y, Nicholas H, Boué J (1986) Clastogen-induced chromosomal breakage as a marker for first trimester prenatal diagnosis of Fanconi anemia. Hum Genet 73: 86-88

Chan JYH, Becker FF, German J, Ray JH (1987) Altered DNA ligase I activity in Bloom's syndrome cells. Nature 325: 357-359

Digweed M, Zakrzewski-Lüdcke S, Sperling K (1988) Fanconi's anaemia: correlation of genetic complementation group with psoralen/UVA response. Hum Genet 78: 51-54

Duckworth-Rysiecki G, Cornish K, Clarke C, Buchwald M (1985) Identification of two complementation groups in Fanconi anemia. Somatic Cell Mol Genet 11: 35-41

Friedrich W, Ebell W, Blütters-Sawatzki R, Junker A, Hübener KH, Schroeder-Kurth T, Kohne E, Kleihauer E (1987) Die Behandlung der Fanconi-Anämie durch Knochenmarktransplantation. Monatsschr Kinderheilkd 135: 253-258

Gebhart E, Kysela D, Matthee H, Nikol M (1985) Cytogenetic analyses utilizing various clastogens in two sibs with Fanconi anemia, their relatives, and control individuals. Hum Genet 69: 309-315

Gillis S, Mochizuki DY, Coulon PJ, Hefeneider SH, Rambthun CA, Gillis AE, Frank MB, Henney CS, Watson JD (1982) Molecular characterization of Interleukin-2. Immunol Rev 63: 167-209

Hand R, German J (1977) Bloom's syndrome: DNA replication in cultured fibroblasts and lymphocytes. Hum Genet 38: 297-306

Hirsch-Kauffmann M, Schweiger M, Wagner EF, Sperling K (1978) Deficiency of DNA ligase activity in Fanconi's anemia. Hum Genet 45: 25-32

Hong Y, Schroeder-Kurth TM (1986) Effect of Alexan (cytoarabinosid) on FA-cells: relevance for bone marrow transplantation, Abstract. 7th International Congress of Human Genetics, Berlin, part II p 501

ISCN Harnden DG, Klinger HD in collaboration with Cytogenet Cell Genet (eds) (1985) An International system for human cytogenetic nomenclature. Karger, Basel

Kantner G, Schroeder TM, Tariverdian G, Wunder E, Füchsel H-J (1986) Autosomal recessive radius aplasia with 8-methoxypsoralen-UVa sensitivity in lymphocytes (Abstract). 7th international congress of human genetics, Berlin, part II, p 700

Klocker H, Auer B, Hirsch-Kauffmann M, Altmann H, Burtscher HJ, Schweiger M (1983) DNA repair dependent NAD^+ metabolism is impaired in cells to one patients with Fanconi's anemia, EMBO 2: 303-307

Marx MP, Smith S, Heyns A du P, van Tonder IZ (1983) Fanconi's anemia: a cytogenetic study on lymphocyte and bone marrow cultures utilizing 1, 2, 3, 4-diepoxybutane. Cancer Genet Cytogenet 9: 51-60

Moustacchi E, Diatloff-Zito C (1985) DNA semi-conservative synthesis in normal and Fanconi anemia fibroblasts following treatment with 8-methoxypsoralen and near ultraviolet light or with X-rays. Hum Genet 70: 236-242

Moustacchi E, Papadopoulo D, Diatloff-Zito C, Buchwald M (1987) Two complementation groups of Fanconi's anemia differ in their phenotypic response to a DNA cross-linking treatment. Hum Genet 75: 45-47

Ray JH, German J (1981) The chromosome changes in Blooms's syndrome, ataxia-telangiectasia, and Fanconi's anemia. In: Arrighi FE, Rao PN, Stubblefield E (eds) Genes, chromosomes and neoplasia. Raven, New York, p 351-378

Sasaki MS (1975) Is Fanconi's anemia defective in a process essential to the repair of DNA cross links? Nature 257: 501-503

Sasaki MS, Tonomura A (1973) A high susceptibility of Fanconi's anemia to chromosome breakage by DNA cross-linking agents. Cancer Res 33: 1829-1836

Schroeder TM (1982) Genetically determined chromosome instability syndromes. Cytogenet Cell Genet 33: 119-132

Schroeder TM, German J (1974) Bloom's Syndrome and Fanconi's anemia: Demonstration of two distinctive patterns of chromosomal disruption and rearrangement. Humangenetik 25: 299-306

Schroeder TM, Kurth R (1971) Spontaneous chromosomal breakage and high incidence of leukemia in inherited disease (analytical review). Blood 37: 96-112

Schroeder TM, Stahl-Maugé CH (1979) Mutagenetic effects of isonicotinic acid and hydracide in Fanconi anemia. Hum Genet 52: 309-321

Schroeder TM, Anschütz F, Knopp A (1964) Spontane Chromosomenaberrationen bei familiärer Panmyelopathie. Humangenetik 1: 194-196

Schroeder TM, Drings P, Beilner P, Buchinger G (1976) Clinical and cytogenetic observations during a six-year period in an adult with Fanconi's anemia. Blut 34: 119-132

Schuler D, Kiss A, Fabian F (1969) Chromosomal peculiarities and "in vitro" examinations in Fanconi's anemia. Humangenetik 7: 314-322

Taylor AMR, Metcalfe JA, Oxford JM, Harnden DG (1976) Is chromatid-type damage in ataxia-telangiectasia after irradiation at G_0 a consequence of defective repair? Nature 260: 441-443

Taylor AMR, Rosney CM, Campbell JB (1979) Unusual sensitivity of ataxia telangiectasia cells to bleomycin. Cancer Res 39: 1046-1050

Wang HG, Fedoroff S (1972) Banding in human chromosomes treated with trypsin. Nature 235: 52-53

Willis AE, Lindahl T (1987) DNA ligase I deficiency in Bloom's syndrome. Nature 325: 355

Willis AE, Weksberg R, Tomlinson S, Lindahl T (1987) Structural alterations of DNA ligase I in Bloom syndrome. Proc Natl Acad Sci USA 84: 8016-8020

Wunder E, Fleischer B (1983) Response of lymphocytes from Fanconi's anemia patients and their heterozygous relatives to 8-methoxypsoralen in a cloning survival test system. Hum Genet 64: 167-172

Zhu TH (1986) Internationales Fanconi-Anämie-Register, I. Phase der Untersuchungen - Erfassung von Patienten, klinische und cytogenetische Differentialdiagnose. Dissertation, University of Heidelberg

Significance of Cellular Sensitivity in a Group of Parents of Fanconi Anemia Patients*

M. P. Marx and S. Smith

Introduction

Since 1964, when Schroeder et al. reported an increased number of chromosomal and chromatid breaks in the lymphocyte cultures of patients with Fanconi anemia (FA), several methods for diagnosis and basic research, making use of various alkylating agents, cloning survival tests, induced sister chromatid exchanges (SCE), and ^{3}H-thymidine uptake and incorporation have been described (Auerbach et al. 1981; Sasaki and Tonomura 1973; Cohen et al. 1982; Cervenka and Hirsch 1983; Shoyab et al. 1981; Wunder and Fleischer 1984; Berger et al. 1980). These tests facilitate a reliable differentiation between patients with FA and those with overlapping clinical features. However, a reliable method for the identification of FA heterozygotes is still hot available.

FA heterozygotes manifest no clinical symptoms of FA. The spontaneous chromosomal aberrations usually present in the cultured cells of FA homozygotes are not observed in those of heterozygotes. The identification of FA heterozygotes, using the usual cell-culture techniques, is thus not possible; more specific methods are required. Various methods have been described and include the use of clastogens such as mitomycin C (MMC), nitrogen mustard, and 1,2,3,4-diepoxybutane (DEB), oxidizing stress, a cloning survival test, and the timing of the cell cycle of lymphocytes. These methods seem to be fairly reliable for the identification of many obligate FA heterozygotes, but with each technique there is an overlap with the results for healthy control persons (Cohen et al. 1982; Cervenka and Hirsch 1983; Dallapicola et al. 1985; Miura et al. 1985).

In our laboratory, we had the opportunity to study 52 obligate carriers of the FA gene. The methods employed were the DEB stress test, SCE evaluation, and cell-cycle analysis. The results provided a reliable system for the diagnosis and identification of FA heterozygotes in the cluster of patients with FA around Bloemfontein in South Africa.

* This work was supported by grants from the Central Research Fund of the University of the Orange Free State and the South African Medical Research Council.

T. M. Schroeder-Kurth A. D. Auerbach G. Obe (Eds.)
Fanconi Anemia, Clinical, Cytogenetic and Experimental Aspects

Material and Methods

Patients. The lymphocyte cultures of 52 parents of patients with FA were cytogenetically analyzed to determine the carrier status within the families investigated and to evaluate the cytogenetic techniques employed for carrier detection. As controls, 46 normal healthy persons of comparable age participated.

Lymphocyte cultures. All test and control whole-blood cultures were established in either TC199 Medium (Gibco, Europe) containing three times the normal concentration of glutamine (300 mg/liter) or Ham's F10 medium (Gibco, Europe) supplemented with fetal calf serum. Harvesting and slide preparation followed a routine protocol.

DEB Studies. DEB (Merck, FRG) was added to the cultures 48 h before harvesting, at three different concentrations: 0.01 μg/ml, 0.1 μg/ml, and 1 μg/ml.

SCE Studies. Bromodeoxyuridine (BUdR; Sigma, FRG) was added to the cultures at a final concentration of 0.01 mg/ml medium. DEB was added 48 h later at a final concentration of 0.1 μg/ml. Slides were differentially stained in acridine-orange (Sigma) and examined under a microscope using a UV light source.

Criteria for Chromosome and SCE analysis. Achromatic areas greater in width than a chromatid were counted as breaks. Exchange configurations, partial endoreduplications, dicentrics, and ring chromosomes were scored as rearrangements. Rearrangements were scored as one break per chromosome involved. Gaps were excluded in calculating breakage rates (Auerbach et al. 1981).

Cells were scored as first, second, or third division metaphases, based on the fluorescing pattern of the chromosomes. SCE frequencies were calculated as exchanges per metaphase.

At least 100 well-spread metaphases per patient per test were analyzed. The types of aberrations, number of SCEs, and generation of mitoses were noted.

Statistical Analysis. The different means for the groups were compared using Student's *t* test.

Results

DEB Studies: Chromosomal Aberrations

The results of our DEB studies are shown in Table 1. The mean spontaneous breakage rate in normal subjects was 0.017 with a range of 0.01-0.05. The addition of 0.01 μg/ml DEB to lymphocyte cultures had no significant effect on the breakage rate, but 0.1 μg/ml and 1 μg/ml induced a significant ($p < 0.01$), dose-dependant breakage rate.

The spontaneous breakage rates of FA heterozygotes did not differ significantly from those in the control group ($p > 0.5$). The addition of DEB at doses

Table 1. Chromosomal breakage in lymphocyte cultures of controls, parents of FA patients, and of FA homozygotes

Subject	n	Spontaneous breakage		DEB-induced breakage					
				0.01 μg/ml		0.10 μg/ml		1.0 μg/ml	
		Mean ±1SD	Range	Mean ±1SD	Range	Mean ±1SD	Range	Mean ±1SD	Range
Controls	46	0.017 ±0.011	0.01-0.05	0.025 ±0.01	0.01-0.04	0.048 ±0.08	0.01-0.07	0.077 ±0.06	0.051-0.08
Parents of FA patients	52	0.065 ±0.021	0.019-0.710	0.338 ±0.106	0.2-0.52	0.993 ±0.134	0.73-1.05	1.341 ±0.181	0.97-1.36
FA homozygotes	42	0.763 ±0.214	0.46-1.28	1.548 ±0.216	1.20-1.96	2.590 ±0.231	2.19-2.90	6.050 ±0.749	2.25-768

which do not induce chromatid aberration in normal cells separated the two groups. At 0.01 μg/ml, 0.1 μg/ml, and 1 μg/ml DEB, there was a highly significant increase ($p < 0.001$) in the breakage rate in the cells of FA heterozygotes compared to that in controls. It is important to note that there was at least a tenfold higher chromosomal breakage rate in each of the tests with heterozygote lymphocytes than in those of the control group (Fig. 1). The results from 42 patients with FA are included in Table 1 for comparison.

Chromatid and/or chromosomal breaks were the most common spontaneous chromosomal aberrations observed in untreated cultures from FA heterozygotes. In controls, occasional breaks and gaps were the only types of chromosomal damage.

In FA heterozygotes, the number of cells with chromosomal aberrations and the degree of chromosomal damage increased significantly with an increase in the concentration of DEB (Table 2). It should also be noted that no chromatid exchange configurations, commonly induced by DEB in the cells of FA heterozygotes were seen in control cells.

SCE Studies

Cell Cycle Studies. The results of the cell-cycle studies are presented in Table 3. The percentages of first, second, and third division metaphases were found to be distinctly different in FA heterozygote cell cultures when compared to those observed in controls, indicating a slower cell cycle in heterozygotes. This distinction became even more evident when 0.1 μg/ml DEB was added to cultures containing BUdR. The greatly increased percentage of first mitoses and the decreased percentage of second and third mitoses was especially noteworthy.

SCE Frequencies. Cells of FA heterozygotes as well as those of controls showed a significant increase ($p > 0.001$) in the number of SCEs observed. There was an enormous increase in the number of SCEs in the cells of FA heterozygotes, which was significantly higher ($p > 0.001$) than that observed in control cultures (76 compared with 22, Table 4, Fig. 2). In the cells of FA heterozygotes, chromatid translo-

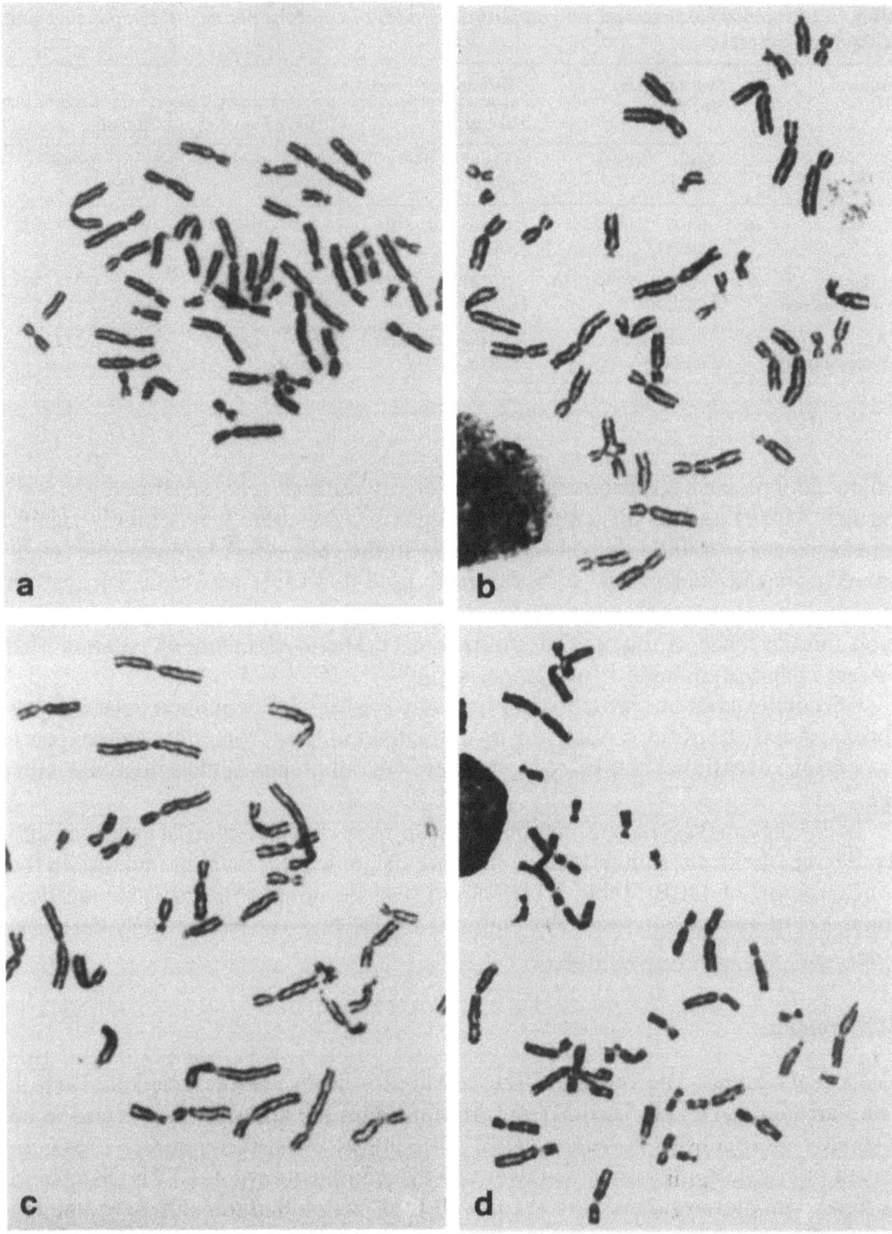

Fig. 1a–d. Examples of chromosomal damage in lymphocyte cultures from FA heterozygotes **a** spontaneous, **b** after the addition of 0.01 μg/ml DEB, **c** after the addition of 0.1 μg/ml DEB, **d** after the addition of 1.0 μg/ml DEB

Table 2. Percentage of cells with chromosomal aberrations at different concentrations of DEB in lymphocyte cultures

DEB concentration (μg/ml)	Cells affected (%)	
	FA heterozygotes (*n* = 52)	Controls (*n* = 46)
0.01	5	1
0.10	19	6
1.0	26	6

Table 3. Percentage of first, second, and third division mitoses

Breakage	*n*	Cells (*n*)	1st mitoses (%)	Aberrations (*n*)	2nd mitoses (%)	Aberrations (*n*)	3rd mitoses (%)	Aberrations (*n*)
Controls								
Spontaneous	46	5250	22.2	0.00	67	0.01	10.8	0.011
Induced by 0.10 μg/ml DEB	41	5010	20	0.02	64	0.07	16	0.13
Parents of FA patients								
Spontaneous	52	5052	38	0.01	57	0.01	5	0.02
Induced by 0.10 μg/ml DEB	52	4270	51	0.87	43	0.92	6	1.02

Chromosomal aberrations were only occasionally observed in cultures from FA heterozygotes, and were concentrated in a few cells, showing a large number of aberrations.

Table 4. Mean number of SCEs per cell

	n	Spontaneous			0.10 μg/ml		
		Cells (*n*)	Mean ±1SD	Range	Cells (*n*)	Mean ±1SD	Range
Controls	22	1980	6.7240 ±0.749	4.28-15	1876	22.00 ± 7.14	17.8-48
Parents of FA patients	30	1650	8 ±4.07	5.2-17.4	1372	76 ±29.74	48.2-141

The mean number of spontaneous SCEs observed in cultures from FA homozygotes of the same order as those in FA heterozygotes. No sister chromatid differentiation was observed after the addition of DEB to the lymphocyte cultures of FA homozygotes, indicating that these cells either do not incorporate BUdR after the addition of DEB or that the cells do not progress further than the first cell cycle.

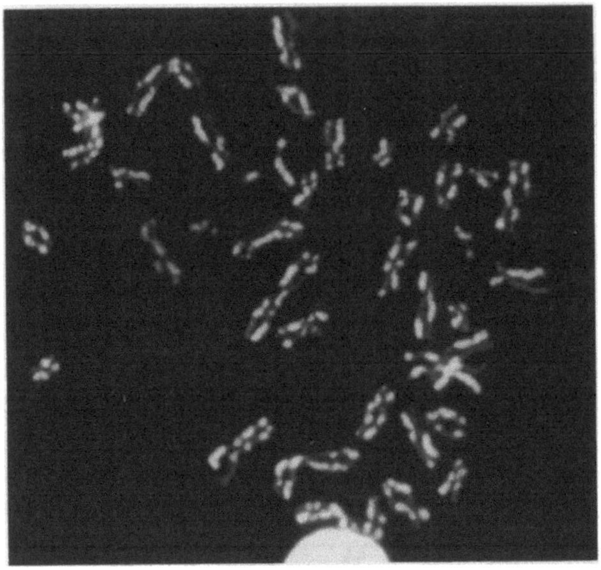

Fig. 2. Increased number of SCEs observed in cells from FA heterozygotes after treatment with 0.1 μg/ml DEB

cations were not observed in second and third division metaphases, and chromosomal breaks were occasionally seen in cells showing elevated SCE frequencies.

Discussion

A reliable method for the detection of FA heterozygotes would be very useful for genetic counseling, particularly in a population with a frequent occurrence of the FA gene. It is thus important to develop an accurate method for the identification of FA heterozygotes. This has been attempted, using a variety of techniques based on the treatment of cell cultures with a number of alkylating and oxidizing agents. Clone survival after treatment with cross-linking agents, spontaneous and induced SCEs, and cell-cycle progression have been studied to this end. The addition of DEB at nontoxic concentrations was found to be a valuable method for identifying carriers of the FA gene (Marx et al. 1983; Auerbach and Wolman 1978), but other investigators could not support these findings (Cohen et al. 1982; Cervenka and Hirsch 1983).

It has repeatedly been shown that FA heterozygotes have the same frequency of chromosomal aberrations in untreated cultures as controls (Auerbach et al. 1981; Cervenka and Hirsch 1983; Marx et al. 1983; Schroeder 1982; Latt et al. 1975). In a study of 52 obligate carriers of the FA gene the addition of three concentrations of DEB to cell cultures from FA heterozygotes induced an elevated level of chromosomal breakage. This makes a clear separation between heterozygotes and controls possible (Table 1). Chromatid exchange configurations typically found in the cell cultures from FA heterozygotes were not observed in control cultures. In contrast with the results of other investigators, false-negative, or false-positive results were found.

Our studies on cell-cycle kinetics substantiated the prolonged cell cycle of FA heterozygote cells described by Dutrillaux et al. (Dutrilleux et al. 1982). This was seen in the higher percentage of first mitoses and the lower percentage of second and third mitoses observed in the cells of FA heterozygotes compared with those of controls. This became even more evident when DEB was added to cultures containing BUdR (Table 2). A further finding was the total absence of any complex chromatid exchange configurations in second or third mitoses.

The number of SCEs found after the addition of DEB to cultures containing BUdR was greatly elevated in both the cells of controls and of FA heterozygotes (Table 3). FA heterozygote lymphocyte cultures, however, had a significantly higher number ($p < 0.001$) of SCEs compared with controls (Fig. 2). This finding is consistent with that reported by Novotna et al. (1979).

We conclude that the cells of FA heterozygotes have a longer cell cycle than those of controls and exhibit a greatly increased level of SCEs and chromatid abnormalities after treatment with DEB. FA heterozygotes may be clearly identified by employing both the DEB stress test and by analyzing cell-cycle kinetics, including evaluating the number of SCEs after the addition of DEB to cultures containing BUdR. Since the FA families in our study seemed to belong to a cluster, representing a distinct FA mutation close to Bloemfontein, our results cannot be generalized (see Smith et al., this volume).

References

Auerbach AD, Wolman SR (1978) Carcinogen induced chromosome breakage in Fanconi's anemia heterozygous cells. Nature 271: 70-71

Auerbach AD, Adler BA, Chaganti RSK (1981) Prenatal and postnatal diagnosis and carrier detection of Fanconi anemia by a cytogenetic method. Pediatrics 67: 128-134

Berger R, Bernheim A, Le Coniat M, Vecchione D, Schaison G (1980) Sister chromatid exchanges induced by nitrogen mustard in Fanconi anemia. Application to detection of heterozygotes and interpretation of results. Cancer Genet Cytogenet 2: 259-267

Cervenka J, Hirsch B (1983) Cytogenetic differentiation of Fanconi anemia, idiopathic aplastic anemia, and Fanconi anemia heterozygotes. Am J Hum Genet 15: 211-223

Cohen MM, Simpson SJ, Honig GR, Maurer HS, Niklas JW, Martin AO (1982) The identification of Fanconi anemia genotypes by clastogenic stress. Am J Hum Genet 34: 794-810

Dallapicola B, Porfirio B, Mokini V, Alumena G, Isacchi G, Grandini E (1985) Effect of oxidants and antioxidants on chromosomal breakage in Fanconi anemia lymphocytes. Hum Genet 69: 62-65

Dutrillaux B, Aurias A, Dutrillaux AM, Buriot D, Prieur M (1982) The cell cycle of lymphocytes in Fanconi anemia. Hum Genet 62: 327-332

Latt SA, Hetten G, Jourgens LA, Buchanan GR, Gerald PS (1975) Induction by alkylating agents of sister chromatid exchanges and chromatid breaks in Fanconi's anemia. Proc Natl Sci USA 72: 4066-4070

Marx PM, Smith S, Heyns A du P, van Tonder IZ (1983) A cytogenetic study on lymphocyte and bone marrow cultures utilizing 1,2;3,4-diepoxybutane. Cancer Genet Cytogenet 9: 51-60

Miura K, Morimoto K, Koizuma A (1983) Proliferation kinetics and mytomycin C-induced chromosome damage in Fanconi's anemia lymphocytes. Hum Genet 63: 19-23

Novotná B, Goetz P, Surkova WI (1979) Effects of alkylating agents on lymphocytes from controls and from patients with Fanconi's anemia. Hum Genet 49: 41-50

Sasaki MS, Tonomura A (1973) A high susceptibility of Fanconi's anemia to chromosome breakage by DNA cross-linking agents. Cancer Res 33: 1829-1836
Schroeder TM (1982) Genetically determined chromosome instability syndromes. Cytogenet Cell Genet 33: 119-132
Schroeder TM, Anschütz F, Knopp A (1964) Spontane Chromosomenaberrationen bei familiärer Panmyelopathie. Humangenetik 30: 317-323
Shoyab M, Gunnell M, Lubiniecki AS (1981) Reduced uptake and incorporation of ^{3}H-thymidine in Fanconi anemia fibroblasts. Hum Genet 57: 296-299
Wunder E, Fleischer B (1984) Response of lymphocytes from Fanconi's anemia patients and their heterozygous relatives to 8-methoxy-psoralene in a cloning test system. Hum Genet 64: 167-172

Chromosomal Studies in Fanconi Anemia Heterozygotes

B. Dallapiccola and B. Porfirio

Introduction

There is evidence that slight phenotypic manifestations of disease in individuals who are heterozygous for autosomal recessive diseases might be the rule, rather than the exception (Vogel 1984). Therefore, analysis of heterozygotes appears to be the simplest and most straightforward strategy for a deeper understanding of the actions of genes influencing multifactorial susceptibility to disease. Also, in a rare condition like Fanconi anemia (FA), with homozygotes numbering about 1 in 300000 (Swift 1971), heterozygotes are common (1 in 300), as shown by a simple analysis according to the Hardy-Weinberg law. If only a small fraction of FA heterozygotes suffer from increased susceptibility to disease, and even if this susceptibility leads to overt disease only in combination with particular environmental conditions, heterozygotes probably account for a major proportion of the inter-individual variation in susceptibility to disease.

In principle, if heterozygous carriers of the gene for FA are predisposed to a particular disorder, that disorder will be found in excess among the close blood relatives of patients with the syndrome. It is also likely that the disorder found in heterozygotes is of the same nature as the one commonly found in homozygotes. On the other hand, diagnosis of heterozygotes is significant for practical reasons, in particular for the genetic counseling of the close relatives of patients with autosomal recessive diseases.

The association of FA with an increased risk of cancer has been studied systematically in FA heterozygotes. In 1971, Swift examined the family history of eight FA patients and reported that among heterozygotes there was an excess of cancer deaths. Three relatives died from acute leukemia as compared with the one death expected. Assuming that these three relatives were FA heterozygotes, it was suggested that carriers of the FA gene account for 5% of all acute leukemia deaths. This hypothesis was plausible due to the very high frequency of acute leukemia in patients with FA (Alter et al. 1981). However, a later study of 25 additional FA families showed no overall elevated incidence of cancer among relatives, and fewer cases of leukemia than expected (Swift et al. 1982). The same conclusion was drawn from a subsequent study on nine additional FA families (Potter et al. 1983).

Therefore, the suggestion that heterozygotes for FA show a higher frequency of malignancy than controls has not received adequate support. The evidence provided by the first study could be explained by a biased selection of families with

T. M. Schroeder-Kurth A. D. Auerbach G. Obe (Eds.)
Fanconi Anemia, Clinical, Cytogenetic and Experimental Aspects

cancer, chance association due to small numbers, the erroneous designation of leukemic patients as FA heterozygotes, or the genetic heterogeneity of this condition. Similarly, an increased frequency of diabetes in FA heterozygotes has been claimed (Swift 1971), but no rationale for this association exists at present.

Gmyrek and Syllm-Rapoport (1964) drew attention to several case reports of relatives of FA patients who had hematological abnormalities or limb malformations. In fact, a significant excess of persons with multiple malformations, especially genitourinary or limb anomalies, was found in the 25 FA families examined by Welshimer and Swift (1982). Since the genitourinary system and the limbs are frequent sites of abnormality in FA homozygotes (Schroeder et al. 1976a), the findings in blood relatives have been regarded as an indication of the predisposition of FA heterozygous carriers to such malformations. Similar conclusions were put forward by Hamel (1986), who described a family identified as a result of cytogenetic confirmation of FA in two siblings whose parents had urinary tract abnormalities. Follow-up studies in the mother's family revealed a remarkable frequency of ureteropelvic obstructions, which were detected in nine additional family members. Whether the presence of urinary tract malformations is related to the presence of the FA trait remains to be determined. Admittedly, it is not possible at present to identify heterozygous carriers of the FA gene at the clinical level, nor to conclude that FA heterozygosity has definite clinical consequences.

Despite the tremendous progress of biochemical and molecular genetics, the primary defect of FA is still unknown. Thus, no reliable direct laboratory test for FA heterozygote detection is available. Nevertheless, extensive, promising investigations have been carried out over the last 10 years, which have tested the susceptibility of FA heterozygous cells to chromosome breakage in vitro. In this chapter such studies are reviewed.

The Diepoxybutane Test

The first attempt to distinguish FA heterozygous individuals from normal individuals was reported by Todaro et al. (1966), who found an increased susceptibility of FA homozygous and heterozygous fibroblasts to in vitro transformation by the oncogenic simian virus 40. However, similar results have been obtained with cell strains from several other syndromes. It was also stated that obligate heterozygotes may be characterized by spontaneous chromosome breakage (Meme et al. 1980), but this is not usually the case (Schroeder and Stahl-Maugé 1979).

In 1978, Auerbach and Wolman described the higher than normal sensitivity of FA heterozygotes to chromosome breakage induced by diepoxybutane (DEB) in fibroblasts. Exposure to 10 ng/ml DEB medium for 6 days resulted in an approximatively fourfold increase in the breakage rate in these cells, as compared with the baseline breakage rates. A similar, although more dramatic effect, had already been reported by the same authors in FA homozygous cells (Auerbach and Wolman 1976). The chromosomal aberrations induced by DEB were similar to those which occurred spontaneously in homozygous cells, open chromatid breaks being the most common. The results obtained by the use of this in vitro stress system were considered adequate to distinguish FA homozygous, FA heterozygous, and normal fibroblasts on the basis of their response to the clastogenic effect of a dose of DEB, which in normal cells does (Auerbach et al. 1979). A possible cytogenetic characteristic distinguishing members of families affected by FA from controls was the significantly increased frequency of induced triradials and quadriradials. Using the same system, a cytogenetic method was developed for the rapid identification of blood lymphocytes and amniotic fluid cells from affected individuals and fetuses, and of blood lymphocytes from carrier individuals (Auerbach et al. 1981). In particular, treatment with 100 ng/ml DEB resulted in a 175-fold increase in the chromosome-breakage rate of affected patients, while lymphocytes from FA heterozygotes showed a fourfold increase compared with that in control lymphocytes. Results confirming the evidence provided by Auerbach et al. (1981) come from different laboratories (Dallapiccola et al. 1983; Gebhart et al. 1985). However, there were reports to show that the DEB-induced chromosome breakage rate was similar in particular heterozygous and normal individuals, severely limiting the use of the test (Fig. 1).

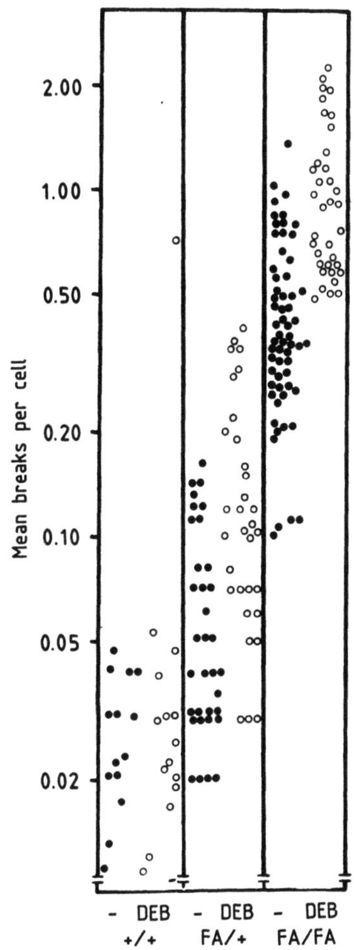

Fig. 1. Effect of 10 ng/ml DEB on chromosome breakage in control subjects *(+/+)*, FA patients *(FA/FA)*, and FA heterozygotes *(FA/+)*. Each point represents the mean number of breaks per cell in an individual experiment based on the scoring of 100 metaphases

Table 1. Spontaneous and DEB-induced breakage rates in two families who requested genetic counseling due to having a child affected by an undiagnosed form of aplastic anemia

	Spontaneous breaks/cell[a]	DEB-induced breaks/cell[a, b]
Family 1		
Father	0.13	0.34
Mother	0.06	0.15
Family 2		
Father	0.10	0.41
Mother	0.04	0.19
Son	0.12	2.00

[a] On the basis of 100 metaphases.
[b] 10 ng/ml DEB was added 24 h after the initiation of the culture.

Nevertheless, the potential use of the DEB test in the genetic counseling of families at risk for aplastic anemia has been suggested by Alimena et al. (1983). These authors reported on a patient without associated somatic malformations and with spontaneous levels of chromosome breakage at the upper limits of the normal range, who developed acute non-lymphatic leukemia (ANLL) following a phase of pancytopenia. The patient died before a DEB test on his lymphocytes could be performed. A definite diagnosis of FA was established retrospectively on the basis of the DEB-test results for the proband's parents (Table 1, family 2). In fact, the striking clastogenic effect of DEB allowed unambiguous differentiation of these parents from controls.

Since then, we have examined another family with a child affected by aplastic anemia. Cytogenetic studies on the patient, performed in another laboratory, had provided inconclusive data. Based on the DEB-test results only, we suggested that the healthy parents were heterozygotes for the FA mutation (Table 1, family 2). The patient was reinvestigated by us, and both spontaneous and DEB-induced breakage rates were consistent with the diagnosis of FA (Dallapiccola et al. 1983).

In contrast with the generally hold view that there is an overlap of breakage rates between obligate heterozygotes and controls, after DEB stress, Marx et al. (1983) found this test accurate and clearcut. According to the cumulative experience of these authors with 54 members of FA families, no overlap in the breakage rates was found with those in controls (Marx and Smith, this volume). These results were attributed to the genetic homogeneity of the sample, from the Orange Free State region of South Africa, which was thought to have a very specific variant of FA with a high spontaneous breakage rate. In addition, it was suggested that technical factors, in particular the influence of the growth medium, were responsible for such unique sensitivity to the test.

An opposite conclusion was reached by Cohen et al. (1982a) who found a lack of correlation between DEB sensitivity and the FA genotype. According to these authors, after DEB stress, two of their five FA homozygotes did not exhibit the expected increase in chromosome breakage, while three of their four individuals with some clinical manifestations of FA (non-FA subjects) did. Furthermore, significant differences in the chromosome breakage rate between FA heterozygotes and controls could not be found over a wide range of DEB doses. Paradoxically, at the highest concentrations, both the mean and the variance of controls were greater than those of the FA heterozygotes. Thus, no discrimination between these two groups was possible using DEB-induced chromosome damage. Similarly, clastogenic treatment could not separate FA heterozygotes from controls in long-term lymphoid cell lines (Cohen et al. 1982b). However, it has to be emphasized that the criteria used for the clinical diagnosis of patients were not those that have been widely accepted (Auerbach et al. 1985).

Also, Cervenka and Hirsch (1983) have reported overlaps in breakage rates of controls and of obligate FA heterozygotes following DEB stress. These conclusions also apply to the results of chromosome breakage studies of cultured untreated and DEB-treated amniocytes and chorionic villi cells from fetuses at risk for FA, diagnosed prenatally as unaffected (Auerbach et al. 1985, 1986; Dallapiccola et al. 1985). In fact, the range of baseline and DEB-induced breakage levels in amniocytes of unaffected fetuses (0.00-0.12 break/cell and 0.00-0.14, respectively) was well within the range of the controls (0.00-0.02 and 0.00-0.06 break/cell). Likewise, the range of spontaneous and induced breaks in trophoblast cells in controls (0.02-0.10 and 0.02-0.14 break/cell, respectively) and in unaffected fetuses (0.00-0.12 and 0.00-0.10 break/cell) was similar.

Therefore, although as a group FA heterozygotes have a higher mean response than normal, DEB clastogenicity cannot be used reliably for the identification of individual heterozygotes. The genetic heterogeneity of FA could account for the controversial results with respect to the chromosome damage induced by DEB.

At present, the clinical usefulness of the DEB stress test is not in question. In fact, the hypersensitivity of FA homozygous cells to the clastogenic effect of this compound has been recommended as a necessary prerequisite for inclusion in the International Fanconi Anemia Registry (IFAR). On the other hand, the identification of heterozygous gene carriers is a more complicated issue, which ideally should be pursued by in vitro testing with a suitable battery of clastogens.

Sister Chromatid Exchange Analysis

The introduction of differential sister chromatid staining techniques has allowed sister chromatid exchange (SCE) analysis, which is widely used to test the mutagenicity of chemical agents. The level of spontaneously occurring SCE in FA is normal (Latt et al. 1975). However, analyses of chemically induced SCE in the cells led to contradictory results.

In FA lymphocytes Latt et al. (1975) found that 10-30 ng/ml mitomycin C (MMC) and, to a lesser extent, 250 μg/ml ethylmethane sulfonate (EMS) induced less than half the frequency of SCE detected in identically treated control lymphocytes. In most of these experiments, the alkylating agents were present on the last day of culture. In other cultures, MCC was present over all 3 days of growth, with essentially the same results. These findings have been corroborated by Cervenka et al. (1981), who cultured normal and FA lymphocytes in the presence of 20 ng/ml MMC.

In contrast with the lower frequency of MMC-induced SCE in FA lymphocytes, FA fibroblasts responded almost normally to SCE induction by 10 ng/ml MMC, given 2 days prior to harvest (Latt et al. 1975). Furthermore, lymphocytes from the parents of patients with FA exhibited a normal SCE response after MMC or EMS treatment.

On the other hand, Novotná et al. (1979) reported that FA lymphocytes responded normally to SCE induction by MMC, added 24 h after the cultures were started at concentrations ranging from 40 to 160 ng/ml. An increased frequency of chromosome breaks was not found except at the highest dose, which seems unusual for FA cells. Likewise, Sasaki (1980) found that the SCE response of FA lymphocytes treated with 5-50 ng/ml MMC added 24 h before harvest was close to normal.

Kano and Fujiwara (1981, 1982) studied FA fibroblast cell lines and found them to be hypersensitive to MMC with respect to SCE induction. Clearly, procedural details, such as the duration of cell culture and harvest, and the treatment schedule, might have significant effects on the results (e.g., Morimoto et al. 1985). Interpretation of the different results obtained in various studies on MMC-induced SCE in FA has not yet been completed. Finally, it should not be overlooked that the blood samples and fibroblast cell lines used in the different studies generally originated from different individuals. In view of the existence of complementation groups in FA (Zakrzewski and Sperling 1980; Duckworth-Rysiecki et al. 1985, this volume), the different responses of FA cells to MMC could be a reflection of the genetic heterogeneity of the disease.

Other chemicals have also been tested for their SCE-inducing abilities in FA. Berger et al. (1980) found that FA lymphocytes demonstrate an increased frequency of SCE in comparison with normal lymphocytes following exposure to nitrogen mustard (HN_2). When nitrogen mustard was added at low concentrations, it was possible, during the whole culture time, to distinguish between FA homozygotes, FA heterozygotes, and controls. In this analysis, the frequency of SCE was the same as in the controls. Furthermore, FA homozygous and normal lymphocytes showed a similar frequency of SCE following exposure to higher concentrations of nitrogen mustard.

Porfirio et al. (1983) investigated the distribution of SCE in the lymphocytes of normal individuals FA heterozygotes, and FA homozygotes after treatment with DEB. It was found that the pattern of response to DEB allows FA heterozygotes to be distinguished from normal subjects. In particular, 10 ng/ml DEB was less effective or completely ineffective in inducing SCE both in homozygous and heterozygous lymphocytes. This dose led to remarkably enhanced SCE rates in the cells of controls (Table 2). The frequency of SCE increased in a dose-dependent manner following treatment with very low doses of the mutagen (10-100 ng/ml), which failed to induce structural chromosomal aberrations in normal lymphocytes. In contrast, cells from both FA patients and FA heterozygotes showed a significantly enhanced breakage rate in DEB-treated cultures compared with the rate in control cultures.

The possibility of bromodeoxyuridine (BrdU) having an effect on the frequency of SCE, chromosomal aberrations, and cell-cycle kinetics should, however, not be overlooked. The induction of SCE with BrdU was shown to be due to at least

Table 2. Spontaneously occurring and 10 ng/ml DEB-induced SCE rates in lymphocytes from normal subjects, patients with FA, and FA heterozygotes

Subjects		Indiv. experiments	SCE per cell ± SD[a]	
	n	*n*	Spontaneous	DEB-induced
+/+	12	12	6.91 ± 2.55	12.00 ± 3.53
FA/FA	7	11	6.78 ± 3.24	7.86 ± 3.46
FA/+	10	13	6.88 ± 2.95	8.16 ± 3.26

+/+, Controls; FA/FA, patients with FA; FA/+, FA heterozygotes
[a] Pooled data based on the 25-50 cells scored in each experiment.

two factors: the substitution of thymidine by the DNA (Mazrimas and Stetka 1978) and the high concentrations of BrdU, which presumably perturb the nucleotide metabolism (Davidson et al. 1980). BrdU was also found to have an effect on mitotic activity (Lambert et al. 1976). FA cells have both an impaired nucleotide metabolism (Shoyab et al. 1981) and a low mitotic index, especially after exposure to cross-linking agents (Weksberg et al. 1979). The results reported by Porfirio et al. (1983) were obtained by using the lowest possible concentration of BrdU compatible with sister chromatid differentiation. Latt et al. (1975) used deoxycytidine to counteract the toxic effect of BrdU, and this led to an increased proportion of second division metaphases in the FA lymphocytes. However, the possibility of disproportionate changes in the types of cells completing two cycles of replication before harvest at metaphase was not ruled out.

Even though BrdU labeling has provided a valuable opportunity, in the cytogenetics of FA to control cell-proliferation kinetics (Miura et al. 1983; Dutrillaux et al. 1982), the controversial results obtained with this method are disappointing. It seems that SCEs are not as reliable a marker for the identification of FA individuals as structural chromosomal aberrations.

Disturbance of the Oxygen Metabolism

A possible disturbance of the oxygen metabolism in patients with FA has been reported. Nordenson (1977) found that the spontaneous levels of chromosomal aberrations in FA lymphocytes in vitro were significantly reduced by the addition of superoxide dismutase (SOD) and catalase - the substrates of which are superoxide radicals and hydrogen peroxide, respectively. Joenje et al. (1981) compared the frequency of spontaneous chromosomal aberration in FA lymphocytes with that in normal lymphocytes cultured in oxygen concentrations ranging from 5% to 45%. The frequency of chromosomal aberration in normal lymphocytes remained unchanged, whereas the frequency of chromosomal aberrations in the lymphocytes of each of four patients with FA increased significantly with increasing oxygen concentrations. In addition, FA cells were sensitive to the clastogenic effect of heavy water (D_2O) (Joenje et al. 1983). In fact, heavy water supports superoxide and singlet oxygen (normal products of oxygen metabolism in the cell) for longer than normal water (H_2O) does. In vivo treatment with bovine SOD was reported to have a positive but temporary effect in two FA patients, as judged by decreased chromosomal aberrations in cultured lymphocytes and an increase in the number of blood cells in venous blood (Izakovic et al. 1985). Furthermore, MMC-induced chromosome breakage was reduced by exogenous SOD and catalase (Raj and Heddle 1980), and was enhanced by high oxygen tension (Joenje and Oostra 1983).

These data indicate that the expression of the FA mutation may be modulated by the action of oxygen or the oxygen metabolism. However this idea is based only on indirect evidence, and the possibility of an abnormality in the free radical scavenging system and/or increased production of oxygen-reactive species in FA cells remains to be demonstrated. Increased production of superoxide ion has indeed been reported in FA red blood cells (Scarpa et al. 1985). Confirmation of this result in the nucleated cells would support the hypothesis that chromosomal aberrations are generated by activated oxygen species.

Decreased erythrocyte-SOD activity in FA was reported by Joenje et al. (1978, 1979) and later confirmed by other investigators (Okahata et al. 1980; Mavelli et al. 1982). Abnormally low levels of SOD were also found in the white blood cells of patients with FA (Yoshimitsu et al. 1984). However, different studies have provided contradictory results and confirmed neither a consistent SOD defect in FA (Brown and Harnden 1978; Scarpa et al. 1985) nor the ability of high oxygen tension to induce damage at the DNA level in FA fibroblasts, as determined by alkaline elution (Seres and Fornace 1982).

At present, there is no support for the idea that the primary defect of the disease is in the free radical scavenging system. However, the possibility that this defect could be a secondary consequence of the FA mutation cannot be excluded.

The current understanding of the involvement of the system of protection and repair against genetic damage by oxygen species in FA has provided additional means for approaching the identification of FA heterozygotes (Dallapiccola et al. 1985). Thus, the modifications of the pattern of chromosome breakage following in vitro treatment with oxidants and antioxidants have been studied. In fact, the arguments discussed above do not disagree with the idea that oxidative stress or the exogenous supply of electron donors could ultimately result in a modification (increase and decrease, respectively) of the spontaneous yields of chromosome breakage in FA lymphocyte cultures. Peripheral blood lymphocytes from eight FA patients, 14 FA heterozygotes, and nine normal subjects were tested for their susceptibility to chromosome breakage induction by DEB and by two peroxides (Dallapiccola et al. 1985). The addition of 10 ng/ml DEB to normal lymphocytes had no effect on the breakage rate. Likewise, oxidative stress by hydrogen peroxide as well as butyl hydroperoxide resulted in breakage yields comparable to those in DEB-treated cultures. There was a high rate of spontaneous chromosome breaks in FA homozygotes. Furthermore, DEB, as well as the two peroxides, dramatically increased chromosome damage (Fig. 2). Interestingly, whereas FA heterozygotes displayed baseline-breakage levels within the normal range, the addition of both DEB and the two peroxides to the cultures increased the breakage rate, allowing a clear distinction of this group of subjects from controls. A consistent finding both in FA homozygotes and heterozygotes was the inter-individual and intra-individual variability of spontaneous and chemical induced chromo-

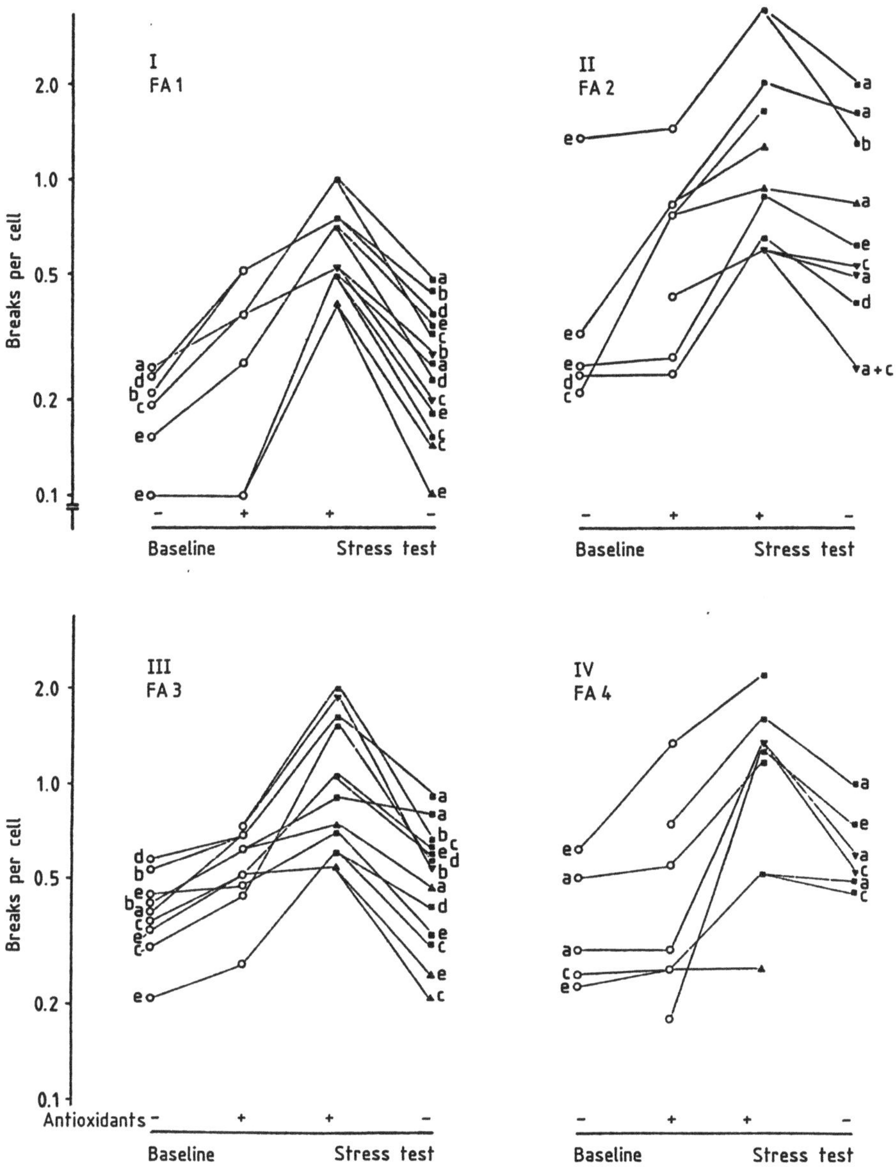

Fig. 2. Spontaneously occurring and DEB- or peroxide-induced chromosome breakage in four representative subjects with FA: effect of antioxidants. For each patient, spontaneous breakage rates *(Baseline)* were compared with those found after: treatment with a variety of antioxidants (*left* side of each panel; *a*, sodium ascorbate; *b*, glutathione; *c*, 1-cysteine; *d*, α-mercaptopropionylglycine; *e*, 2-mercaptoethanol); treatment DEB (■), butyl hydroperoxide (▲) and hydrogen peroxide (▼) *(Stress test)*; combined treatment of stressing agents with antioxidants (*right* side of each panel). Multiple experiments were carried out on each patient using blood samples taken on separate days. Interconnected points represent results obtained on the same day

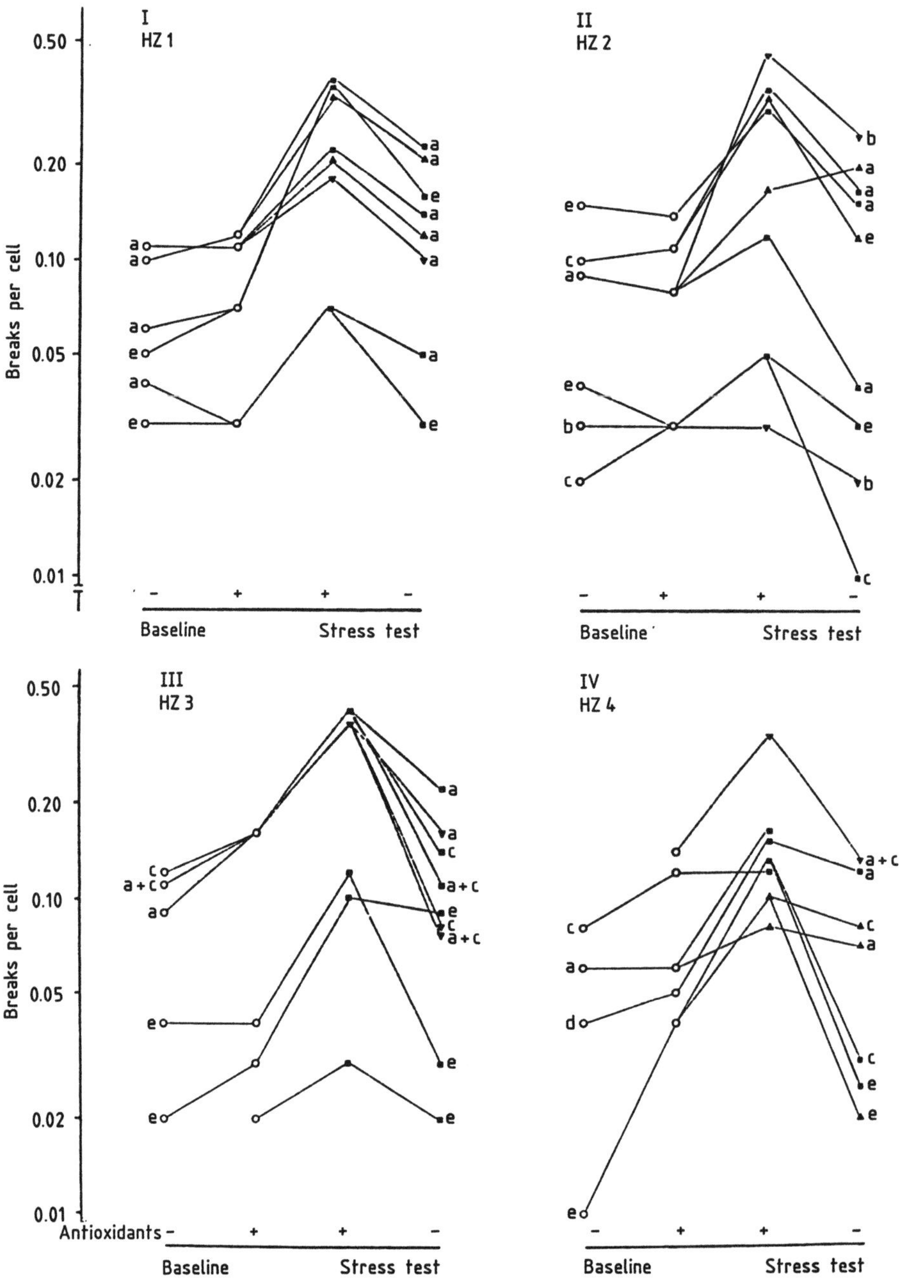

Fig. 3. Spontaneously occurring and DEB- or peroxide-induced chromosome breakage in four representative FA heterozygotes: effect of antioxidants. For each subject, spontaneous breakage rates *(Baseline)* were compared with those found after: treatment with a variety of antioxidants (same as in Fig. 2; *left* side of each panel); treatment with DEB or with peroxides (*Stress test;* for symbols see Fig. 2); combined treatment of stressing agents with antioxidants (*right* side of each panel). Multiple experiments were carried out on each subject using blood samples taken on separate days. Interconnected points represent results obtained on the same day. Variations within the lower log cycle are not statistically different

some breakage (Berger et al. 1977; Schroeder et al. 1976b). A clear separation of heterozygotes from controls was therefore not possible in individual cases, unless multiple blood samples were taken on different occasions and tested for hypersensitivity to various clastogens (Fig. 3).

In this context, we (Dallapiccola et al. 1985) also made use of a previously recognized effect on human lymphocyte chromosomes, namely the prevention of chemically induced breakage by the addition of antioxidants to cell cultures (Shamberger et al. 1973; Gebhart and Becher 1976). A partial suppression of the chromosomal instability was obtained by treating FA lymphocytes with a battery of antioxidants. In this study, the most consistent protective effect was achieved using 1-cysteine, 2-mercaptoethanol, glutathione (GSH), and α-mercaptopropionylglycine, a sulfhydryl group being the main structural feature of these chemicals. GSH functions in the maintenance of sulfhydryl groups of other molecules and protects cells against the detrimental effects of free radicals and reactive oxygen species that are formed during metabolism. Moreover, GSH together with GSH S-transferase participates in the detoxification of a variety of foreign compounds (Meister 1983). For example, Boyland and Williams (1965) demonstrated that DEB is enzymatically conjugated with GSH. In this respect, it is also noteworthy that increased GSH S-transferase activity and fast decay of GSH have been found in FA erythrocytes (Dallapiccola et al. 1984). These results would suggest that the consistently high levels of GSH S-transferase could be responsible for the faster depletion of cellular GSH. This, in turn, would explain the increased susceptibility of FA cells to mutagens and carcinogens and might also be a critical parameter for endogenous chromosome breakage in these patients.

Available data on FA heterozygotes also point to antioxidants having a protective effect against DEB- and peroxide-stressed lymphocytes. However, this phenomenon could be seen only when the induced rates of chromosome breaks were sufficiently high, which was not always the case (Dallapiccola et al. 1985). Nevertheless, cytogenetic characterization of both FA homozygotes and heterozygotes by oxidizing stress could be valuable in finding a method for the identification of FA mutation according to the clastogenic effects of alkylating agents.

Conclusion

In the last decade, efforts to develop in vitro tests for the identification of FA heterozygotes have not been successful. No study has provided accurate and reliable results with obligate heterozygotes. Even the DEB test - which gives reproducible results in the diagnosis of FA homozygotes and also shows a rather distinct clastogenic effect in a proportion of heterozygotes - does not meet widely accepted criteria for a screening test in the population. The other laboratory tests, which are also based on the presumed ability of different chemicals to induce differential yields of breaks and/or SCE in FA heterozygotes and controls, provide even less satisfactory results.

There is an urgent need to improve laboratory tests for the study of FA heterozygotes. It is likely that cloning of the FA gene will circumvent the difficulties related to the use of indirect approaches for analysis of this mutation at the cellular level.

References

Alimena G, Avvisati G, De Cuia MR, Gallo E, Novelli G, Dallapiccola B (1983) Retrospective diagnosis of a Fanconi's anemia patient by diepoxybutane (DEB) test results in parents. Haematologica 68: 97-103

Alter BP, Parkman R, Rappeport JM (1981) Bone marrow failure syndromes. In: Nathan DG, Oski FA (eds) Hematology of infancy and childhood, 2nd edn. Saunders, Philadelphia, pp 168-249

Auerbach AD, Wolman SR (1976) Susceptibility of Fanconi's anaemia fibroblasts to chromosome damage by carcinogens. Nature 261: 494-496

Auerbach AD, Wolman SR (1978) Carcinogen-induced chromosome breakage in Fanconi's anaemia heterozygous cells. Nature 271: 69-70

Auerbach AD, Warburton D, Bloom AD, Chaganti RSK (1979) Prenatal detection of the Fanconi anemia gene by cytogenetic methods. Am J Hum Gent 31: 77-81

Auerbach AD, Adler B, Chaganti RSK (1981) Prenatal and postnatal diagnosis and carrier detection of Fanconi anemia by a cytogenetic method. Pediatrics 67: 128-135

Auerbach AD, Sagi M, Adler B (1985) Fanconi anemia: prenatal diagnosis in 30 fetuses at risk. Pediatrics 76: 794-800

Auerbach AD, Zhang M, Ghosh R, Pergament E, Verlinsky Yuri, Nicolas H, Boué J (1986) Clastogen-induced chromosome breakage as a marker for first trimester prenatal diagnosis of Fanconi anemia. Hum Genet 73: 86-88

Berger R, Bussel A, Schenmetzler C (1977) Somatic segregation in Fanconi anemia. Clin Genet 11: 409-415

Berger R, Bernheim A, Le Coniat M, Vecchione D, Schaison C (1980) Sister chromatid exchanges induced by nitrogen mustard in Fanconi's anemia. Application to the detection of heterozygotes and interpretation of the results. Cancer Genet Cytogenet 2: 259-267

Boyland E, Williams K (1965) An enzyme catalysing the conjugation of epoxides with glutathione. Biochem J 94: 190-197

Brown KW, Harnden DG (1978) Erythrocyte superoxide dismutase in ataxia-telangiectasia and Fanconi's anaemia. Lancet 11: 1260-1261

Cervenka J, Hirsch BA (1983) Cytogenetic differentiation of Fanconi anemia, idiopathic aplastic anemia, and Fanconi anemia heterozygotes. Am J Med Genet 15: 211-223

Cervenka J, Arthur D, Yasis C (1981) Mitomycin C test for diagnostic differentiation of idiopathic aplastic anemia and Fanconi anemia. Pediatrics 67: 119-127

Cohen MM, Simpson SJ, Honig GR, Maurer HS, Nicklas JW, Martin AO (1982a) The identification of Fanconi anemia genotypes by clastogenic stress. Am J Hum Genet 34: 794-810

Cohen MM, Fruchtman CE, Simpson SJ, Martin AO (1982b) The cytogenetic response of Fanconi's anemia lymphoblastoid cell lines to various clastogens. Cytogenet Cell Genet 34: 230-240

Dallapiccola B, Mokini V, Porfirio B, Alimena G, Isacchi GC, Gandini E (1983) Studio citogenetico e familiare delle pancitopenie associate ad instabilità cromosomica. In: Tura S, Zaccaria A, Dallapiccola B (eds) Citogenetica Oncologica. Esculapio, Bologna, pp 85-105

Dallapiccola B, Magnani M, Novelli G, Mandelli F (1984) Increased glutathione S-transferase and fast decay of reduced glutathione in Fanconi's anemia. Acta Haematol 71: 143-144

Dallapiccola B, Porfirio B, Mokini V, Alimena G, Isacchi G, Gandini E (1985) Effect of oxidants and antioxidants on chromosomal breakage in Fanconi anemia lymphocytes. Hum Genet 69: 62-65

Davidson RL, Kaufman ER, Dougherty CP, Ouellette AM, Di Folco C, Latt SA (1980) Induction of sister chromatid exchanges by bromodeoxyuridine in DNA. Nature 284: 74-76

Duckworth-Rysiecki G, Cornish K, Clarke CA, Buchwald M (1985) Identification of two complementation groups in Fanconi anemia. Somatic Cell Genet 11: 35-43

Dutrillaux B, Aurias A, Dutrillaux A, Buriot D, Prieur M (1982) The cell cycle of lymphocytes in Fanconi's anemia. Hum Genet 62: 327-332

Gebhart E, Becher R (1976) Comparative studies on the specificity of anticlastogenic action in human lymphocytes in culture. Hum Genet 32: 49-64

Gebhart E, Kysela D, Matthee H, Nikol M (1985) Cytogenetic analyses utilizing various clastogens in two sibs with Fanconi anemia, their relatives, and control individuals. Hum Genet 69: 309-315

Gmyrek D, Syllm-Rapoport I (1964) Zur Fanconi Anämie (FA). Analyse von 129 beschriebenen Fällen. Z Kinderheilkd 91: 297-337
Hamel BCJ (1986) Urinary tract abnormalities in a family with Fanconi anaemia (Abstract). 7th International congress of human genetics, Berlin. p 699
Izakovic V, Strbakova, Kaiserova E, Krizan P (1985) Bovine superoxide dismutase in Fanconi anaemia. Therapeutic trial in two patients. Hum Genet 70: 181-182
Joenje H, Eriksson AW, Frants RR, Arwert F, Houwen B (1978) Erythrocyte superoxide dismutase deficiency in Fanconi's anemia. Lancet 1: 204
Joenje H, Frants RR, Arwert F, de Bruin GJM, Kostense PJ, van de Kamp JJP, de Koning J, Erikkson AW (1979). Erythrocyte superoxide dismutase deficiency in Fanconi's anaemia established by two independent methods of assay. Scand J Clin Lab Invest 39: 759-764
Joenje H, Arwert F, Eriksson AW, de Koning H, Oostra AB (1981) Oxygen dependence of chromosomal aberrations in Fanconi's anaemia. Nature 290: 142-143
Joenje H, Oostra AB (1983) Effect of oxygen tension on chromosomal aberrations in Fanconi anaemia. Hum Genet 65: 99-101
Joenje H, Oostra AB, Wanamarta AH (1983) Cytogenetic toxicity of D_2O in human lymphocyte cultures. Increased sensitivity in Fanconi's anemia. Experientia 39: 782-784
Kano Y, Fujiwara Y (1981) Roles of DNA interstrand crosslinking and its repair in the induction of SCE and a higher induction in Fanconi's anemia cells. Mutat Res 81: 365-375
Kano Y, Fujiwara Y (1982) Higher inductions of twin and single sister chromatid exchanges by cross-linking agents in Fanconi's anemia cells. Hum Genet 60: 233-238
Lambert B, Hansson K, Lindsten J, Sten M, Werelius B (1976) Bromodeoxyuridine-induced sister chromatid exchanges in human lymphocytes. Hereditas 83: 163-174
Latt SA, Stetten G, Juergens LA, Buchanan GR, Gerald PS (1975) Induction by alkylating agents of sister chromatid exchanges and chromatid breaks in Fanconi's anemia. Proc Natl Acad Sci USA 72: 4066-4077
Marx MP, Smith S, Heyns A du P, van Tonder IZ (1983) Fanconi's anemia: a cytogenetic study on lymphocyte and bone marrow cultures utilizing 1,2:3,4 diepoxybutane. Cancer Genet Cytogenet 9: 51-60
Mavelli I, Ciriolo MR, Rotilio G (1982) Superoxide dismutase, glutathione peroxidase in oxidative hemolysis. A study of Fanconi's anemia erythrocytes. Biochem Biophys Res Commun 106: 286-290
Mazrimas JA, Stetka DG (1978) Direct evidence for the role of incorporated BudR in the induction of sister chromatid exchanges. Exp Cell Res 117: 23-30
Meister A (1983) Selective modification of glutathione metabolism. Science 220: 472-477
Meme JS, Gripenberg U, Kahkonen M (1980) Fanconi's anemia: chromosome breakage in a large African family. Hereditas 93: 255-260
Miura K, Morimoto K, Koizumi A (1983) Proliferative kinetics and mitomycin C-induced chromosome damage in Fanconi's anemia lymphocytes. Hum Genet 63: 19-23
Morimoto K, Sato-Mizuno M, Koizumi A (1985) Sister-chromatid exchanges and cell-cycle kinetics in human lymphocyte cultures exposed to alkylating mutagens: apparent deformity in dose-response relationships. Mutat Res 152: 187-196
Nordenson I (1977) Effect of superoxide dismutase and catalase on spontaneously occurring chromosome breaks in patients with Fanconi's anemia. Hereditas 86: 147-150
Novotná B, Goetz P, Surkova NI (1979) Effects of alkylating agents on lymphocytes from controls and from patients with Fanconi's anemia. Hum Genet 49: 41-50
Okahata S, Kobayashi Y, Usui T (1980) Erythrocyte superoxide dismutase activity in Fanconi's anaemia. Clin Sci 58: 173-175
Porfirio B, Dallapiccola B, Mokini V, Alimena G, Gandini E (1983) Failure of diepoxybutane to enhance sister chromatid exchange levels in Fanconi's anemia patients and heterozygotes. Hum Genet 63: 117-120
Potter NC, Sarmousakis C, Frederick PL (1983) Cancer in relatives of patients with aplastic anemia. Cancer Genet Cytogenet 9: 61-66
Raj AS, Heddle JA (1980) The effect of superoxide dismutase, catalase and L-cysteine on spontaneous and on mitomycin C-induced chromosomal breakage in Fanconi's anaemia and normal fibroblasts as measured by the micronucleus method. Mutat Res 78: 59-66
Sasaki MS (1980) Chromosome aberration formation in relation to DNA repair in human cells.

In: Generoso WM, Shelby MD, de Serres FJ (eds) DNA repair and mutagenesis in eukaryotes. Plenum, New York, pp 285-313

Scarpa M, Rigo A, Momo F, Isacchi G, Novelli G, Dallapiccola B (1985) Increased rate of superoxide ion generation in Fanconi anemia erythrocytes. Biochem Biophys Res Commun 130: 127-132

Schroeder TM, Tilgen D, Krueger J, Vogel F (1976a) Formal genetics of Fanconi's anemia. Hum Genet 32: 257-288

Schroeder TM, Drings P, Beilner P, Buchinger G (1976b) Clinical and cytogenetic observations during a six-year period in an adult with Fanconi's anaemia. Blut 34: 119-132

Schroeder TM, Stahl-Maugé C (1979) Mutagenic effects of isonicotinic acid hydracide in Fanconi's anemia. Hum Genet 52: 309-321

Seres DS, Fornace AJ (1982) Normal response of Fanconi's anaemia cells to high concentrations of O_2 as determined by alkaline elution. Biochim Biophys Acta 698: 237-242

Shamberger RJ, Baughman FF, Kalchert SL, Willis CE, Hoffman GC (1973) Carcinogen-induced chromosomal breakage decreased by antioxidants. Proc Natl Acad Sci USA 70: 1461-1463

Shoyab M, Gunnell M, Lubiniecki AS (1981) Reduced uptake and incorporation of ^{3}H-thymidine in Fanconi anemia fibroblasts. Hum Genet 57: 296-299

Swift M (1971) Fanconi's anemia in the genetics of neoplasia. Nature 230: 370-373

Swift M, Caldwell RJ, Chase C (1982) Reassessment of cancer predisposition of Fanconi anemia heterozygotes. INCI 65: 863-867

Todaro GJ, Green H, Swift MR (1966) Susceptibility of human diploid fibroblasts to transformation by SV40 virus. Science 154: 1252

Vogel F (1984) Clinical consequences of heterozygosity for autosomal recessive diseases. Clin Genet 25: 381-415

Weksberg R, Buchwald M, Sargent P, Thopmson MW, Siminovitch L (1979) Specific cellular defects in patients with Fanconi anemia. J Cell Physiol 101: 311-324

Welshimer K, Swift M (1982) Congenital malformations and developmental disabilities in ataxia-telangiectasia, Fanconi anemia, and xeroderma pigmentosum families. Am J Hum Genet 34: 781-793

Yoshimitsu K, Kobayashi Y, Usui T (1984) Decreased superoxide dismutase activity of erythrocytes and leukocytes in Fanconi's anemia. Acta Haematol (Basel) 72: 208-210

Zakrzewski S, Sperling K (1980) Genetic heterogeneity of Fanconi anemia demonstrated by somatic cell hybrids. Hum Genet 56: 81-84

Part III

Investigations of the Defect in Fanconi Anemia Cells

BrdU-Hoechst Flow Cytometry Links the Cell Kinetic Defect of Fanconi Anemia to Oxygen Hypersensitivity*

H. Hoehn, M. Kubbies, D. Schindler, M. Poot, and P. S. Rabinovitch

The BrdU-Hoechst Cell Kinetic Assay

When resting human cells are activated in media containing BrdU, thymidine residues are replaced by the halogenated analogue during semiconservative DNA replication. BrdU substitution leads to diminished fluorescence if these cells are stained with the fluorochrome Hoechst 33258. This is a principle familiar to cytogeneticists employing the differential metaphase staining technique for sister chromatid exchange (SCE) analysis (Latt 1973). By measuring the amount of Hoechst dye quenching after BrdU incorporation in a flow cytometer, one can literally count the number of times a cell has divided in the presence of BrdU (Kubbies and Rabinovitch 1983). The use of a second, BrdU-independent dye (e.g., ethidium bromide) permits the simultaneous recording of quenched and unquenched fluorescence (the latter, of course, reflecting the regular 2 c to 4 c oscillations of DNA content as cells replicate and divide). Figure 1 shows examples of such a bivariate (Hoechst fluorochrome vs. ethidium bromide) fluorescence analysis. The informational content of this type of analysis is unique since it resolves cell-cycle phase fractions throughout three successive cell cycles. By electronic framing, rotation, and projection onto the Hoechst axis, the component phases of each individual cell cycle can be separately displayed: they are then amenable to analysis by conventional curve fitting techniques (bottom panels in each figure). In the example of a 72 h phytohemagglutinin (PHA)-stimulated peripheral blood-lymphocyte culture from a healthy donor (Fig. 1 a), the cell cycle distribution of a total of 91944 cells was recorded and analyzed by curve fitting. In Table 1 these data are compared with analogous results from a second healthy donor, and from two patients with Fanconi anemia (FA).

Impaired Growth of Fanconi Anemia Cells is due to a G_2 Phase Defect

As shown in Fig. 1 b, the bivariate-flow analysis of PHA-stimulated FA lymphocytes yields a 72-h cell-cycle distribution quite different from that of the normal donor. Most notably, the G_2-phase clusters of the first and second cycle are more

* Supported by Deutsche Forschungsgemeinschaft grant Ho 849/2 - 1 and National Institutes of Health grant AG - 01751

T. M. Schroeder-Kurth A. D. Auerbach G. Obe (Eds.)
Fanconi Anemia, Clinical, Cytogenetic and Experimental Aspects

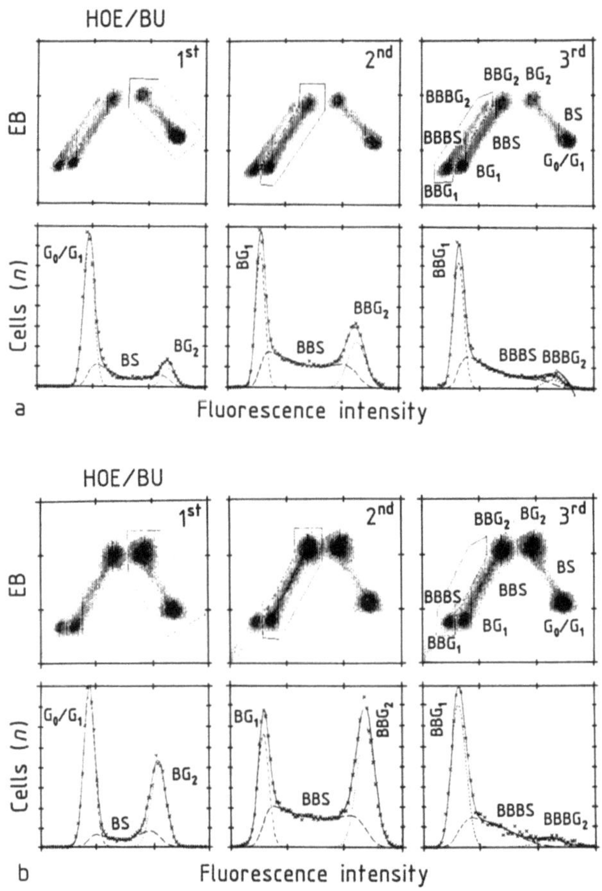

Fig. 1a, b. Bivariate flow cytometric analysis of replicative heterogeneity within human diploid lymphocyte cultures harvested 72 h after PHA stimulation. The cell cycle and cell cycle compartment distributions of cells from **a** a 10-year-old healthy lymphocyte donor, **b** an 8-year-old patient with clinical and cytogenetic evidence of FA. The *bottom panels* in each part are curve-fitted Hoechst *(HOE)* fluorescence data limited to individual cell cycles. See text for interpretation. *EB*, ethidium bromide

prominent in the lymphocytes of patients with FA than in normal lymphocytes. This is confirmed by the quantitative analysis of the rotated projections of individual cell-cycle data onto the Hoechst axis (bottom panels): in the donor, both the first and second cycle distributions show greatly elevated G_2-phase amplitudes. Table 1, summarizes the data from several such analyses. It shows that 33.7%–37.0% of the 72-h populations of the two patients with FA were found in the G_2 phases of the first and second cycles. In contrast, the first plus second G_2-phase compartments of the normal cells amount to only around 10% of the total. This strong predominance of G_2- over G_1-phase cells in 72-h lymphocyte cultures is typical for FA donors: using single-parameter flow analysis (assay of Hoechst fluorescence only), we showed that the combined 72-h G_2/G_1 ratios of the fractions from the cell cycle were greater than 2.0 in four FA patients, but be-

Table 1. Cell cycle and cycle compartment distributions of normal and Fanconi anemia lymphocytes 72 h after PHA stimulation

Cell cycle	1st cycle			2nd cycle			3rd cycle		
Normal 1	38.3			37.2			24.5		
Normal 2	26.8[a]			26.9			40.6		
FA 1	54.5			38.5			7.0		
FA 2	40.7			45.5			13.8		
Compartment	G_0/G_1	S	G_2	G_1	S	G_2	G_1	S	G_2
Normal 1	21.9	12.8	3.6	11.4	18.5	7.3	11.3	11.7	1.5
Normal 2	18.5	5.0	3.3	8.6	11.5	6.7	18.6	17.3	4.7
FA 1	26.1	10.1	18.3	7.9	15.1	15.4	4.1	2.5	0.4
FA 2	18.9	6.9	14.9	8.2	15.2	22.1	6.8	5.2	1.8

Numbers are percentages of the total number of cells analyzed

[a] In normal donor 2, 5.7% of cells had already progressed into the fourth cycle.

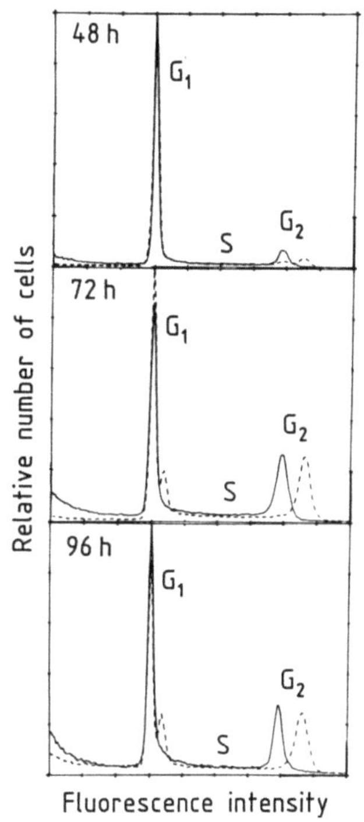

Fig. 2. Conventional, single parameter flow cytometric analysis of BrdU-effects on the proliferation of FA lymphocytes. The *unbroken lines* denote Hoechst staining of FA cells grown in the absence of BrdU. The *broken lines* denote mithramycin staining of FA cells grown in the presence of 65 μM/liter BrdU. The fluorescence of the latter dye is slightly enhanced, rather than quenched, by BrdU substitution. Note that the respective G_2 phase histogram peaks rise, and remain elevated, in identical fashion. This proves that BrdU itself does not provoke the G_2 accumulations seen in FA cells

low 1.0 in 57 non-FA donors, including patients with nonhereditary forms of anemia (Schindler et al. 1985). The flow cytometric findings of G_2-phase accumulations in FA lymphocytes fully agree with previously reported cell-kinetic data obtained by the conventional SCE-staining technique (Dutrillaux et al. 1982). Together, these observations define G_2-phase accumulations as the hallmark of cell-cycle progression in the FA genotype.

Experiments conducted by conventional flow cytometry (Fig. 2) show that the

G_2-phase accumulations described occur irrespective of whether FA lymphocytes are exposed to BrdU. Therefore, the base analogue itself cannot be responsible for the G_2-phase defect in the lymphocytes. As a result of our current experience with more than 200 BrdU-Hoechst lymphocyte assays, we can state with confidence that the G_2-phase accumulations described are germane to FA cells. Most importantly, they do occur spontaneously, i.e., in the absence of any treatment with cross-linking agents (Latt et al. 1982).

Since so many cells accumulate in the G_2 compartments of the first and second cycle following activation, one might expect that only a comparatively small percentage of FA lymphocytes manages to enter the third cell cycle within the 72-h culture period. Table 1 shows this to be the case. The accumulation in the G_2 phases of either the first or the second cycle prevents a considerable portion of cells from patients with FA from further division; a deficit of net growth is the result. Are there additional factors that might account for the poor growth performance of these cells? The answer is clearly no: if the G_0/G_1-phase fractions of the first cycle are studied as a measure of the nonactivated-cell fraction (Table 1), it becomes clear that there is no systematic difference between FA and normal cells with respect to the initial mitogen response. The growth deficit of FA lymphocyte cultures therefore cannot be due to improper cell activation; it is caused solely by a G_2-phase defect of cells that respond to the PHA stimulus in the same way as normal cells.

G_2 Phase Defect of Fanconi Anemia Cells Consists of G_2 Phase Prolongation and G_2 Phase Arrest

Whereas a single measurement 72 h after PHA exposure assigns the disturbance of FA cell-cycle progression to the G_2 phase, a single measurement does not answer the question whether the G_2-phase accumulations observed result from increased G_2-phase transit times (G_2-phase prolongation), or from a complete blockage of cells in the G_2 phase (G_2-phase arrest). In order to answer this question, we conducted studies in which the type of analysis shown in Fig. 1 was repeated up to ten times during the course of a 96-h stimulation experiment. This sequential analysis allowed measurement of the flow of activated cells throughout the various compartments of three consecutive cell cycles (Kubbies et al. 1985a). If the number of cells remaining in a given compartment was then plotted as a function of time after stimulation, the resulting curves show an excellent fit to the recently modified cell-kinetic ("transition probability") model of Smith and Martin (Rabinovitch 1983). There are several advantages of treating the BrdU-Hoechst flow data in this fashion (Fig. 3): first, minimum compartment transit times can easily be derived by computing the distances between the x-axis intercepts of pairs of successive curves, each denoting the time course of cell exit from a given compartment. Second, the number of cells incapable of exit from a given compartment can be measured by comparing the plateau phases of two successive exit curves. If all cells that enter also leave a given compartment, then the extrapolated plateau levels of the two curves delimiting that compartment must coincide. If, however, a proportion of cells is permanently halted after entry into such a compartment,

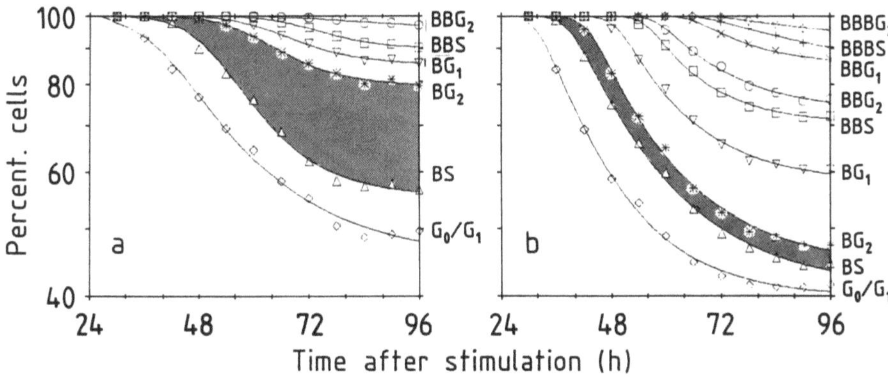

Fig. 3a, b. Cell cycle compartment exit curves constructed by fitting sequential BrdU-Hoechst flow cytometric data to the modified Smith-Martin cell-kinetic model (Kubies et al. 1985b). Note the difference in the size of the shaded equivalents of first-cycle G_2 compartment transits in FA (**a**) and normal (**b**) lymphocytes. See text for explanation of symbols and the distinction between compartment prolongation and compartment arrest seen in these curves

then the two delimiting curves will plateau at different levels, the difference being the number of cells arrested within that compartment. Third, the slopes of the fitted curves yield the transition probability; this is a complex but informative measure of growth capacity. Finally, the part of these exit curves that is strictly exponential can be used to estimate mean compartment durations, as the mean length of an exponential process is the inverse of the transition probability (Kubbies et al. 1985a).

The application of this comprehensive scheme of cell-cycle analysis in patients with FA showed that both the slow down of compartment transit and complete compartment arrest caused the characteristic G_2-phase accumulations in FA-lymphocyte cultures (Kubbies et al. 1985b). In the examples given in Fig. 3, the minimum duration of the first cycle of the G_2 phase in the FA sample was 10.7 h, as opposed to 5.2 h for the normal sample. In addition, the exit curves delimiting the G_2 compartment of the FA sample (BS and BG_2) show a much greater final distance between their computed plateau levels than do the corresponding curves of the normal donor. This means that 19.5% of the cycling FA cells were arrested after entry into the G_2 compartment of the first cell cycle. In the normal donor, this figure is only 2.7%, and G_2 phase arrest in excess of 5% has never been observed in young or young adult (<40 years) non-FA lymphocyte donors. As G_2-phase defects can be induced by a variety of agents in normal cells, it seemed reasonable, at this stage of our studies, to ask the question below.

Can Cell-Cycle-Active Drugs Mimic the Endogenous Cell-Cycle Disturbance of FA Cells in Normal Cells?

In order to answer this question, 72-h lymphocyte cultures from normal donors were exposed to a variety of standard agents that are known to interfere with cell proliferation at specific points in the cell cycle. Special emphasis was placed on

Table 2. Summary of cell-kinetic effects exerted by cell-cycle-active agents in human lymphocyte cultures

Disease/agents	Cell-cycle parameters				
	G_0/G_1 lag	G_0/G_1 arrest	S/G_2 arrest	Cell decay	Third cycle
Fanconi anemia	Normal	Normal	↑↑↑	↑↑	↓↓↓
Cross-linking agents[a]	↑↑	↑↑	↑	↑↑	↓
Bleomycin	↑↑	↑↑	↑↑	↑↑	↓
Mitotic spindle inhibitors[b]	Normal	↑↑	↑↑	Normal	↓
DNA synthesis inhibitors[c]	Normal/↑	↑	Normal	↑	↓
RNA synthesis inhibitors[d]	Normal/↑↑	Normal/↑↑	Normal	↑	↓
Protein synthesis inhibitors[e]	↑↑		Normal	↑	↓

↑, increased; ↓, decreased

[a] Mitomycin C, diepoxybutane.

[b] Colcemid, vinblastine.

[c] Aphidicolin, ara-C, hydroxyurea, FUDR.

[d] α-Amanitine, cyclosporin.

[e] Cycloheximide.

drugs whose known or presumed target is the G_2 segment of the cell cycle, and to which FA cells are known to be hypersensitive. Much to our surprise, even substances such as mitomycin C and diepoxybutane failed to produce a pattern of cell-cycle disturbance that mimics in complete detail the picture of the spontaneous disturbance seen in FA lymphocytes. Table 2 presents a qualitative summary of these results. It shows that the cross-linking agents (a) increase the initial lag period following activation, and (b) increase the number of nonresponding cells, i. e., the G_0/G_1 fraction. Both these effects are very different from those observed in FA cells.

An additional agent reported to induce G_2-phase-specific cell-cycle defects is oxygen (Balin et al. 1978). We therefore tested the effects of various oxygen concentrations on normal lymphocyte growth. The results of these tests were, however, disappointing. The proliferation of both FA and normal lymphocytes was found to be insensitive to manipulations of oxygen supply during the 72-h-test periods. Surprisingly, parallel work with FA fibroblast cultures yielded definitive evidence for the increased sensitivity of this cell type towards ambient oxygen.

Near-Normal Growth and Cloning is Restored in FA Fibroblast Cultures by Reduction of Ambient Oxygen

The poor growth performance of FA fibroblast cultures is a well-documented experience shared by many workers in the field (e.g., Weksberg et al. 1979). Our laboratories have a long-standing interest in the impaired growth of fibroblast-like cells from a number of human genetic disorders, particularly Werner's syndrome (Salk et al. 1985). We therefore included FA fibroblasts in our systematic studies, testing the effects of ambient, reduced, and elevated oxygen culture conditions on the growth performance of human mutant cells. The parameters tested in these long-term studies were (a) growth velocity, (b) in vitro lifespan, (c) cloning effi-

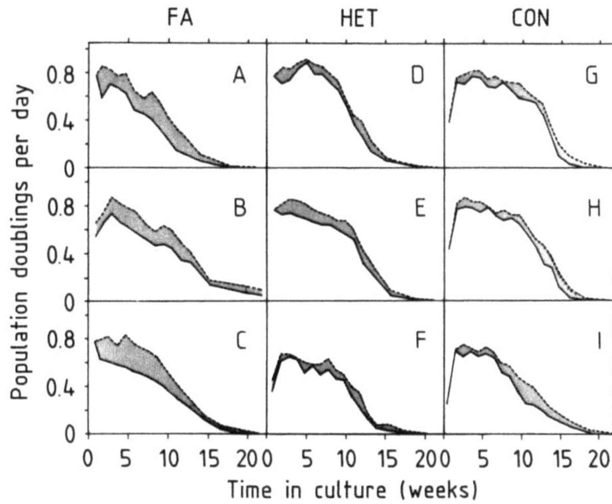

Fig. 4 A–I. Growth velocity of **A–C** FA, **D–F** heterozygote *(HET)*, and **G–I** control *(CON)* fibroblast cultures at ambient *(unbroken lines)* and 5% *(broken lines)* oxygen conditions. Cells (5×10^4) were plated into a 25 cm^2 tissue-culture flask and passaged at weekly intervals. Population doublings per day were based on weekly cell counts *B*, one round of replications; *BB*, two rounds of replication in the presence of BrdU; *BBB*, three rounds of replication

Table 3. Percentages of growth differences at low (5% v/v) compared with ambient (20% v/v) oxygen culture conditions

	Fanconi anemia	Heterozygotes	Controls
Life span/cumulative population doubling			
A	39.0	13.8	14.2
B	30.1	18.5	13.8
C	37.7	18.6	20.7
$\bar{x} \pm SD$	35.6±4.8	17.0±2.7	16.2±3.9
Cloning efficiency			
A	364.1	63.3	52.3
B	506.6	39.6	35.2
C	276.0	40.2	44.3
$\bar{x} \pm SD$	382.2±116.4	47.7±13.5	43.9±8.6
Colony diameter			
A	125.6	21.8	26.4
B	136.4	20.8	27.4
C	151.4	22.1	32.8
$\bar{x} \pm SD$	137.8±13.4	21.6±0.7	28.9±3.4

ciency, and (d) colony diameters. As an example, we show the result of growth-velocity testing, comparing 5% and 20% (v/v) oxygen atmospheres (Fig. 4).

Growth velocity was assessed by weekly cell counts during serial passage of three homozygous, three obligate heterozygous, and three unrelated control strains. Figure 4 shows the growth velocity of all strains, plotted as population doublings per day, to be inferior at ambient oxygen (solid lines) to growth at 5%

oxygen (v/v, dotted lines). However, as indicated by a comparison of the shaded areas, the FA group shows the greatest improvement. The visual impression of disproportional improvement of FA-cell growth as a result of long-term exposure to low oxygen was confirmed by the quantitative analysis of several other growth and cloning parameters. As shown in Table 3, the percentage extension of the total lifespan of FA cells exposed to 5% oxygen was twice that observed in the heterozygote and control strains. An even more marked improvement of the FA cells over the other strains was evident from the cloning data: at 5% oxygen, the FA strains tested showed a six- to nine-fold improvement in cloning over that in the heterozygote and control strains. Figure 5 shows representative cloning dishes

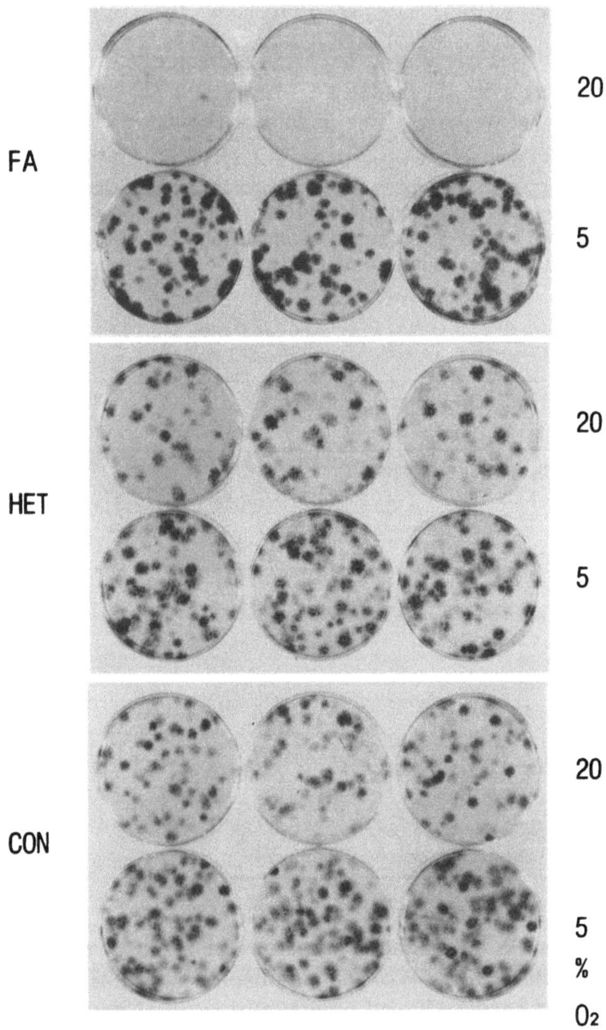

Fig. 5. Representative cloning dishes of FA, heterozygote *(HET)*, and control *(CON)* strains exposed to 20% and 5% (v/v) oxygen. In each dish, 200 cells were plated, incubated for 12-day periods, fixed, and stained with crystal violet. Half original size

which illustrate this effect. FA fibroblasts, which clone very poorly in ambient oxygen conditions, reached 94% of the overall cloning efficiency of the heterozygote strains when exposed to only 5% oxygen. It should be noted that the greater benefit of low oxygen in the cloning, as opposed to in the mass culture assays, is not unexpected, as it is known that oxygen deprivation exerts its greatest growth-promoting effect at low cell densities (Taylor et al. 1978).

Note also that the data in Table 3 suggest no differences between heterozygote and control strains that could be interpreted in terms of a heterozygote manifestation of the low-oxygen effect.

Low Oxygen Improves the Growth of FA Fibroblasts by Mitigation of Their G_2 Phase Defect

Our unpublished work with varying oxygen culture conditions provides evidence for the interaction of two separate mechanisms that are responsible for the improved growth of FA cells at reduced oxygen: first, as depicted in Fig. 6, exposure to low levels of oxygen decreases the noncycling (G_0/G_1) cell fraction; in other words, low-oxygen conditions promote the recruitment of resting cells into the cell cycle. This effect is universal, affecting FA, heterozygote, and control strains alike.

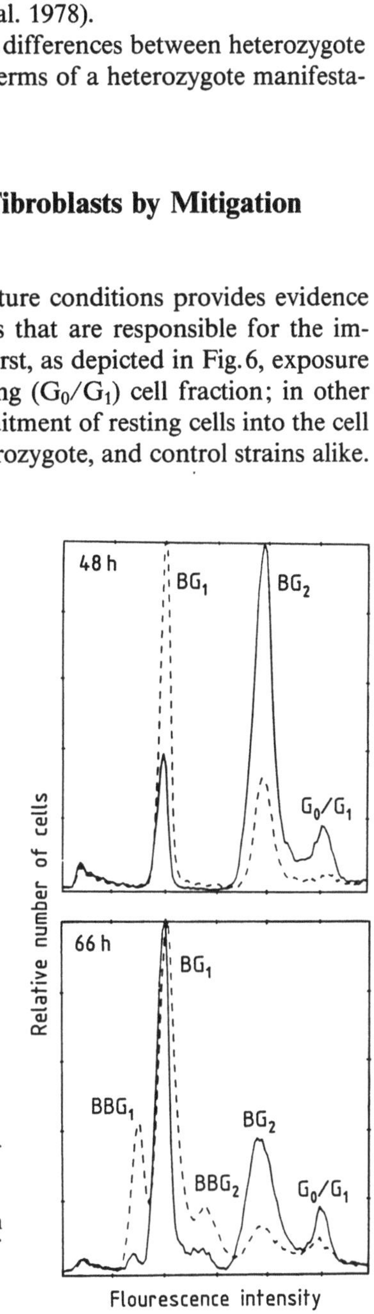

Fig. 6. One-parameter BrdU-Hoechst flow histograms (Hoechst fluorescence only) of FA fibroblast cultures exposed to ambient *(unbroken lines)* and 5% *(broken lines)* oxygen. Owing to the quench effect, BrdU-substituted (replicating) cells displayed less fluorescence than noncycling cells (G_0/G_1 fraction). The prefixes *B* and *BB* denote, respectively, one and two rounds of replication in the presence of BrdU. Note the reduced amplitudes of both the G_0/G_1 and the BG_2 compartments at 48 and 66 h after stimulation. Also note the much higher amplitude of the BBG_1 phase cells in the low as opposed to the ambient oxygen culture. See text for further details

It explains the overall improvement in growth velocity, lifespan, cloning efficiency, and colony diameter seen in all of the strains tested. More relevant in the context of FA, a second oxygen related effect appeared to act selectively during the G_2 phase of the FA cell cycle. In general, G_2 phase accumulations are not as striking in FA fibroblasts as they are in FA lymphocytes. The reason for the more subtle expression of the G_2 phase defect in FA fibroblasts as opposed to in FA lymphocytes is seen in the fact that human diploid fibroblasts and FA fibroblasts in particular, do not grow as well as lymphocytes; they also show less synchrony following mitogen stimulation. In single-parameter BrdU-Hoechst studies with FA fibroblast cultures exposed to 5% oxygen, we nevertheless observed highly significant reductions in their abnormally elevated G_2 phase fractions (Schindler et al. 1985). As illustrated in Fig. 6, these reductions were seen following, stimulation of previously quiescent FA cultures, both at early and at later stages. The 66-h comparison of the low oxygen (broken lines) and the ambient oxygen (solid lines) histograms also showed that reduction of amplitude of the BG_2 compartment improved the overall proliferation of these cells: whereas 10% of the cells exposed to low oxygen managed to enter the third cycle (BBG_1) at 66 h, this applied to only 1%-2% of those in the sister culture exposed to ambient oxygen.

These growth studies first of all confirm the beneficial effect of low oxygen culture conditions on the growth of normal human diploid fibroblasts (Packer and Fuehr 1977). They also provide the first evidence that FA fibroblasts benefit from the reduction of atmospheric oxygen to a greater extent than normal cells (Schindler and Hoehn 1988). Knowing that the greater benefit seen in FA cells results from a reduction of their pathologically elevated G_2 cell fractions, factors which reversibly delay or arrest cells in the G_2 phase of the cell cycle must therefore play a key role in the expression of the genetic defect in FA. We believe that our studies have identified one such factor, ambient oxygen, as being responsible for the G_2 defect and for the poor growth of FA fibroblast-like cells.

Induction of an FA-Like G_2 Phase Defect by Elevated Oxygen in Normal Fibroblast Cultures

The "ambient oxygen sensitivity theory" suggested by Joenje et al. (1981) and our data requires that the G_2 phase be the most oxygen-sensitive stage of the human diploid fibroblast cell cycle. So far, our BrdU-Hoechst studies of the cell cycle of normal human fibroblasts fully confirm previous evidence for selective interference of elevated oxygen tension with cell-cycle progression during the G_2 phase (Latt 1973). As an illustration of this effect, Fig. 7 shows that the G_2 fractions from the first cycle of normal fibroblasts increased as the oxygen supply was raised to higher than ambient levels: the left two panels represent distributions of normal fibroblasts exposed to either 5% or 20% oxygen. At 60 h after serum stimulation, these cultures displayed around 38% of their first-cycle cells in their BG_2 compartments. However, a sister culture exposed to 35% (v/v) oxygen accumulated 71.6% of its first-cycle population in BG_2. If one compares the G_0/G_1 clusters of the ambient and elevated oxygen panels, one hardly notes any difference. The computed data confirm that the recruitment of the G_0/G_1 cell fraction into the cell cycle is

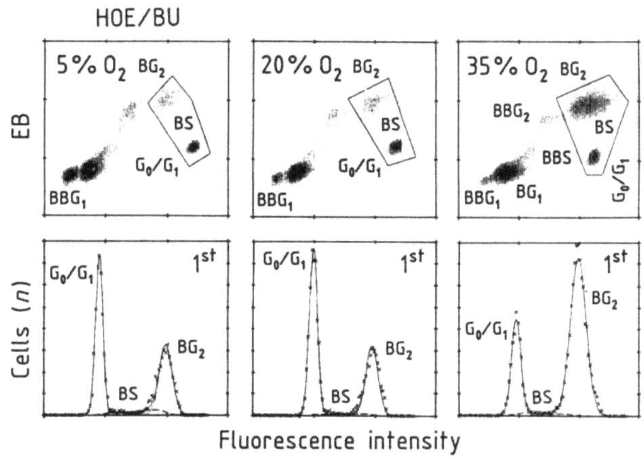

Fig. 7. Bivariate ethidium bromide *(EB)* vs. Hoechst/BrdU *(HOE/BU)*-flow cytometric analysis of FA sister cultures exposed to 5%, 20%, and 35% oxygen for 60 h after stimulation of a quiescent (serum-deprived) culture. The quantitative analysis is limited to the first-cycle cells only. Note nearly identical proportions of (G_0/G_1 and BG_2 phase cells at low and ambient, but strongly elevated BG_2 phase fractions at 35% oxygen. The *bottom panels* show the rotated projections of the first-cycle signals onto the Hoechst axis. The quantitative data derived by curve fitting are given in the text

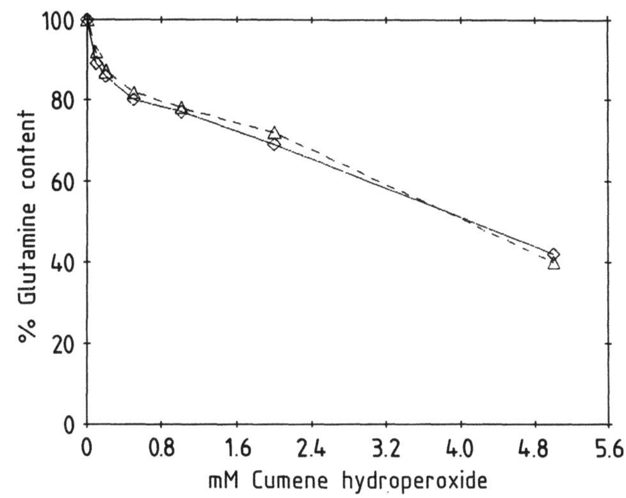

Fig. 8. Cellular reduced glutathione content (vertical axis) as a function of cumene hydroperoxide concentration (horizontal axis). The glutathione content of FA (◇, *unbroken line*) and normal (△, *broken line*) fibroblasts was determined by a newly developed flow cytometric assay (Poot et al. 1986). The 100% glutathione levels corresponded to 18.9 ± 2.1 n*M* glutathione per mg protein for FA cells ($n = 4$), and to 20.4 ± 2.2 n*M* glutathione per mg protein for normal cells ($n = 6$)

only minimally affected by exposure to high oxygen. The cell cycle disturbance provoked by elevated oxygen thus resembles in surprising detail the spontaneously altered cell cycle pattern of FA cells. In contrast to normal cells, which require exposure to higher than ambient oxygen in order to manifest a G_2 phase disturbance, FA fibroblasts express their G_2 phase defect under ambient oxygen conditions; at lower than ambient oxygen levels, they loose at least part of this defect, and show near-normal growth. Are FA fibroblast then, as postulated by a number of authors, defective in the detoxification of oxygen?

Primary Detoxification of Oxygen is Normal in FA Fibroblasts

The first toxic product of oxygen metabolism is superoxide, which can be detoxified by superoxide dismutase (SOD). The reported activities of this enzyme in the erythrocytes of patients with FA range from normal to severely reduced (Scarpa et al. 1985). As the rate of superoxide formation depends on the rate of oxygen consumption, these activities are related to hemoglobin content, which is quite often lowered in patients suffering from FA. Clearly, the crucial information needed is that relating to the steady state level of superoxide. This agent in itself is rather unreactive, but it can be converted into the extremely reactive hydroxyl radical (Bors et al. 1980). The latter reacts with lipids to form lipid peroxides; these in turn need to be detoxified by glutathione peroxidase. The activity of this enzyme is normal in FA erythrocytes, as is their resistance to oxydative hemolysis (Mavelli et al. 1982). In FA fibroblasts, both the steady state level of reduced glutathione and the capacity for de novo synthesis of this compound are normal (Poot et al. 1986). Figure 8 shows the glutathione content of fibroblasts from a patient with FA and from a healthy individual incubated with cumene peroxide, a model lipophilic hydroperoxide. Evidently, the glutathione system of both cell strains had the same response towards this peroxide. Hence, the capacity to detoxify lipophilic peroxides is not likely to be impaired in FA fibroblasts. All available evidence therefore suggests that the most common free radical scavenging pathways, representing the primary line of defence against oxygen damage, are not grossly defective in FA cells.

Conclusion

Our experimental data show that FA lymphocytes and fibroblasts have a distinctive G_2 phase defect, consisting of both G_2 phase transit delay and complete blockage. This defect is expressed in ambient oxygen culture conditions, when normal cells show no inhibition of cell cycle progression. It is mitigated by exposure to low oxygen. A very similar, if not identical, G_2 defect can be induced in normal fibroblasts by exposure to higher than ambient oxygen. Cross-linking agents induce a cell-kinetic disturbance that includes a defective G_0/G_1 phase exit. Such a pattern is neither observed in FA nor inducible in normal cells by exposure to higher than ambient oxygen levels. As FA fibroblasts have no recognizable defect in primary oxygen detoxification, we postulate that their hypersensitivity to ambient oxygen is due to a reduced ability to cope with oxygen damage at the chromatin and/or DNA levels. In the light of our findings, enzymes that repair oxygen damage at the chromatin and DNA levels (Hollstein et al. 1984) are prime candidates for the elusive genetic defect in this fascinating, and highly challenging disease.

References

Balin AK, Goodman DPB, Rasmussen H, Cristofalo VJ (1978) Oxygen-sensitive stages of the cell cycle of human diploid cells. J Cell Biol 78: 390

Bors W, Saran M, Czapski G (1980) In: Bannister HW, Bannister JV (eds) Biological and clinical aspects of superoxide and superoxide dismutase. Elsevier/North Holland, New York, p 337

Dutrillaux B, Aurias A, Dutrillaux AM et al. (1982) The cell cycle of lymphocytes in Fanconi anemia. Hum Genet 62: 327

Joenje H, Arwert F, Eriksson AW, De Koning H, Oostra AB (1981) Oxygen-dependence of chromosomal aberrations in Fanconi's anaemia. Nature 290: 142

Hollstein MC, Brooks P, Linn S, Ames BN (1984) Hydroxymethyluracil DNA glycosylase in mammalian cells. Proc Natl Acad Sci USA 81: 4003

Kubbies M, Rabinovitch PS (1983) Flow cytometric analysis of factors which influence the BrdUrd-Hoechst quenching effect in cultivated human fibroblasts and lymphocytes. Cytometry 3: 276

Kubbies M, Schindler D, Hoehn H, Rabinovitch PS (1985a) Cell cycle kinetics by BrdU-Hoechst flow cytometry: an alternative to the differential metaphase labelling technique. Cell Tissue Kinet 18: 551

Kubbies M, Schindler D, Hoehn H, Schinzel A, Rabinovitch PS (1985b) Endogenous blockage and delay of the chromosome cycle despite normal recruitment and growth phase explain poor proliferation and frequent edomitosis in Fanconi anemia cells. Am J Hum Genet 37: 1022

Latt SA (1973) Microfluorometric detection of deoxyribonucleic acid replication in human metaphase chromosomes. Proc Natl Acad Sci USA 70: 3395

Latt SA, Kaiser TN, Lojewski A et al. (1982) Cytogenetic and flow cytometric studies of cells from patients with Fanconi's anemia. Cytogenet Cell Genet 33: 133

Mavelli I, Ciriolo MR, Rotilio G et al (1982) Superoxide dismutase, glutathione peroxidase and catalase in oxidative hemolysis. Biochem Biophys Res Commun 106: 286

Packer L, Fuehr K (1977) Low oxygen concentration extends the lifespan of cultured human diploid cells. Nature 267: 423

Poot M, Verkerk A, Koster JF, Jongkind JF (1986) De novo synthesis of glutathione in human fibroblasts during in vitro ageing and in some metabolic diseases as measured by a flow cytometric method. Biochim Biophys Acta 833: 580

Rabinovitch PS (1983) Regulation of human fibroblast growth rate by both noncycling cell fraction and transition probability is shown by growth in 5-bromodeoxyuridine followed by Hoechst 33258 flow cytometry. Proc Natl Acad Sci USA 80: 2951

Salk D, Bryant E, Hoehn H, Johnston P, Martin GM (1985) In: Salk D, Fujiwara Y, Martin GM (eds) Werner's syndrome and human aging. Plenum, New York, p 305

Scarpa M, Rigo A, Momo F et al. (1985) Increased rate of superoxide ion generation in Fanconi anemia erythrocytes. Biochem Biophys Res Commun 130: 127

Schindler D, Kubbies M, Hoehn H, Schinzel A, Rabinovitch PS (1985) Presymptomatic diagnosis of Fanconi's anaemia. Lancet I: 937

Schindler D, Hoehn H (1988) Fanconi anemia mutation causes cellular. Susceptibility to ambient oxygen. Am J Hum Gent (in press)

Taylor WG, Camalier RF, Sanford KK (1978) Density-dependent effects of oxygen on the growth of mammalian fibroblasts in culture. J Cell Physiol 95: 33

Weksberg R, Buchwald M, Sargent P, Thompson MW, Siminovitch L (1979) Specific cellular defects in patients with Fanconi anemia. J Cell Physiol 101: 311

Oxygen Metabolism and Chromosomal Breakage in Fanconi Anemia*

H. Joenje and J. J. P. Gille

Introduction

The physiological basis of the enhanced chromosomal instability in Fanconi anemia (FA) cells, discovered more than two decades ago by Schroeder and coworkers, is still poorly understood. Nordenson (1977) was the first to report the protective effect of superoxide dismutase (SOD) and catalase on the frequency of chromosomal aberrations in FA lymphocyte cultures, and to suggest that either cellular overproduction of "activated" oxygen species such as superoxide radicals ($O_2^{\cdot -}$), hydrogen peroxide (H_2O_2), and hydroxyl radicals ($OH^{\cdot}$) or a deficient cellular detoxification process might be primarily responsible for the chromosomal instability in FA. This finding has subsequently promoted an experimental approach that complements investigations at the level of DNA repair.

Endogenous Antioxidant Defenses

Several laboratories have demonstrated a 20%–40% deficiency of CuZnSOD in FA erythrocytes, based on activity levels per g hemoglobin (Joenje et al. 1978, 1979; Okahata et al. 1980; Mavelli et al. 1982; Yoshimitsu et al. 1984). This deficiency, though moderate, may be considered as quite substantial in view of the fact that the activity of most enzymes, including the antioxidant enzyme glutathione peroxidase (Mavelli et al. 1982) tends to be elevated in FA erythrocytes, which is a more commonly observed phenomenon in bone marrow dysfunction (Jalbert et al. 1975).

Although Brown and Harnden (1978) and Scarpa et al. (1985) reported normal levels of erythrocyte SOD in FA on a per cell basis, it should be pointed out that FA erythrocytes usually tend to be macrocytic (Gmyrek and Syllm-Rapoport 1964) and therefore contain more hemoglobin per cell. We think erythrocyte SOD levels are preferably to be expressed as units per g hemoglobin, since (a) in several vertebrates, erythrocyte SOD has been found to be remarkably constant when based on the amount of hemoglobin rather than on the number of cells (Maral et

* Part of these investigations were supported by the Foundation for Fundamental Biological Research (BION) which is subsidized by the Netherlands Organization for the Advancement of Pure Research (ZWO), and by the Netherlands Cancer Foundation.

T. M. Schroeder-Kurth A. D. Auerbach G. Obe (Eds.)
Fanconi Anemia, Clinical, Cytogenetic and Experimental Aspects

al. 1977), and (b) the main source of superoxide in the erythrocyte probably results from the formation of methemoglobin from hemoglobin (Wever et al. 1973). Scarpa et al. (1985) calculated that FA erythrocytes are characterized by a 2.3-fold increase in the flux of superoxide. In spite of this "prooxidant state" there is no indication, however, that FA erythrocytes are more fragile than red blood cells of normal individuals. Nor is there any evidence that the erythrocyte abnormality is somehow responsible for the chromosomal aberrations in whole blood lymphocyte cultures, even though it is known that the presence of erythrocytes tends to lower the level of aberrations in lymphocyte cultures. Our attempts to correlate chromosomal breakage in FA to a diminished antioxidant capacity of blood plasma, as measured by the capacity to inhibit spontaneous autoxidation of a calf-brain homogenate (assay of Stocks et al. 1974a, b), did not reveal any difference between FA and normal blood plasma specimens, as the following results show:

FA patients ($n=5$, $\pm$SD)	61 $\pm$ 4%
Normal value (mean $\pm 2 \times$ SD)	66 $\pm$ 11%

SOD in FA erythrocytes, though deficient, is indistinguishable from the wild-type enzyme by gel electrophoresis and isoelectric focusing, and has a normal activity per unit of enzyme antigen, so that there is no evidence for a mutation in the CuZnSOD gene in FA (Joenje et al. 1979). Therefore, the erythrocyte SOD deficiency appears to be the result of a disturbed regulation in this cell type.

In order to relate cellular SOD deficiency to chromosomal breakage it would be useful to observe the deficiency in nucleated FA cells as well. Yoshimitsu et al. (1984) recently reported FA leukocytes to be deficient in CuZnSOD but not in the mitochondrial enzyme MnSOD. Abeliovich and Cohen (1978) found normal levels of total SOD in FA fibroblasts, as determined at a specific point in time after trypsinization of the cells. However, evaluation of the cellular "antioxidant status" is complicated by the fact that the antioxidant enzyme system consists of many components, while a deficiency in one component might be compensated by overproduction of certain other components. In addition to enzymatic factors such as CuZnSOD, MnSOD, catalase, and glutathione peroxidase, low molecular weight components, such as glutathione should also be taken into account. In fibroblasts there is an additional complication due to the fact that all components of the antioxidant defense system tend to follow a characteristic pattern of changes as a function of time during a single passage, which makes comparison of cell strains at a specific point in time virtually meaningless. Gille et al. (1987) recently compared CuZnSOD, MnSOD, catalase, and glutathione peroxidase as well as reduced glutathione in two FA and two control fibroblast strains over a period of several weeks following trypsinization. No significant differences were observed in the patterns of CuZnSOD and glutathione, whereas FA fibroblasts appeared to contain more MnSOD, catalase, and glutathione peroxidase, especially when incubated for relatively long periods. Therefore, the observation by Yoshimitsu et al. (1984) of a CuZnSOD deficiency in FA leukocytes indicates that such a deficiency may be unique to cells from the hemopoietic system. On the other hand, the enhanced MnSOD, catalase, and glutathione peroxidase levels in FA fibroblasts might be indicative for a "prooxidant state" of this cell type (Cerutti 1983), somehow leading to an increased level of certain protective enzyme activities. Definite proof for a prooxidant state in FA fibroblasts requires an accurate estimate of the actual fluxes of endogenous reactive oxygen generated in these cells.

Cellular Response to Oxidative Stress

An additional approach to characterize the nature of the chromosomal instability in FA is to study the effects of various kinds of oxidative stress on FA cells. Joenje et al. (1981) and Joenje and Oostra (1983) reported that chromosomal breakage frequencies observed in 3-day lymphocyte cultures from patients with FA are dependent upon the oxygen tension during cultivation, in the range 3%–45% O_2.

This effect of oxygen tension should not be confused with the well known "oxygen effect" in radiobiological systems, where the presence of extremely hypoxic environments (i.e., less than 10^{-3}% O_2) protects against damage from ionizing radiation; the sensitizing effect of oxygen in such systems is saturated at relatively low oxygen tensions, 2%–3% O_2, which is well below the range in which the effect described here is observed. In addition, no radiation is involved in the clastogenic response of FA cells to oxygen.

The fact that chromosomal breakage rates in FA tend to be decreased at oxygen tensions lower than 20% O_2 strongly suggests that "spontaneous" chromosomal aberrations commonly observed in FA cells in vitro are in fact due to the relatively hyperoxic condition presented by an air-equilibrated environment. Since the oxygen tension existing in most tissues in situ is in the range 1%–5% O_2, it follows that the number of chromosomal aberrations occurring in vivo should be considerably lower than that observed in cultured cells. This is in agreement with the results obtained by Schmid (1967).

Just as seen with background breakage frequencies in standard lymphocyte cultures, a relatively large variation in oxygen sensitivity is observed from case to case and also in individual cases when analyzed on different occasions, so that the response to oxygen per se is not a reliable criterium for diagnosis of FA (Joenje and Oostra 1983). Part of the inconsistency might be due to the presence of clastogen-resistant cells that may develop in some unusual cases. For example, patient ST in Joenje and Oostra (1983), who exhibited a normal spontaneous aberration rate and no oxygen response, has now been identified as being completely clastogen-resistant in the lymphocyte culture test (Kwee et al. 1983; see also Arwert and Kwee, this volume; Auerbach, Rogatko and Schroeder-Kurth; Schroeder-Kurth et al., this volume). Another source of variation may originate from the rather strong antimitotic effect of high oxygen tension, which may prevent the most heavily affected cells from entering metaphase. There is indeed evidence that FA have a tendency to accumulate in the G_2 phase of the cell cycle (Kubbies et al. 1985), a phenomenon which, according to Hoehn et al. (this volume) is sensitive to oxygen tension.

In earlier studies, no effect of oxygen tension on chromosomal breakage was observed in 3-day cultures from healthy individuals. Using a culture medium with increased pH-buffering capacity, longer incubation times (4–7 days), and higher levels of oxygen (up to 60%), Joenje and Oostra (1986) recently showed that nor-

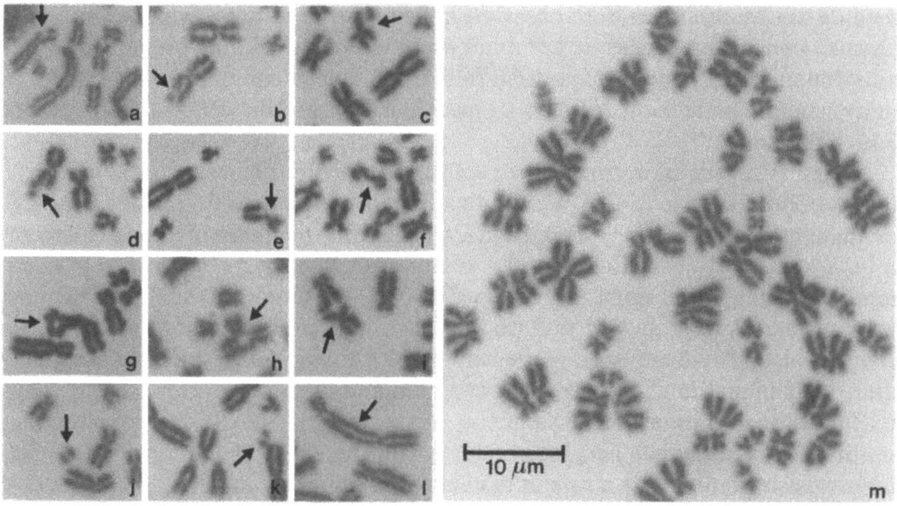

Fig. 1 a–m. Oxygen-induced cytogenetic abnormalities observed in normal human lymphocyte cultures chronically exposed (5–7 days) to 50%–60% oxygen. The pattern of aberrations closely resembles that observed in FA lymphocytes cultured for 3 days under air-equilibrated conditions (20% oxygen). **a, b** chromatid gaps; **c–f** chromatid breaks; **g–i** chromatid interchanges; **j, k** acentric fragments; **l** dicentric chromosome; **m** endoreduplicated cell with 40 diplochromosomes

mal human lymphocyte cultures also exhibit an increased chromosomal breakage rate in response to oxygen. Also, a remarkable increase in the frequency of endoreduplication was observed, a phenomenon that is seen in FA cultures already under standard (normoxic) culture conditions (Fig. 1). Thus in their response towards oxygen, the difference between FA and normal cells is not an absolute, but a relative one.

The observations discussed so far are consistent with the notion that FA cell types are deficient in some process intimately related to oxygen metabolism which in a normal cell affords protection against the cytogenetic toxicity of hyperoxia. The deficient process in FA may effect either the complex system that prevents excessive fluxes of endogenous reactive molecules (activated oxygen species, lipid peroxides, and aldehydes; see Dallapiccola et al. 1984, 1985) or the cellular components that determine the cells' capacity to tolerate oxygen-induced damage. This "tolerance" may involve either a repair process for damaged DNA, chromatin, or some other target, or another process enabling the cell to compensate for such damage. At the biochemical level, no DNA damage has thus far been identified as a result of cellular exposure to hyperoxia, as determined by the technique of alkaline elution (Seres and Fornace 1982). Further research will be required to elucidate to actual mechanisms involved.

One of the most striking features of FA cells is their extreme sensitivity to both the killing and chromosome-breaking effects of polyfunctional alkylating agents like mitomycin C. Joenje and Oostra (1983) showed that FA lymphocytes, after treatment with a low dose of mitomycin C in the G_0 phase of the cell cycle, are much more sensitive to the clastogenic effect of oxygen than without such treatment. A similar effect has been observed in lymphocyte cultures from normal individuals when using higher concentrations of mitomycin C, *cis*-platinum, or diepoxybutane (H. Joenje et al., unpublished data). This phenomenon may suggest a more general connection between oxygen metabolism and cellular tolerance to cross-link damage.

The toxic effects of hyperoxia are usually ascribed to the excessive production of superoxide radicals ($O_2^{\cdot -}$), which, through dismutation and Fenton chemistry, are thought to give rise to H_2O_2 and OH, respectively, the latter of which is known to be a particularly harmful agent. In addition, singlet oxygen ($^1O_2$) may play an important role (DiGuiseppi and Fridovich 1984). To find out which species may be of primary importance in the generation of chromosomal aberrations in FA, Joenje et al. (1986) determined the sensitivity of FA lymphocytes to the clastogenic effect of paraquat and streptonigrin, two compounds that are supposed to exert toxicity through intracellular production of $O_2^{\cdot -}$ (Fridovich 1978). No abnormal sensitivity was observed. This result, along with the effect of D_2O in FA (see below) suggests that $^1O_2$ has a role in the clastogenic process in FA.

Effects of Antioxidants

Several laboratories have documented an ameliorating effect of antioxidants on chromosomal aberrations in FA, which in principle could be the basis for treatment of the disease. A protective effect in lymphocyte cultures has been reported for SOD and catalase (Nordenson 1977), and for low molecular weight antioxidants such as glutathione and vitamin C (Dallapiccola et al. 1985). In a limited clinical trial, Izakovic et al. (1985) found a transient suppressing effect on the chromosomal breakage frequency in lymphocytes from two patients receiving SOD therapy. Nagasawa and Little (1983) found a remarkable protective effect of SOD on mitomycin C-induced cell killing of FA fibroblasts, whereas fibroblasts from controls were not protected. Using micronucleus formation as a measure for chromosomal breakage, Raj and Heddle (1980) observed a protective effect of SOD, catalase, and L-cysteine on spontaneous and mitomycin C-induced chromosomal breakage in FA, which was considered by the authors as "nonspecific" since a similar difference (in terms of percentage reduction) was observed in normal fibroblasts. However, as pointed out by Nagasawa and Little (1983), the absolute reductions were significantly greater in FA fibroblasts.

In contrast to these rather encouraging results, our laboratory has failed so far to observe a consistent ameliorating effect of a variety of antioxidants in FA lymphocyte cultures, including SOD (Table 1; cf. Auerbach et al. 1984). The discrepancy may be due to the fact that in the studies by Nordenson (1977) and Dallapiccola et al. (1985), medium 199 was used, whereas in our laboratory Ham's F10 medium is routinely used. One of the differences is that medium 199 is relatively low in folic acid content and is known to lead to higher spontaneous levels of chromosomal breakage than Ham's F10 medium (Keck and Emerit 1979). The conflicting data could thus be explained by assuming that the excess chromosomal damage observed with medium 199 is susceptible to treatment with antioxidants. A similar reasoning may apply to the protective effect against chromosomal break-

Table 1. Effect of antioxidants on spontaneous chromosomal breakage in FA-lymphocyte cultures[a]

Addition[b]	Final concentration	Metaphases with aberration(s) %	
		Minus	Plus
Superoxide dismutase + catalase	50 μg/ml of each	36	41
Nordihydroguaiaretic acid	10 μ*M*	22	24
Vitamin E	100 μg/ml	36	35
	20 μg/ml	22	19
	20 μg/ml	21	17
	10 μg/ml	36	37
Vitamin C	20 μg/ml	18	14
	20 μg/ml	19	35
Beta-carotene	50 μ*M*	21	23
	50 μ*M*	18	18
	50 μ*M*	19	27
Selenium (as sodium selenite)	0.1 μ*M*	21	18
	0.1 μ*M*	18	18
	0.1 μ*M*	19	17
	0.1 μ*M*	36	15
	2.5 μ*M*	18	16
	2.5 μ*M*	19	17
L-cystein	0.1 m*M*	18	16
	0.1 m*M*	19	12
Reduced glutathione	0.1 m*M*	18	25
	0.1 m*M*	19	23
Butylated hydroxytoluene	25 μg/ml	22	18

[a] Cultures were grown for 72-96 h at 20%-40% oxygen in the absence or presence of the indicated antioxidants, which were added at the time of culture initiation.
[b] Replicates were analyzed on separate occasions.

age in FA lymphocytes by cocultivation with normal lymphocytes (Nordenson et al. 1980), a phenomenon which could not be reproduced in our laboratory either (H. Joenje and A. B. Oostra, unpublished data). The above assumption should be tested experimentally.

A general difficulty in interpreting the absence of a protective effect of an antioxidant added to intact cells is that one usually does not know whether the critical cellular target is accessible to the compound. To overcome this problem, Joenje et al. (1983) have tested the effect of D_2O on chromosomal breakage in FA. D_2O as a solvent supports a drastically increased lifetime of $^1O_2$ and to a lesser extent of superoxide, and is rapidly exchanged with H_2O molecules in intact cells. The exposure of lymphocyte cultures to a medium in which H_2O is replaced by D_2O appeared to induce chromosomal breakage, to which FA lymphocytes were particularly sensitive. This indicates that $^1O_2$ or $O_2^{\cdot -}$ present at some stage in the aqueous compartment of the cell, may be involved in the generation of chromosomal

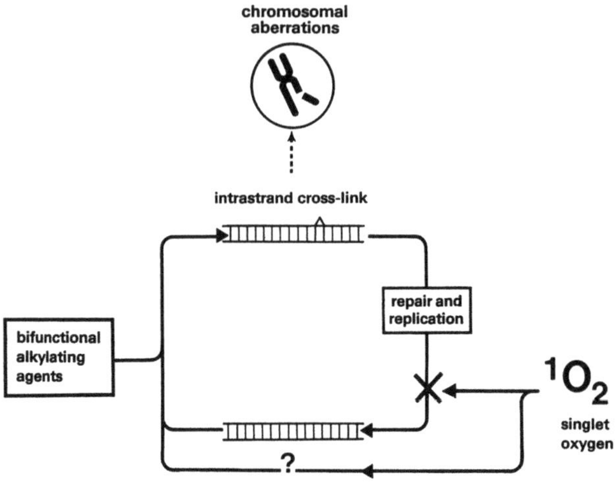

Fig. 2. Possible role of singlet oxygen ($^1O_2$) in the generation of chromosomal aberrations in FA. The evidence for a specific sensitivity of FA cells to the intrastrand type of DNA cross-links was reported by Poll et al. (1985)

breakage in FA. Since the normal sensitivity of FA cells to paraquat and streptonigrin (Joenje et al. 1986) indicates that $O_2^{\cdot -}$ is unlikely to act as an intermediate, $^1O_2$ is left as the most plausible candidate for inducing chromosomal breakage in FA. This extremely reactive oxygen species, which is known to be formed during normal metabolic reactions, has been shown to cross-link proteins (Goosey et al. 1980) and nucleic acids (Dubbelman et al. 1982) and is able to abolish the biological activity of DNA (Lafleur et al. 1987). To reconcile the involvement of $^1O_2$ with the effects of oxygen tension and polyfunctional alkylating agents in FA, we propose, as a working hypothesis, that in FA cells some function of the DNA repair/replication machinery normally involved in removal of cross-link damage is specifically sensitive to a $^1O_2$-driven process (Fig. 2). The FA mutation may effect this repair/replication function either by making it hypersensitive to normal fluxes of $^1O_2$ or by causing an abnormally high flux of $^1O_2$ for which the repair/replication function is intrinsically sensitive. Alternatively, $^1O_2$ may act directly on the DNA to produce a specific type of cross-link damage that is not well tolerated by an FA cell. Further research is required to elucidate the relationship between oxygen metabolism and chromosomal breakage in FA.

References

Abeliovich D, Cohen MM (1978) Normal activity and nucleoside phosphorylase, superoxide dismutase and catalase in skin fibroblast cultures from ataxia-teleangiectasia patients. Isr J Med Sci 14: 284–287

Auerbach AD, Sagi M, Carter DM (1984) Enhancement of carcinogen-induced chromosome breakage and sister chromatid exchange by 13-*cis*-retinoic acid. In: Hollaender A, Tice R (eds) International symposium on sister chromatid exchange: twenty-five years of experimental research. Plenum, New York, pp 333–341

Brown KW, Harnden DG (1978) Erythrocyte superoxide dismutase in ataxia-teleangiectasia and Fanconi's anaemia. Lancet 2: 1260

Cerutti P (1983) Prooxidant states and tumor promotion. Science 221: 375-381

Dallapiccola B, Magnani M, Novelli G, Mandelli F (1984) Increased activity of glutathione S-transferase and fast decay of reduced glutathione in Fanconi's anemia erythrocytes. Acta Haematol (Basel) 71: 143-144

Dallapiccola B, Porfirio B, Mokini V, Alimena G, Isacchi G, Gandini E (1985) Effect of oxidants and antioxidants on chromosomal breakage in Fanconi anaemia lymphocytes. Hum Genet 69: 62-65

DiGuiseppi J, Fridovich I (1984) The toxicology of molecular oxygen. CRC Crit Rev Toxicol 12: 315-342

Dubbelman TMAR, Van Steveninck AL, Van Steveninck J (1982) Hematoporphyrin-induced photooxidation and photodynamic cross-linking of nucleic acids and their constituents. Biochim Biophys Acta 719: 47-52

Fridovich I (1978) The biology of oxygen radicals. Science 201: 875-880

Gille JJP, Wortelboer HM, Joenje H (1987) Antioxidant status of Fanconi anemia fibroblasts. Hum Genet 77: 28-31

Gmyrek D, Syllm-Rapoport I (1964) Zur Fanconi Anaemie (FA). Analyse von 129 beschriebenen Fällen. Z Kinderheilkd 91: 297-337

Goosey JD, Zigler JS, Konoshita JH (1980) Crosslinking of lens crystallins in a photodynamic system: a process mediated by singlet oxygen. Science 208: 1278-1280

Izakovic V, Strbakova E, Kaiserova E, Krizan P (1985) Bovine superoxide dismutase in Fanconi anaemia. Therapeutic trial in two patients. Hum Genet 70: 181-182

Jalbert P, Leger J, Bost M, Bachelot C, Mouriquand C, Sele B, Frappat P (1975) Fanconi's anaemia: cytochemical and biochemical aspects. Nouv Rev Fr Hematol 15: 551-566

Joenje H, Eriksson AW, Frants RR, Arwert F, Houwen B (1978) Erythrocyte superoxide dismutase deficiency in Fanconi's anaemia. Lancet 1: 204

Joenje H, Frants RR, Arwert F, De Bruin GJM, Kostense PJ, Van de Kamp JJP, De Koning J, Eriksson AW (1979) Erythrocyte superoxide dismutase deficiency in Fanconi's anaemia established by two independent methods of assay. Scand J Clin Lab Invest 39: 759-764

Joenje H, Arwert F, Eriksson AW, De Koning H, Oostra AB (1981) Oxygen-dependence of chromosomal aberrations in Fanconi's anaemia. Nature 290: 142-143

Joenje H, Oostra AB (1983) Effect of oxygen tension on chromosomal aberrations in Fanconi anaemia. Hum Genet 65: 99-101

Joenje H, Oostra AB, Wanamarta AH (1983) Cytogenetic toxocity of D_2O in human lymphocyte cultures. Increased sensitivity in Fanconi's anemia. Experientia 39: 782-784

Joenje H, Oostra AB (1986) Oxygen-induced cytogenetic instability in normal human lymphocytes. Hum Genet 74: 438-440

Joenje H, Nieuwint AWM, Oostra AB, Arwert F, De Koning H, Roozendaal KJ (1987) Cytogenetic toxicity of paraquat and streptonigrin in Fanconi's anemia. Cancer Genet Cytogenet 25: 37-45

Keck M, Emerit I (1979) The influence of culture medium composition on the incidence of chromosomal breakage. Hum Genet 50: 277-283

Kubbies M, Schindler D, Hoehn H, Schinzel A, Rabinovitch PS (1985) Endogenous blockage and delay of the chromosome cycle despite normal recruitment and growth phase explain poor proliferation and frequent endomitosis in Fanconi anemia cells. Am J Hum Genet 37: 1022-1030

Kwee ML, Poll EHA, Van de Kamp JJP, De Koning H, Eriksson AW, Joenje H (1983) Unusual response to bifunctional alkylating agents in a case of Fanconi anaemia. Hum Genet 64: 384-387

Lafleur MVM, Nieuwint AWM, Aubry JM, Kortbeek H, Arwert F, Joenje H (1987) DNA damage by chemically generated singlet oxygen. Free Rad Res Commun 2: 343-350

Maral J, Puget K, Michelson AM (1977) Comparative study of superoxide dismutase, catalase and glutathione peroxidase levels in erythrocytes of different animals. Biochem Biophys Res Commun 77: 1525-1535

Mavelli I, Ciriolo MR, Rotilio G, De Sole P, Castorino M, Stabile A (1982) Superoxide dismutase, glutathione peroxidase and catalase in oxidative hemolysis. A study of Fanconi's anemia erythrocytes. Biochem Biophys Res Commun 106: 286-290

Nagasawa H, Little JB (1983) Suppression of cytotoxic effect of mitomycin-C by superoxide dismutase in Fanconi's anemia and dyskeratosis congenita fibroblasts. Carcinogenesis 4: 795-799
Nordenson I (1977) Effect of superoxide dismutase and catalase on spontaneously occurring chromosome breaks in patients with Fanconi's anemia. Hereditas 86: 147-150
Nordenson I, Bjoerksten B, Lundh B (1980) Prevention of chromosomal breakage in Fanconi's anemia by cocultivation with normal cells. Hum Genet 56: 169-171
Okahata S, Kobayashi Y, Usui T (1980) Erythrocyte superoxide dismutase activity in Fanconi's anaemia. Clin Sci 58: 173-175
Poll EHA, Arwert F, Joenje H, Wanamarta AH (1985) Differential sensitivity of Fanconi anaemia lymphocytes to the clastogenic action of *cis*-diamminedichloroplatinum (II) and trans-diamminedichloroplatinum (II). Hum Genet 71: 206-210
Raj AS, Heddle JA (1980) The effect of superoxide dismutase, catalase and L-cystein on spontaneous and on mitomycin induced chromosomal breakage in Fanconi's anemia and normal fibroblasts as measured by the micronucleus method. Mutat Res 78: 59-66
Scarpa M, Rigo A, Momo F, Isacchi G, Novelli G, Dallapiccola B (1985) Increased rate of superoxide ion generation in Fanconi anemia erythrocytes. Biochem Biophys Res Commun 130: 127-132
Schmid W (1967) Familial constitutional panmyelocytopathy, Fanconi's anemia (FA) II. A discussion of the cytogenetic findings. Semin Hematol 4: 241-249
Seres DS, Fornace AJ (1982) Normal response of Fanconi's anemia cells to high concentrations of O_2 as determined by alkaline elution. Biochim Biophys Acta 698: 237-242
Stocks J, Gutteridge JMC, Sharp RJ, Dormandy TL (1974a) Assay using brain homogenate for measuring the antioxidant activity of biological fluids. Clin Sci Mol Med 47: 215-222
Stocks J, Gutteridge JMC, Sharp RJ, Dormandy TL (1974b) The inhibition of lipid autoxidation by human serum and its relation to serum proteins and alpha-tocopherol. Clin Sci Mol Med 47: 223-233
Wever R, Oudega B, Van Gelder BF (1973) Generation of superoxide radicals during the autoxidation of mammalian oxyhaemoglobin. Biochim Biophys Acta 302: 475-478
Yoshimitsu K, Kobayashi Y, Usui T (1984) Decreased superoxide dismutase activity of erythrocytes and leukocytes in Fanconi's anemia. Acta Haematol (Basel) 72: 208-210.

Cellular Effects of Fanconi Anemia Genes and Their Correction by Microinjection*

E. Wunder, B. Fleischer, M. Gök, and Vijayalaxmi

Introduction

The great variation in the severity and pattern of clinical symptoms in nonconsanguinous patients with Fanconi anemia (FA) has puzzled most observers who have examined sizable groups of such patients. In addition to their hematological problems and usually rather small stature, they may present with diverse malformations of the skeleton (radius and thumb dysplasia being the most characteristic) and of many inner organs. It seems that this genetic condition can affect embryonal development at different sites and without precise targeting to any tissue or organ system. There are also cases without any recognizable malformation, and these patients come to medical attention only because of their pancytopenia.

Hematopoietic failure also shows strong individual variation in the age of onset and the course of the disease: it may start at birth or at any time later in life until about the third decade; episodes of hematopoietic failure are irregular and it generally varies in severity between hardly noticeable and severely disabling.

In view of all the phenotypic variations it is not easy to determine common factors that may relate them to underlying molecular disturbances; the only contention that can be made from clinical observations is that this genetic trait interferes with basic cellular functions which, under specific growth conditions during development and in hematopoiesis, control the proliferation and/or the differentiation of cells.

A first hint that true genetic variation contributes to the high phenotypic variability of the disease came from a comparison of nonconsanguinous families affected by FA: the age of onset of pancytopenia and the extent of the malformations within one sibship were similar, but they differed largely between sibships (Schroeder et al. 1976). Secondary processes and ambient exogenous factors may, in the individual organism, influence the clinical manifestation of the genetic condition to some degree. Because cells are closer to the origin of disturbances, cell behavior presumably reflects differences of the condition in unrelated patients more precisely, and could be a valuable source of further genetic and molecular information concerning underlying mutations.

The best known cellular manifestation is endogenous chromosome fragility in lymphocytes after short-term culture (Schroeder et al. 1964); since chromosome

* This study was largely supported by the Deutsche Forschungsgemeinschaft.

T. M. Schroeder-Kurth A. D. Auerbach G. Obe (Eds.)
Fanconi Anemia, Clinical, Cytogenetic and Experimental Aspects

breakage rates vary with time in the same individual, this manifestation, although genetic in origin, may be influenced by ambient factors in the organism.

The hypersensitivity of cells from patients with FA to treatment with bivalent mutagens is a further consequence of the defect. If fresh lymphocytes are derived from one individual on different occasions and are treated in vitro with 8-methoxypsoralen (8-MOP) plus long-wave ultraviolet light (UVA) under defined conditions, their clone survival rate can be easily reproduced, as we found in previous studies. While homozygous FA cells always demonstrated more sensitivity to the treatment than controls, the degree of hypersensitivity differed considerably among nonconsanguinous patients (Wunder and Fleischer-Reischmann 1983). In order to determine the range of values in homozygous and compare this with that in obligate heterozygotes and controls, this study was extended to large cohorts; one goal was to see whether, by this parameter, groups of FA mutations that showed clearly different degrees of hypersensitivity could be recognized.

The hypersensitive reaction to cross-linking agents allows precise measurement of the cellular reaction under defined in vitro stress conditions based on the damage caused. The molecular origin of this impaired response in FA cells is at present little understood. It may be related to a diminished capacity for cellular repair; it is tempting to hypothesize that a specific repair system for this type of DNA damage exists in humans and that FA is caused by mutations of genes pertaining to this mechanism. The analogous xeroderma pigmentosum (XP), another rare recessive human genetic disease, has brought evidence, that a UV excision repair system exists in man, which is indispensable for the protection of DNA against light damage. Several complementation groups, supposedly representing different mutated genes that are involved in this protection mechanism, indicate heterogeneity in XP. Comparison of FA with the paradigm of human "reparatoses" shows some differences, however. In XP, an early step in the excision repair of UV light damage in DNA provides a good explanation of the pathological events in the organism, which occur in the skin after exposure to sunlight. In contrast, the symptoms in patients with FA are apparent without any exposure to exogenous mutagens.

Accordingly, the abnormal endogenous functions in FA cells that appear under the near-physiologic conditions of in vitro cell culture may well correspond to manifestations in the organism such as disturbed hematopoiesis and malformations, which also stem from endogenously imbalanced functions. A second goal of our studies was therefore to study FA cells for such endogenous anomalies. The in vitro cloning efficiency of lymphocytes was assessed as an indicator, while the spontanous somatic mutation rate of lymphocytes was determined in order to monitor endogenous mutational events in vivo. Furthermore, specificity of the mutagen response with regard to DNA damage was assayed by comparison of the response toward treatment with cross-linking and noncrosslinking psoralens. Finally an attempt was made to correct the defect by supplementing mutant cells with the missing gene product or other component: replication recovery after treatment with 8-MOP plus UVA was restored by microinjection of extracts from functionally normal cells.

Cloning Efficiency of Phytohemagglutinin Stimulated Normal, Heterozygous, and Homozygous FA Lymphocytes

The cloning of peripheral blood lymphocytes is a more recent technique than that of fibroblasts. Lymphocyte growth depends not only on growth factors in the serum, but also on lymphokines, which are generated by mononuclear blood cells after stimulation (Pick 1987).

The cloning efficiency of FA +/+, FA +/−, and normal (−/−) T cells was tested using two different methods:

1. The phytohemagglutinin (PHA)-stimulated cells were suspended in complete medium containing agar and then placed in sterile glass capillaries as described previously (Wunder and Fleischer 1983). After incubation for 7-8 days, the number of clones was counted under a microscope.
2. Cloning efficiency was assessed under optimal growth conditions, with lymphocyte growth factors added in excess and in the presence of feeder cells. Stimulated cells were distributed at low density in 96-well microtiter plates; crude T cell growth factor (TCGF) plus interleukin-2 were added and highly γ-irradiated Daudi cells included. After 15 days of incubation, the number of wells in which cells were growing was determined, and cloning efficiency calculated according to Albertini et al. (1982).

As can be seen from Fig. 1 a (left part) and b, the cloning efficiency of homozygous cells without growth optimization was considerably decreased. The mean was about 30% less than the mean cloning efficiency in normal cells, and the distribution of individual values was homogenous. The heterozygous cells gave intermediate values.

This result is in agreement with the recent findings of Kubbies et al. (1985), which were made using a different method. Using BrdU-Hoechst flow cytometry, FA +/+ and normal lymphocytes were proliferated after stimulation with PHA and cultivation at the same cell density as used during the initial phase of our first method. The results of this study indicate that in FA +/+, cell recruitment, i.e., lymphoblastic transformation in response to PHA stimulation, occurs at a normal rate. Further proliferation of these cells was diminished by the arrest of about 24% of the growing cells during the first two cycles; concomitantly, the duration of the G_2 phase was markedly extended.

In comparison, under optimal growth conditions, as shown in the right part of Fig. 1 a, there are only minimal differences between the cloning efficiency of FA and normal cells. From the results, it seems that this endogenous impairment in FA lymphocytes can be compensated by adding appropriate growth factors, implying that these are involved in the impairment of proliferation and possibly cell cycle regulation by FA mutations.

Effect of FA Genes on Spontaneous Somatic Mutation Rates

The FA trait causes disturbances in postembryonic life, mainly in the bone marrow (apparent through periodical episodes of pancytopenia), the bone marrow also being predisposed to malignant transformation in patients with FA. Since the

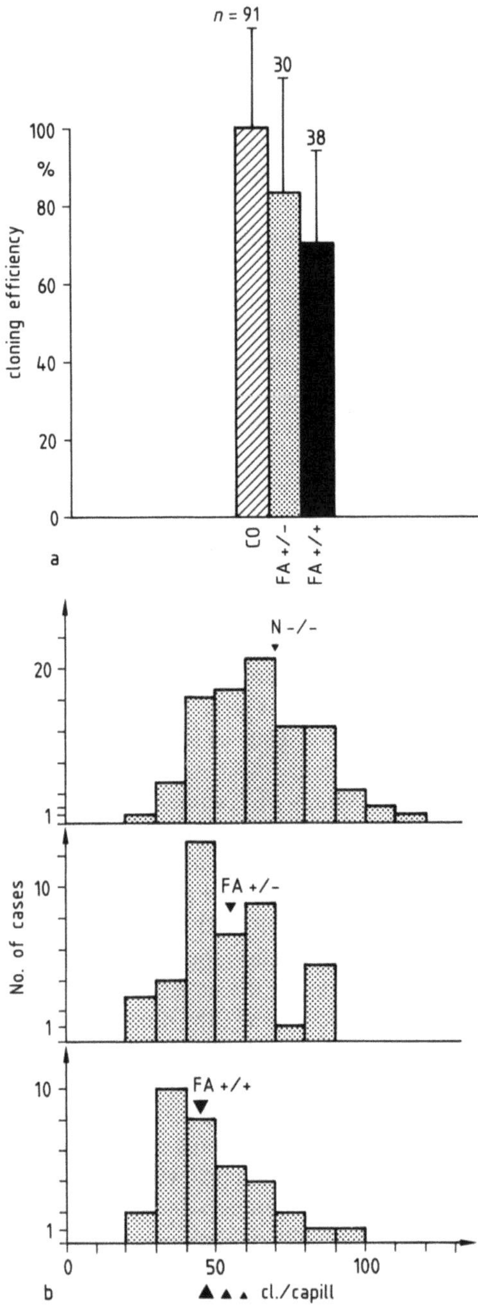

Fig. 1 a, b. The cloning efficiency of fresh peripheral lymphocytes after stimulation with PHA. **a** *(left)* Growth in agar, RPMI medium, and fetal calf serum (FCS) for 7-8 days without additional growth factors or feeder cells. *Columns* show mean values of 20 nonconsanguinous patients with FA *(FA^{++})* and 27 obligate heterozygotes (their parents, *FA^{+-}*), relative to 80 controls (*CO;* mean of controls, 100%). The *bars* above the columns indicate the standard deviation of the means. If the same case was examined twice, the mean of the two values was used. For technical details see

somatic mutation of genes which control cell differentiation plays a key role in this process, the question arises whether in blood cells, along with endogenous chromosome damage, increased spontaneous somatic mutation rates occur which could be monitored in suitable indicator genes.

In a first attempt to answer this question, the *H*ypoxanthine-*G*uanine-*P*hosphoribosyl-*t*ransferase (HGPRT) gene was chosen. The functional loss of enzyme activity was assessed and the spontaneous somatic mutation rates of thioguanine-resistant peripheral lymphocytes were compared in normal, heterozygous, and homozygous individuals (for technical details, see Vijayalaxmi et al. 1985). The results (Fig. 2) showed differences between nonconsanguinous individuals with FA; from a total of seven patients (including two previously studied patients), five had increased spontaneous somatic mutation rates, while two others did not. All obligate heterozygous parents showed rates within the range of age-matched controls. In the homozygous group, the mean value of the spontaneous somatic mutation rate was significantly elevated. For the two homozygous individuals who showed rates close to the mean of controls, two interpretations are possible: they either represent extreme values of a uniform distribution with overlap into the normal range, or the FA phenotype splits into two groups with regard to this parameter, one with increased and one with normal mutation rates.

Calculation showed that the estimated rate of spontaneous chromosome breaks with the potential to create terminal deletions at Xq, where the HGPRT locus is found, could account for the total increase in the mutation rate monitored in this way. That spontaneous point mutations, rearrangements, microdeletions, etc.,

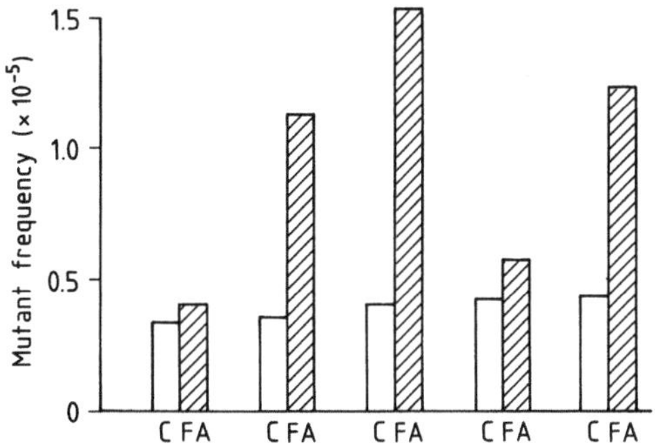

Fig. 2. Determination of the frequency of thioguanine-resistant peripheral lymphocytes, which is indicative of spontaneous somatic mutations; this was determined in five nonconsanguinous patients with FA *(FA)* and age-matched controls *(C)*. PHA-stimulated cells were cloned in microtiter wells containing feeder cells, growth factors, complete medium, and thioguanine. (From Vijayalaxmi et al. 1985)

Wunder and Fleischer (1983). *(right)* Growth in microtiter wells that contain, besides RPMI medium and FCS, γ-irradiated feeder cells (Daudi; 40 Gy), crude TCGF and interleukin-2. *Columns* show mean relative values of five nonconsanguinous patients with FA and five obligate heterozygotes (their parents) relative to ten controls. The *bars* indicate standard deviations of the mean. For technical details see Vijayalaxmi et al. (1985). **b** Distribution of the numbers of clones per capillary in the groups shown in **a** *(left)*. *Arrowheads* show means

are also increased, and contribute to inactivation of this indicator gene in the FA condition, is therefore less likely.

Effect of FA Genes on Cloning Survival of Lymphocytes After Treatment with a Cross-linking Psoralen

The influence of FA genes on the cellular response after mutagenic stress was investigated by treating PHA-stimulated lymphocytes with psoralens and UVA. After treatment, cells were suspended in agar, placed into open glass capillaries, and incubated for 7-8 days in 5% oxygen and 5% carbon dioxide at 37 °C; the proportion of surviving clones versus the proportion of clones from the untreated cells of the same donor was determined. As described elsewhere (Wunder and Fleischer 1983), the variation in the number of clones within different capillaries filled with identically treated cells was very small, indicating the high level of accuracy achieved with the method.

If psoralens are added to the medium, they rapidly pass through the cellular membranes, intercalating selectively into the DNA double helix, and after photoactivation with UVA form covalent adducts, which have a genotoxic effect (Vijayalaxmi and Wunder 1985). A special advantage of the psoralen familiy of mutagens, besides precise damage targeting, is the well-known chemical structure of DNA adducts, which react with thymidine in adenine-thymine-(AT)-rich regions (Sage and Moustacchi 1987). They first form monoadducts and if another thymidine is present in the opposite strand, at the adjacent position, bivalent psoralens such as 8-MOP can form cross-links in a second reaction.

After exposure to this mutagen, lymphoblasts from all patients with FA showed pronounced hypersensitivity, as shown in Fig. 3 a (left side) and b. The values showed an even distribution and the mean survival rate was about half of that seen in normal cells. There was also a wide range of interindividual differences among nonconsanguinous normal probands; a slight sex difference was seen, females being more sensitive, but age was apparently not a significant factor. (Further details will be published elsewhere.)

The mean of values found in heterozygous probands lay between that of controls and patients with FA. Thus, it can be concluded that just a slight decrease of the level of functional gene products of FA loci increases mutagen sensitivity under these experimental conditions. Response to this mutagen in our cohort showed no distinguishable classes in the degree of hypersensitivity that might be indicative for different types of underlying FA mutants.

Effect of FA Genes on Cloning Survival of Lymphocytes After Treatment with a Monovalent Psoralen

The hypersensitivity of FA cells to treatment with 8-MOP plus UVA corresponds to their hypersensitivity to other bivalent mutagens. These drugs are chemically completely different, and have in common only their ability to form DNA cross-links. Thus it may seem that the mutant cells are specifically unable to deal with

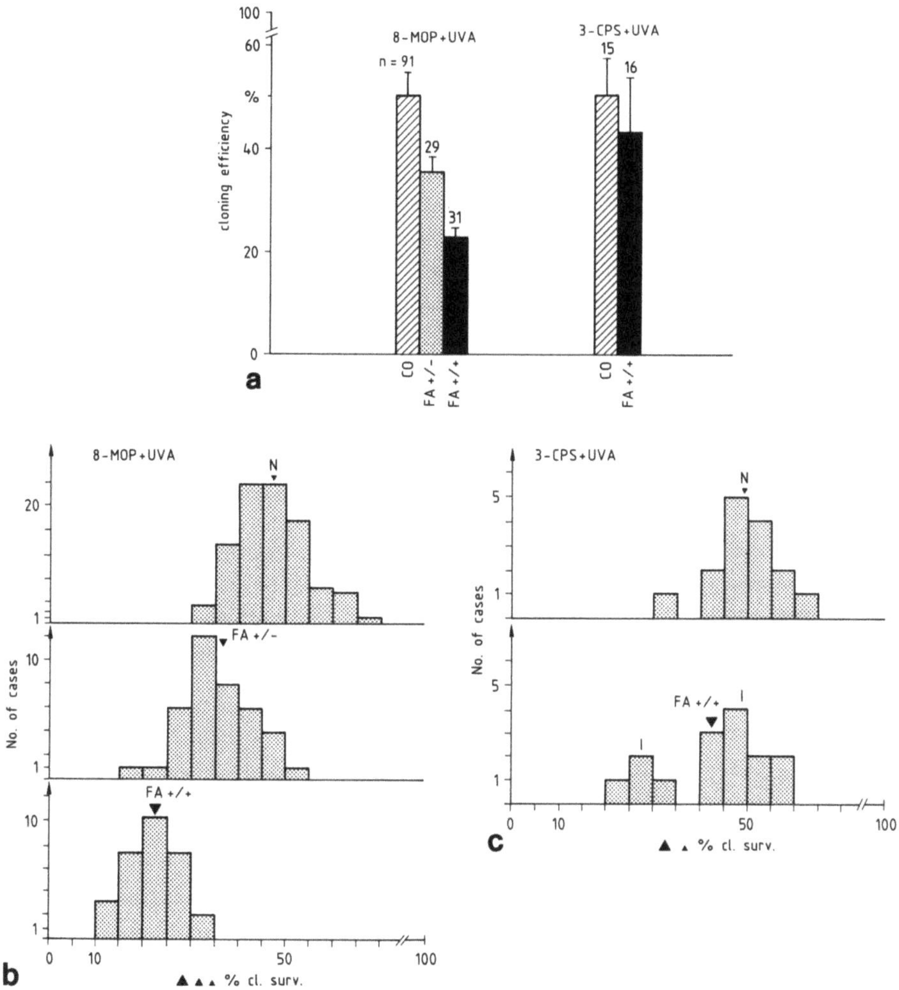

Fig. 3 a–c. The cloning survival rates of PHA-stimulated lymphocytes after treatment with (**a** *left*, **b**) bivalent 8-MOP plus UVA (0.02 μg/ml; 6 kJ/m^2) in 22 nonconsanguinous patients with FA, 28 obligate heterozygotes and 80 normal controls, and (**a** *right*, **c**) after treatment with monovalent 3-CPS plus UVA (equitoxic dose) in 14 of the nonconsanguinous patients with FA and 15 controls. If the same individual was tested twice, the mean of the two values was used. **a** *Columns* represent the mean of survival rates relative to the value in the untreated cells of the same individual (100%). *Bars* indicate the standard deviation. **b, c** Distribution of values (*arrow heads* show means) from individual probands belonging to the homozygous, heterozygous, and normal control groups. *Upright lines* indicate means of subsets

cross-links; however, because of the dependence of adduct formation on the DNA sequence discussed above, there is always a majority of monoadducts generated along with biadducts (cross-links), and there is no a priori guarantee that the hypersensitivity observed is exclusively due to the cross-links.

In order to analyze this, the cloning survival rates of lymphocytes taken from the same patients were tested after treatment with 3-carbethoxypsoralen (3-CPS), a psoralen analogue, which almost exclusively generates monoadducts. Since this substance tends to generate concomitantly free oxygen radicals during UVA irradiation, treatment was performed under low oxygen pressure (4%).

Our results (Figs. 3 a, right side, and 3 c) showed the mean of the FA cell values to be significantly lower than that of normal cells, indicating that FA genes are involved in the cellular reaction to monoadduct DNA damage. The extent of this impairment in the totalized values of the group with FA tested appeared to be smaller than that seen with 8-MOP plus UVA. The bimodal distribution of values, with a smaller fraction showing pronounced hypersensitivity and the remaining cases with values within the normal range, may mark a split phenotype, one subgroup of patients with FA showing increased sensitivity to 3-CPS + UVA monoadducts and the other not.

Correction of Defective Replication Recovery After 8-MOP plus UVA in FA Complementation Group A Cells by Microinjection

Analysis of replicative synthesis rates after treatment with 8-MOP plus UVA at a critical dose also revealed a split phenotype among cells derived from nonconsanguinous patients with FA (Fig. 4 a). After an initial decrease of nucleotide incorporation (phase I), which is common in normal individuals and in all cases of FA,

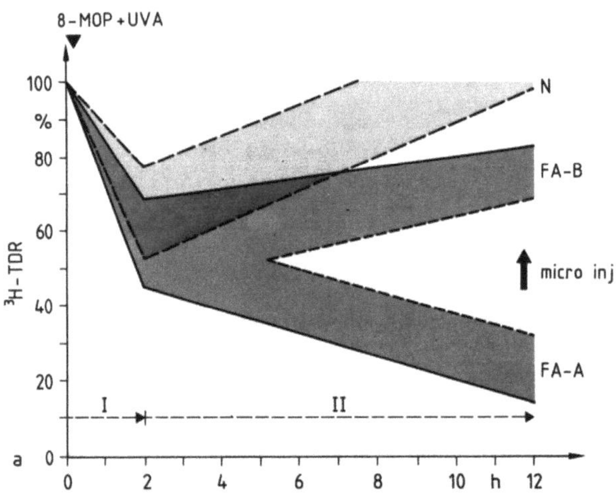

Fig. 4 a. Replicative DNA synthesis rate kinetics after treatment with 0.05 μg/ml 8-MOP plus activation by 6 kJ/m^2 UVA. Schematic capture of ranges as determined by autoradiography in six normal and seven FA skin fibroblast cultures derived from different individuals (scheme modified from Heise 1985). ^{3}H-TdR incorporation was assessed by a pulse for 30 min (for technical details see Gök and Wunder 1987). Phase *I* indicates the initial decrease of replication rates following 8-MOP plus UVA treatment; phase *II* shows recovery in normal cells, which reached pretreatment values after 12 h or sooner, while FA cultures showed a split phenotype: one group showed no recovery at this dose, while the other recovered in a similar way to do normal cells, the former type corresponding to complementation group A *(FA-A)*, the latter to group B *(FA-B)* according to Duckworth-Rysiecki et al. (1985). Phenotypic correction in FA(A) cells after microinjection of extracts involved restituting the recovery phase, as indicated by the *arrow*

adjacent (phase II) cells derived from some patients with FA showed recovery of incorporation similar to that in normal cells, while those from other FA patients lacked this recovery mechanism (Heise 1985; Moustacchi and Diatloff-Zito 1985). It has been shown that this functional difference is related to the complementation group; FA cell cultures without recovery belong to FA complementation group A [FA(A)] while the others belong to FA group B [FA(B)] (Moustacchi et al. 1987) as defined by Buchwald and coworkers (Duckworth-Rysiecki et al. 1985).

This defective function in FA(A) cells can be phenotypically corrected by microinjection of extracts from HeLa cells, as we reported recently (Gök and Wunder 1987); when the fibroblasts were injected prior to 8-MOP plus UVA treatment, they showed normal recovery (Fig. 4b, sections b and c). Injection of less than 20% cell equivalent was sufficient for complete correction. When the cells were injected 15 h prior to mutagen treatment, the function was still restored (Fig. 4b, section d). Thus it is evident that the activity which is missing in FA(A) cells is abundantly present in untreated normal cells and appears to have a rather slow turnover rate inside these cells.

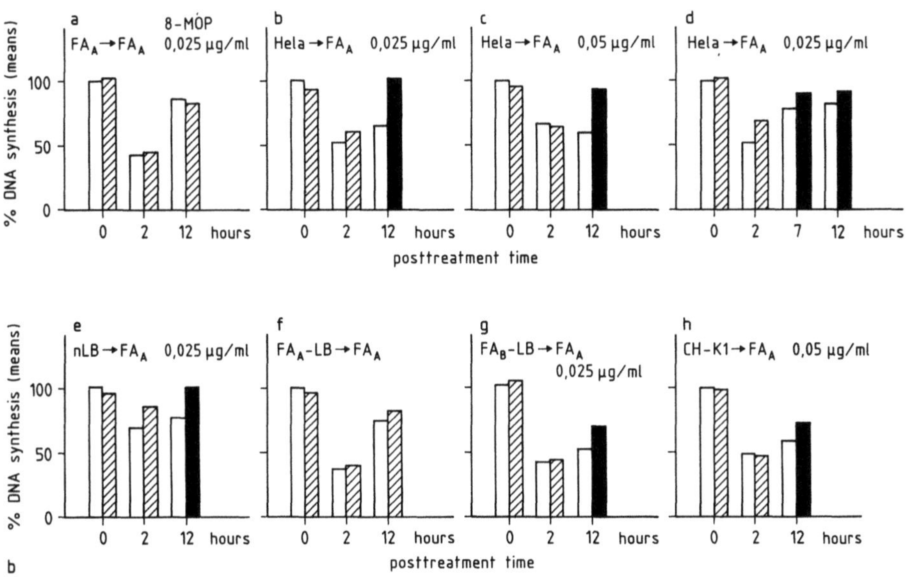

Fig. 4 b. Effect of microinjection of cellular extracts into FA(A) fibroblasts on replication recovery after treatment with 8-MOP plus UVA as illustrated in **a** (drug concentrations as indicated). *Columns* show the mean silver grain count of at least 25 cells relative to pretreatment values of uninjected cells. *Unhatched columns:* cells which were not microinjected. *Hatched columns:* microinjected cells which show no significantly different incorporation rate from that in noninjected but otherwise identically treated cells. *Shaded columns:* microinjected cells with significantly higher values (>95% confidence level) than uninjected and otherwise identically treated cells (internal controls). For technical details see Gök and Wunder (1987). Extracts *a* from FA(A) fibroblasts (negative control), *b-d* from HeLa cells, *e* from a normal human lymphoblastoid line *(nLB)*, *f* from an FA(A) lymphoblastoid line, *g* from an FA(B) lymphoblastoid line *(LB)*, *h* from chinese hamster K1 cells. In *d,* cells were incubated for 15 h prior to *P*soralen-*UVa* light (PUVA) treatment and in all other cases for 2 h

The function in FA fibroblasts can be restored by extracts from normal lymphoblastoid cells as well as by HeLa cell extracts (Fig. 4b, section e), indicating that this activity is not tissue-specific. Extracts prepared from FA(B) lymphoblasts correct recovery to a large degree, while those from FA(A), as expected, do not (Fig. 4b, sections f and g).

This factor is also present in cells from other mammals. Extracts from rodent cells have the potential to correct the defect (Fig. 4b, section h) which indicates some evolutionary conservation of this gene product, as in proteins that interact with specific spatial structures, either with DNA or with other proteins, to form functional complexes (Robson and Garner 1986).

Conclusion

Several endogenous and mutagen-dependent disturbances resulting from FA mutations were examined. While some of them were present in all cases, others were seen only in some of the cases of FA.

In a cohort of 22 nonconsanguinous FA patients, examined cells showed, without exception, decreased cloning survival rates after treatment with 8-MOP plus UVA, confirming that cellular hypersensitivity to this drug can be considered as pathognomonic for the FA trait, i.e., it is found regularly in patients who also display periodic pancytopenia of the FA type. The individual values representing the degree of hypersensitivity of our clinically unambiguous and cytogenetically confirmed cases of FA (all of them were also hypersensitive to DEB) extended over a considerable range and were evenly distributed, so that no phenotypic groups with clearly distinct ranges of hypersensitivity towards this mutagen could be distinguished among the patients examined.

The heterozygote group also showed decreased survival rates, the mean of which lay between that of homozygotes and controls. The reduction of the gene product level by mutation in one allele is evidently sufficient to affect cellular response towards this mutagen, while not precipitating hematological symptoms. Through individual testing, most of the heterozygotes could be identified, while others escaped detection, as their values fell in the zone of overlap with the values of controls.

The effect of FA genes on the cloning efficiency of stimulated lymphocytes, if they are cultured without the addition of growth factors and feeder cells, is also closely related to the gene dose, since the value for heterozygotes lies between that for homozygotes and controls. The observation that growth factors added in excess can compensate this defect shows that these proteins mediate the primary genetic defect to a mechanism involved in the control of proliferation and possibly of the cell cycle. The expression of growth factors after mitogenic stimulation may be insufficient in the cells of patients with FA.

It is possible that this effect is not limited to lymphocytes; proliferation and differentiation of bone marrow stem cells also depend on the adequate production of growth factors and the response to them (Dexter and Spooncer 1987). Although not all growth factors and their receptors in bone marrow stem cells are identical to those in mature lymphocytes, a decrease in proliferation in both of these may indicate that common functions are impaired, either in expression regulation of the respective genes, or in the intracellular transmission of their signals. Functional dissection of these components will be necessary for further, more detailed analysis. The decreased cloning efficiency and extended doubling time in FA fibroblasts (Schindler et al. 1986) may be related to the basic defect in a similar way.

Analysis of our results with regard to the hypothesis of a defect in cross-link repair as the central lesion in FA showed that the data are compatible with a decreased cellular capacity for DNA repair or for other cellular response mechanisms to DNA cross-links that influence cell survival after DNA damage, such as the replication of a damaged DNA template or associated cell cycle regulation. In one subgroup of patients with FA, an abnormal response to psoralen monoadducts was found, indicating that in this group, cross-links can not be the exclusive cause of primary damage in DNA that results in impaired processing. Cellular anomalies appearing without mutagen treatment show that the effects of FA mutations are not restricted to the DNA repair mechanism but also impair independent cellular functions as described above.

In cells ascribed to complementation group A, compensation of the disturbance of replication recovery after treatment with 8-MOP plus UVA by extracts from functionally normal cells shows that this function depends on a gene product that is constitutively expressed in abundant amounts in untreated normal cells. It is expressed independent of cell differentiation and is present in sufficient amounts in FA(B) cells.

Two hypotheses could account for the complex cellular phenotype in FA with endogenous and mutagen response defects, some of which are constantly present, while others are restricted to subgroups. First, the possibility cannot be excluded that more than one gene is involved. Closely neighboring but functionally independent genes can be frequently coinherited in a population and appear as one genetic entity. An example of this was recently found by Lehman et al. (1986) in a comparable genetic disease, ataxia-telangiectasia (AT). In cells from persons with AT increased radiosensitivity is found, and their replicative DNA synthesis is not reduced after irradiation as it is in normal cells. After the transfection of DNA from normal human cells into AT cells, a subline was recovered in which the increased radiosensitivity was restored, but the anomalous lack of reduction in DNA synthesis after irradiation persisted. Alternatively, if there is functional dependence or hierarchical regulation between genes, the inactivation of a downstream gene can leave other functions intact and lead to partial manifestation as compared with inactivation of the master gene.

The second possibility is that the underlying gene or genes code for multifunctional proteins which are involved in different subcellular mechanisms. Recently, several examples of this kind have been found in factors affecting transcription as well as replication, and also in growth factor-related protooncogenes affecting DNA synthesis and expression of sets of genes with special functions in proliferation, differentiation, and embryogenesis (Wagner and Müller 1986; Ohlsson and Pfeifer-Ohlsson 1987). Protooncogenes appear to be especially promising candidates in the further search for a method for the identification of FA genes, since disturbances in all these mechanisms form part of the natural history of this genetic disease. In addition, the involvement of some protooncogenes in cellular response to mutagen treatment is now becoming apparent (R. Becker, personal communication).

In summary, extensive information about the cellular phenotype in FA suggests that various subcellular mechanisms are disturbed. At present, the link between these mechanisms is not clear. Some of these are always impaired, others only in subsets of FA patients. Deficient replication recovery after treatment with 8-MOP plus UVA in complementation group A is a subcellular defective function that can be restored in the living mutant cell by microinjection of cellular extracts. Biochemical characterization of the restituting gene product may be the key to deciphering the underlying mechanisms.

Acknowledgements. We are greatly obliged to Prof. Schroeder-Kurth for referring to us, over a long period of time, FA families, diagnosed by cytogenetic analysis, and for reading the manuscript. We thank Dr. Auerbach as well as Dr. Moustacchi and Prof. Harris, for submitting the cell lines used in this study. Prof. Bisagni generously provided us with 3-CPS from his own synthesis, and we obtained highly purified 8-MOP from Dr. Averbeck. Finally, special thanks are due to Prof. Gruss and Dr. Brahms, who let us use their microinjection facilities.

References

Albertini RJ, Castle KL, Borcherding WR (1982) T-cell cloning to detect the mutant 6-thioguanine-resistant lymphocytes present in human peripheral blood. Proc North Acad Sci USA 79: 6617-6621

Dexter TM, Spooncer E (1987) Growth and differentiation in the hemopoietic system. Annu Rev Cell Biol 3: 423-441

Duckworth-Rysiecki G, Cornish K, Clarke CA, Buchwald M (1985) Identification of two complementation groups in Fanconi anemia. Somatic Cell Mol Genet 11/1: 35-41

Gök MM, Wunder E (1987) Microinjection of normal cell extracts into Fanconi anemia fibroblasts corrects defective scheduled DNA synthesis recovery after 8-methoxypsoralen plus UVA treatment. Hum Genet 75: 350-355

Heise J (1985) Untersuchungen des Mutageneffekts von 8-Methoxypsoralen und UVA bei reparaturkompetenten und reparaturdefizienten menschlichen Zellen. Dissertation, University of Heidelberg

Kubbies M, Schindler D, Hoehn H, Schinzel A, Rabinovitch PS (1985) Endogenous blockage and delay of the chromosome cycle despite normal recruitment and growth phase explain poor proliferation and frequent endomitosis in Fanconi anemia cells. Am J Hum Genet 37: 1022-1030

Lehmann AR, Arlett CF, Burke JF, Green MHL, James MR, Lowe JE (1986) A derivative of an ataxia telangiectasia (A-T)cell line with normal radiosensitivity but with A-T-like inhibition of DNA synthesis. Int J Radiat Biol 49: 639-643

Moustacchi E, Diatloff-Zito C (1985) DNA semi-conservative synthesis in normal and Fanconi anemia fibroblasts treatment with 8-methoxypsoralen and near ultraviolet light or with X-rays. Hum Genet 70: 236-242

Moustacchi E, Papadopoulo D, Diatloff-Zito C, Buchwald (1987) Two complementation groups of Fanconi's anemia differ in their phenotypic response to a DNA-crosslinking treatment. Hum Genet 75: 45-47

Ohlsson RI, Pfeifer-Ohlsson SB (1987) Cancer genes, proto-oncogenes, and development. Exp Cell Res 173: 1-16

Pick E (ed) (1987) Molecular cloning and analysis of lymphokines. Academic, New York (Lymphokines, vol 13)

Robson B, Garner J (1986) Introduction to proteins and protein engineering. Elsevier, Amsterdam, pp 314-344

Sage E, Moustacchi E (1987) Sequence context effects on 8-methoxypsoralen photobinding to defined DNA fragments. Biochem 26 (12): 3307-3314
Schindler D, Kubbies M, Hoehn H, Schinzel A, Rabinovitch PS (1987) Fanconi Anemia Mutation causes cellular susceptibility to ambient oxygen. Annual Meeting of the German and Austrian Societies of Hematology and Oncology, Würzburg, West Germany, Oct. 4-7, 1987. Blut 55 (4): 319
Schroeder TM, Anschütz F, Knopp A (1964) Spontane Chromosomenaberrationen bei familiärer Panmyelopathie. Humangenetik 1: 194-196
Schroeder TM, Tilgen D, Krüger J, Vogel F (1976) Formal genetics of Fanconi's anemia. Hum Genet 32: 257-288
Vijayalaxmi, Wunder E (1985) Comparison of sister-chromatid exchange induced by photoactivated 3-carbethoxypsoralen and 8-methoxypsoralen in human blood lymphocytes. Mutat Res 152: 211-215
Vijayalaxmi, Wunder E, Schroeder TM (1985) Spontaneous 6-thioguanine-resistant lymphocytes in Fanconi anemia patients and their heterozygous parents. Hum Genet 70: 264-270
Wagner EF, Müller R (1986) A role for protooncogenes in differentiation. In: Kahn P, Graf T (ed) Oncogenes and growth control. Springer, Berlin Heidelberg New York, pp 18-26
Wunder E, Fleischer B (1983) Response of lymphocytes from Fanconi's anemia patients and their heterozygous relatives to 8-methoxypsoralen in a cloning survival test system. Hum Genet 64: 167-172

Phenotypic and Genetic Heterogeneity in Fanconi Anemia, Fate of Cross-Links, and Correction of the Defect by DNA Transfection*

E. Moustacchi, D. Averbeck, C. Diatloff-Zito, and D. Papadopoulo

Introduction

The isolation and characterization of mutants unusually susceptible to DNA-damaging agents in prokaryotes and in lower eukaryotes helped considerably in the unraveling of the mystery of the genetic control mechanism and metabolic steps of DNA repair functions (for review see Friedberg 1985). The lack of available mutant cells defective in their response to DNA damage hampered for similar studies in human cells many years. The first indication of a DNA repair defect associated with an inherited human disease was found by Cleaver in 1968. The unusual sensitivity to sun of fibroblasts from a patient with the disease xeroderma pigmentosum (XP) was found to be associated with an excision defect of DNA lesions. This observation stimulated great interest in examination of the response to DNA-damaging agents in the cells from patients with a number of other hereditary diseases, particularly those associated with chromosomal abnormalities and with a high incidence of neoplasia (for reviews see Friedberg et al. 1979; Hanawalt and Sarasin 1986). Since then, a number of diseases other than XP have been shown to be abnormal in their response to DNA-damaging agents. It should be kept in mind, however, that an abnormal sensitivity of cells to killing by physical and/or chemical agents interacting with DNA does not necessarily imply a specific defect in DNA repair. An imbalance in DNA biosynthesis and replication, membrane defect(s) interfering with nuclear function(s), the abnormal production of endogenous metabolic products that damage DNA, or mitochondrial susceptibility to agents may create increased cellular sensitivity.

Fanconi anemia (FA), an inherited disorder in humans (Fanconi 1967; Schroeder et al. 1976; Schroeder 1982), belongs to the class of diseases possibly linked to deficiencies in the processing of DNA lesions. Cells from individuals with FA have, among other features discussed in this book, an increased sensitivity to agents that cause interstrand DNA cross-links such as mitomycin C (MMC) bifunctional nitrogen mustards, diepoxybutane (DEB), and photoactivated psoralens (Sasaki and Tonomura 1973; Auerbach and Wolman 1976; Weksberg et al. 1979; Ishida and Buchwald 1982). These cells are reported to be only marginally

* This work was financially supported by the CNRS (UA 533), the CEA (Saclay, France), the ARC (Villejuif, France), INSERM (contract no. 852017) and the CEE, Brussels (contract no. B16-151-F).

T. M. Schroeder-Kurth A. D. Auerbach G. Obe (Eds.)
Fanconi Anemia, Clinical, Cytogenetic and Experimental Aspects

susceptible to DNA damage induced by monofunctional alkylating agents or by ultraviolet (UV) or ionizing radiation (Sasaki and Tonomura 1973; Finkelberg et al. 1974; Duckworth-Rysiecki and Taylor 1985; Klocker et al. 1985; Lam and Reynolds 1986). On the basis of the more or less specific cellular and chromosomal hypersensitivity of FA to DNA cross-linking agents as well as on the basis of biochemical studies, it was claimed that FA cells are defective in DNA cross-link recognition (Fujiwara et al. 1979; Fujiwara 1982) and/or processing. However, the role and nature of defective DNA repair in this disease is still controversial (Fornace et al. 1979; Kaye et al. 1980; Poll et al. 1984; Gruenert et al. 1985).

We have therefore considered this problem by first attempting to classify the FA cell lines phenotypically, using a parameter related to DNA repair. In XP, nine different complementation groups with different levels of excision repair inhibition of UV-induced lesions have been identified (for review see Friedberg 1985). Several genetic complementation groups have also been found in ataxia telangiectasia (Jaspers and Bootsma 1982; Murnane and Painter 1982) and in Cockayne's syndrome (Lehmann 1982), which are other diseases involving anomalies in the repair processing of DNA damage. These findings, together with the wide spectrum of symptoms (Glanz and Fraser 1982; Duckworth-Rysiecki et al. 1984) and the wide range of the age of onset of hematological problems in FA, suggest that a phenotypic and genetic heterogeneity could underlie the response of DNA cross-linking agents in FA. The results presented here show that this is indeed the case. Subsequently, in order to specify the possible defect in DNA repair, the fate of DNA-induced cross-links in FA cells from genetically and phenotypically well-defined cell lines was compared to that of normal cells using the alkaline elution procedure. Differences among FA cell lines are reported here. Finally, since almost nothing is known about the chromosomal location, expression, and regulation of the genes controlling the sensitivity of human cells to DNA cross-linking agents, a project aiming at the isolation of such genes was initiated. Conditions for DNA-mediated transfer and the expression of wild-type genes in FA cell lines were established. The characterization of the transformed cells obtained will be described here.

Phenotypic and Genetic Classification of FA Cell Lines

The treatment of normal mammalian cells with a variety of DNA-damaging agents results in a dose-dependent reduction in the rate of DNA semiconservative synthesis, as measured by the incorporation of radiolabeled thymidine (Painter 1977). This transient inhibition of DNA synthesis is due to a decreased rate of replicon initiation and/or fork progression caused by the presence of lesions in DNA (for review see Painter 1986). It is followed, in normal cells, by a recovery of the DNA synthesis rate with time, provided that the dose used is not so high as to cause a permanent block (Rudé and Friedberg 1977). This recovery phase is thought to reflect the time needed to repair or bypass DNA lesions. It does not take place after the treatment of excision-deficient XP (Rudé and Friedberg 1977) or of UV-sensitive but excision-proficient Cockayne's syndrome cells with 254 nm UV (Lehmann et al. 1979).

We studied the effect of treatment with 8-methoxypsoralen (8-MOP) plus near-UV radiation (365 nm or UVA) on semiconservative DNA synthesis in 21 FA fibroblast cell lines from patients of different geographic origin compared with two obligate heterozygous cell lines and four normal lines. This study was extended to lymphoblastoid cell lines. 8-MOP was chosen as a cross-linking agent because it is known to photobind almost specifically to the pyrimidine bases in DNA, forming defined monoadducts and interstrand cross-links (for review see Song and Tapley 1979).

Figure 1 A shows how the rate of DNA synthesis in normal human fibroblasts decreased immediately after 8-MOP photoaddition and continued to decrease for about 3-4 h. This decline was followed by a recovery which began 4 h after treatment and reached a maximum at about 10 h. The extent of inhibition, the delay in recovery, and the maximum value attained were dose-dependent. It should be noted that for doses above 4.5 kJ m^{-2} the recovery was not observed in normal fibroblasts. Figure 2 shows that normal lymphoblasts respond in the same manner as fibroblasts. However, the concentration of 8-MOP, using the same UVA incident dose necessary to reach the same level of inhibition is five times lower in lymphoblasts than in fibroblasts. The same difference between cell types is also observed in clonogenic cell survival (Papadopoulo, data not shown). FA heterozygotes cannot be distinguished from normal cells according to the rates of DNA semiconservative synthesis, measured after 8-MOP plus UVA treatment (Fig. 1 B) although they demonstrate a level of clonogenic cell survival which lies between that of normal individuals and that of FA homozygotes (Wunder and Fleischer 1983; Fig. 3).

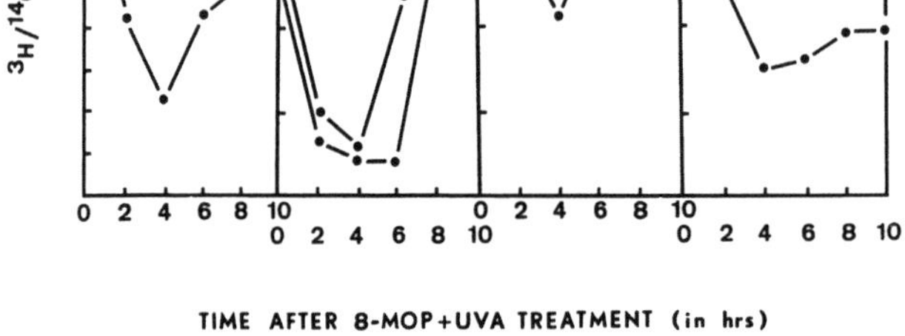

Fig. 1 A–D. Rates of semiconservative DNA synthesis in human fibroblasts as a function of time after treatment with 8-MOP (10^{-5} *M*) and a dose of 3.6 kJ.m^{-2} UVA. Rates of DNA synthesis were measured after 30-min pulses of ^3H-thymidine as a function of time. Cells were prelabeled with ^{14}C-thymidine for 24 h. Rates determined by liquid scintillation spectrometry are expressed as the $^3H/^{14}C$ ratio of treated over untreated samples. For details, see Moustacchi and Diatloff-Zito (1985). Rates **A** in a normal cell line (Jacquot), **B** in two FA heterozygous cell lines (F 311 and F 253), **C** in an FA cell line belonging to complementation group B according to Duckworth-Rysiecki et al. (1985), **D** in an FA cell line belonging to complementation group A according to Duckworth-Rysiecki et al. (1985)

When 21 FA fibroblastic cell lines were examined for DNA synthesis as a function of time after treatment with the highest UVA dose (3.6 kJ m^{-2}, after which a recovery of DNA synthesis was still seen in normal and heterozygous cell lines), two classes of FA lines could be distinguished. The first class included 15 cell lines which were almost indistinguishable from normals; 10 h after treatment they had recovered a normal rate of semiconservative DNA synthesis. A cell line representative of this type of response is shown in Fig. 1C. In the second class, which included six FA cell lines, such a recovery was not observed even 24 h after treatment (see Fig. 1D for a typical response). Figure 2 shows that FA lymphoblasts can also assigned to the same two classes in terms of DNA synthesis.

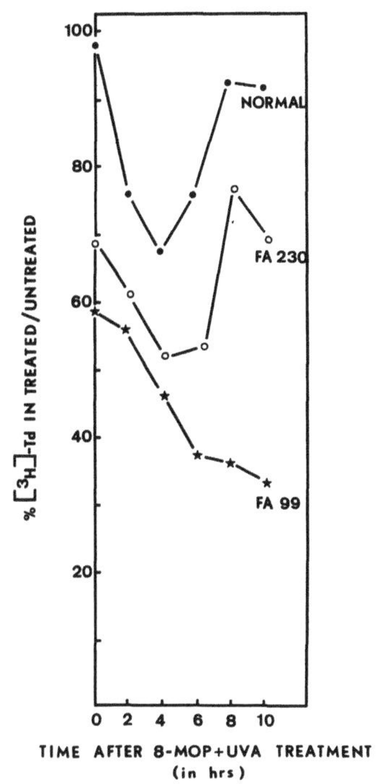

Fig. 2

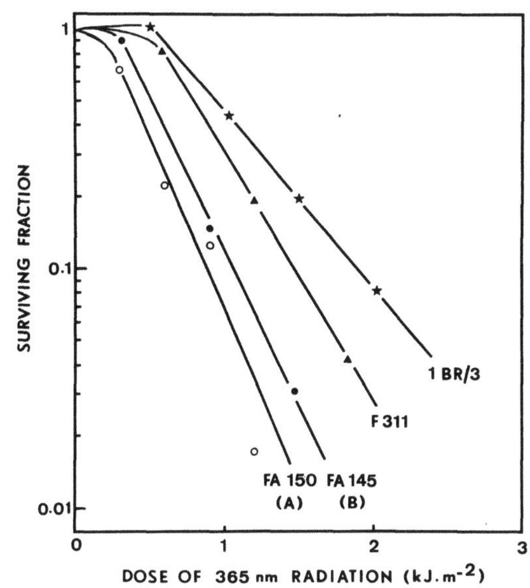

Fig. 3

Fig. 2. Rates of semiconservative DNA synthesis in human lymphoblasts as a function of time after treatment with 8-MOP (5.10^{-6} *M*) and a dose of 1.2 kJ.m^{-2} UVA. A lymphoblastoid strain of normal origin Priess (●) was provided by W. Bodmer (University of Oxford); FA 230 (○) belongs to complementation group B and was derived from the same patient as the fibroblast cell line 1199; FA 99 (★) belongs to group A and was derived from the same patient as the fibroblast cell line 402. Treatment of cells was as in Fig. 1 but labeling of parental DNA with ^{14}C-thymidine was omitted since the same number of cells in suspension, as determined by hemocytometer countings, were treated. For technical details, see Moustacchi et al. (1987)

Fig. 3. Clonogenic cell survival to 8-MOP (10^{-5} *M*) as a function of the UVA dose. 1 BR/3 (★) is the normal cell line, provided by C. Arlett (University of Sussex); FA 150 (○) belongs to complementation group A; FA 145 (●) belongs to complementation group B according to phenotypic classification; the 311 cell line (▲) is an FA heterozygote

Genetic heterogeneity within FA has recently been demonstrated by complementation analysis of somatic cell hybrids constructed from FA lymphoblastoid cell lines. The presence of at least two complementation groups was demonstrated through the measurement of growth inhibition by the DNA cross-linking agent MMC and of spontaneous and MMC-induced chromosomal breakage (Duckworth-Rysiecki et al. 1985). In fact, the two genetic complementation groups A and B in FA correspond to the two phenotypic classes described above. The two fibroblastic cell lines 145 and 1199 and the lymphoblastoid cell line 230 (derived from the same patient as the fibroblast cell line 1199), which belong to complementation group B (Duckworth-Rysiecki et al. 1985), showed a response to 8-MOP plus UVA similar to that of normal cell lines (Fig. 2). In contrast, the two fibroblastic cell lines 156 and 402 and the lymphoblastoid cell line 99 (derived from the same patient as the fibroblast cell line 402), belonging to complementation group A (Duckworth-Rysiecki et al. 1985), did not recover a normal rate of DNA synthesis even 24 h after treatment by 8-MOP plus UVA (Fig. 2).

The recovery of normal rates of DNA synthesis in normal and FA group B cells is not a consequence of an increased proportion of cells synthesizing DNA, as observed after treatment with MMC (Claassen et al. 1986). A recovery similar to that observed in the population of normal cells and not exceeding the values found in untreated cells is observed for at least 12 h after 8-MOP photoaddition when the proportion of cells in S phase is measured by autoradiographic grain counting in individual cells. Our results clearly indicate that the measurement of semiconservative DNA synthesis after cross-linking treatment constitutes a rapid and reliable test allowing classification of FA patients into classes which correlate with the two genetic complementation groups identified by complementation studies (Moustacchi et al. 1987).

Mutants with increased sensitivity to the lethal effects of MMC and 8-MOP photoaddition have been isolated from mouse lymphoma L5178Y cells by a replica-plating technique (Hama-Inaba et al. 1983; H. Hama-Inaba, personal communication). These mutants are not sensitive to UV radiation, X-rays, 4-nitroquinoline-1-oxide, or methylmetane sulfonate. They have been assigned to at least two genetic complementation groups denominated $MC^{S}I$ and $MC^{S}II$ (Hama-Inaba et al. 1983). Apparently such mouse-cell mutants share many features with FA cells. We followed the DNA semiconservative synthesis after 8-MOP photoaddition in normal, $MC^{S}I$, and $MC^{S}II$ mutant cells. As seen in Fig. 4, normal and $MC^{S}II$ cells are almost indistinguishable with respect to this parameter: the inhibition of DNA synthesis is followed by recovery to an almost normal rate. In contrast, lymphoblastoid mutant cells belonging to the complementation group $MC^{S}I$ do not demonstrate such a recovery phase, even 24 h after treatment. This behavior is similar to that of FA cell lines belonging to groups B and A, respectively. In both human and mouse cells, mutants hypersensitive to DNA cross-linking agents demonstrate similar phenotypic patterns with respect to DNA semiconservative synthesis after a DNA-damaging treatment. Thus, it will be of interest to establish, by interspecies somatic hybridization, whether or not there is a similarity between the mouse and human gene mutations.

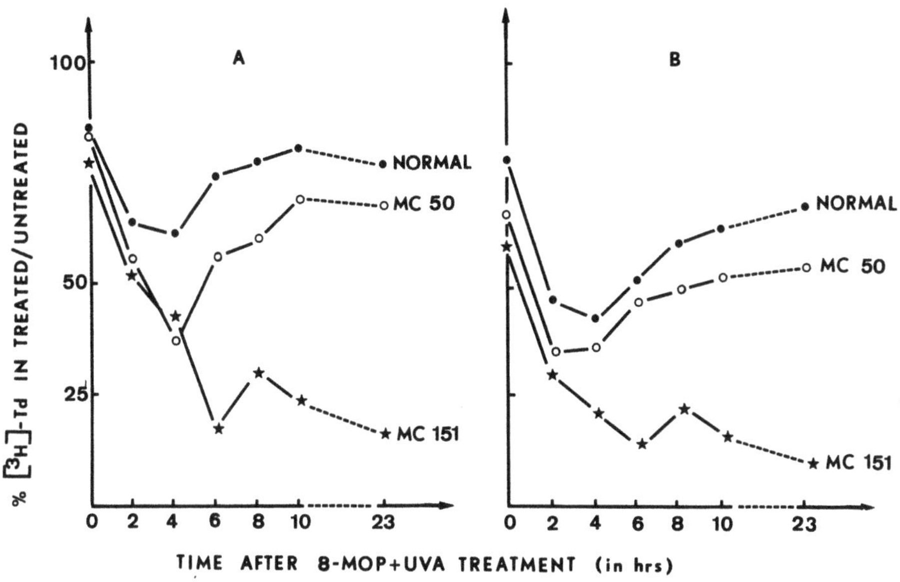

Fig. 4. Rates of semiconservative DNA synthesis in mouse lymphoma cell mutants as a function of time after treatment with 8-MOP (5.10^{-6} *M*) and a dose of **A** 1.2 $kJ.m^{-2}$ or **B** 2.4 $kJ.m^{-2}$ UVA. The normal cell line (●) is L51; MC 50 (○) is a mutant belonging to complementation group $MC^{S}II$ (Hama-Inaba et al. 1983); MC 151 (★) is a mutant belonging to complementation group $MC^{S}I$ (Hama-Inaba et al. 1983). Cells grown in RPMI (5.10^5 cells/ml) plus 10% serum were pulse-labeled for 30 min with 4 μCi/ml ^{3}H-thymidine (specific activity 80 Ci/m*M*) immediately after treatment with 8-MOP (15 min incubation in the dark) and two doses of UVA, and every 2 h during posttreatment incubation. Incorporation of ^{3}H-thymidine was stopped by adding 40 μg/ml of cold thymidine. Cells were collected on GF/C Whatman filters, thoroughly washed with cold phosphate-buffered solution (PBS), 5% trichloracetic acid, and cold methanol. The dried filters were counted in a toluene-based scintillation mixture. Untreated controls were processed in parallel

8-MOP Photoinduced DNA Cross-Links in FA Cells

Both cell survival and induction and repair of DNA cross-links after 8-MOP photoaddition were compared in normal and FA cell lines. In terms of clonogenic cell survival, FA cells belonging to complementation group A were found to be twice as sensitive to 8-MOP photoaddition as normal cells, whereas the level of sensitivity of FA cells from group B lay between the two (Fig. 3). A cell line derived from an obligate heterozygote parent of patient with FA was slightly more sensitive than a normal cell line (Fig. 3). Although Fig. 3 represents only one cell line for normal and heterozygote genotypes, this has been confirmed using two other normal and one other FA heterozygote cell lines (data not shown). In accord with the results obtained by others (Weksberg et al. 1979), the differential sensitivity of FA cells as compared with that of normal cells is less pronounced after the photoaddition of psoralens than after treatment with MMC or DEB. The reason for the difference in the killing efficiency of these different agents is still unknown. DEB is a directly acting agent that reacts mainly at the N7 of guanine, and a cross-link between the N7 of two guanines on two strands of the DNA double helix occurs readily. Interactions of DEB with glutathione synthetase have been reported (Boyland and Williams 1965). MMC requires metabolic activation to reactive species to produce interstrand cross-linking between the O6 of guanines. Moreover, various oxygen species such as superoxide, hydrogen peroxide, and hydroxyl radicals are generated by MMC, leading to a variety of adducts (Pritsos and Sartorelli 1986). In contrast, in the case of psoralens, cross-links and monoadducts are directly photoinduced on pyrimidines and, at least with regard to the cytotoxicity of 8-MOP, an oxygen effect appears to be absent. In summary, the enzymatic composition and metabolic activity of cells can affect the reactivity of MMC or DEB while these parameters do not interfere with the photoreactivity of psoralens. In addition, it has to be borne in mind that, for these three agents, not only the chemical nature of the adducts induced but also the ratio of monoadducts to cross-links, differ greatly. The genetic defect in FA cells is clearly pleiotropic. The hypersensitivity to MMC and DEB, which is extremely useful for the diagnosis of FA or for selection (see below) may reflect differences in both the enzymatic reducing systems and in the capacity for DNA cross-link repair in FA as opposed to in normal cells. This is why, in our repair studies, we preferred to analyze cross-links induced by psoralens plus UVA. Moreover, the pyrimidine-pyrimidine cross-links formed by 8-MOP and UVA are resistant to the periods of alkali treatment necessary for DNA denaturation, whereas the purine-purine MMC-induced cross-links are known to be alkali-labile.

The induction and incision of cross-links were followed by alkaline elution according to Kohn et al. (1976). Normal and FA cells were labeled for 24 h with ^{14}C-thymidine and treated with 8-MOP plus UVA; the size of DNA was reduced by X-ray treatment. An internal standard of ^{3}H-labeled DNA from X-irradiated cells was included in all experiments. The fraction of ^{14}C-labeled DNA retained on the filter indicated the presence of DNA interstrand cross-links. Lower retention following posttreatment incubation indicated the incision of cross-links.

For the same doses of 8-MOP plus UVA, about the same amount of cross-linking was induced in both normal and FA (complementation groups A and B) cell lines, fibroblasts, and lymphoblasts. After 6 h of posttreatment incubation, about 60% of the cross-links were incised in normal fibroblasts, whereas only about 32% of the cross-links were incised in fibroblasts from patients FA 150 and FA 402, belonging to complementation group A (Fig. 5). After 24 h of posttreatment incubation, further incision of cross-links was observed in the FA cells of both groups A and B (Fig. 5, Table 1), the final level remaining, however, below that of normal cells. Lymphoblastoid cell lines derived from the same patients appeared to follow the same pattern as the fibroblasts (Table 1). When a monofunctional agent such as 3-carbethoxypsoralen (3-CPS) was used, there was no change in the elution profile during posttreatment incubation (data not shown). This indicates that in this case the incision of monoadducts did not contribute to the changes in profiles observed after treatment with 8-MOP plus UVA.

FA cells demonstrate a certain capacity for cross-link incision. However, they exhibit slower repair kinetics and lower levels of cross-link incision than normal cells, group A cell lines being more affected than those of group B. It is of interest to note that using a variety of biochemical approaches, XP cells belonging to com-

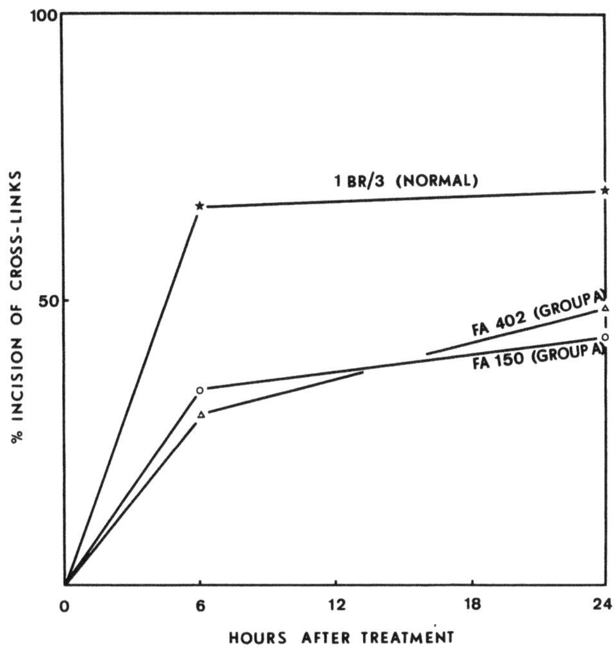

Fig. 5. Incision of induced DNA cross-links in normal and FA cells as a function of incubation time after treatment with 8-MOP (10^{-5} *M*) and a dose of 3.6 kJ.m^{-2} UVA. Data derived from alkaline elution kinetics, determined as a function of the ^{14}C-labeled DNA retained on the filter (Kohn et al. 1976)

Table 1. Percentage of cross-links incised in normal and FA cells after 24 h (fibroblasts) or 6 h (lymphoblasts) of posttreatment incubation as measured by alkaline elution

	Normal (%)	FA group B (%)	FA group A (%)
Fibroblasts	50	39	25
Lymphoblasts	44	34	9

The data represent individual experiments.

plementation group A were found to be completely defective in the incision of both monoadducts and cross-links (Kaye et al. 1980; Gruenert and Cleaver 1985). Therefore the biochemical defect in FA is not comparable to that observed in XP complementation group A.

In summary, at variance with the results of Fujiwara et al. (1979) and Fujiwara (1982), we find that the major defect in FA, even in complementation group A, is not a complete deficiency in cross-link repair. This appears to be true at least in a range of doses of biological significance (survival range approx. 0.01%–1%). This is confirmed by a double irradiation experiment in which, after a first UVA dose, the unbound 8-MOP is washed out and cells are reirradiated. This protocol allows comparison of different amounts of cross-linking for a total constant number of lesions (monoadducts plus cross-links). In this case FA cells are also able to incise cross-links (data not shown).

Analysis of data on semiconservative DNA synthesis and alkaline elution after 8-MOP photoaddition shows that, at least in group A, although cross-links are incised, the DNA initiation and/or elongation is hampered. This indicates that the substrate left for the DNA polymerase after slow incision is unsuitable for polymerizing. Moreover, it has been reported that the frequency of sister chromatid exchange (SCE) induced by 8-MOP plus UVA is higher in the FA cell lines than in normal fibroblasts (Billardon and Moustacchi 1986). SCE production involves the interchange of DNA duplexes between damaged chromatids followed by ligation. Thus, the slower kinetics of incision of cross-links, the absence of recovery of a normal rate of DNA synthesis, and the hypersensitivity to SCE induction by bifunctional psoralens are likely to reflect a diminished capacity of DNA cross-link processing in FA group A cells. At this stage, it is not possible to decide if one of the gene products (or cofactors) needed for completion of the whole incision-excision process is missing or if the regulatory control of a repair pathway is defective in FA cells. That FA group B cells have a repair defect is perhaps even more questionable. In fact, such cells are able to recover a normal rate of semiconservative DNA synthesis, whereas they demonstrate relatively slow cross-link incision kinetics, and they are hypersensitive to SCE induction by 8-MOP photoaddition (Billardon and Moustacchi 1986). This seems to be an enigma like the one in the case of Cockayne's syndrome, in which UV sensitivity is associated with an apparently normal excision-repair capacity (Mayne et al. 1982). It is clear that other molecular methods will have to be applied in order to resolve these problems.

Correction of the Abnormal Response of FA Fibroblasts to DNA Cross-Linking Agents by Transfection with Normal Human DNA

The approach using DNA-mediated human gene transfer into Chinese hamster ovary (CHO) mutant cells, and the selection at the same time of a cotransfected, cloned bacterial gene (Rubin et al. 1983, 1985; Westerveld et al. 1984) allowed the cloning of a human DNA-repair gene (Rubin et al. 1985; Van Duin et al. 1986) and its localization (Rubin et al. 1985). However, up to now, attempts using the direct method of DNA-mediated gene transfer have failed to restore normal repair capacity in defective human fibroblasts (for review see Lehmann 1985). These failures may be due to several factors, including the low capacity of these cells to integrate exogenous DNA (Lehmann 1985), the selection protocol that favors isolation of revertants (Royer-Pokora and Haseltine 1984; Schultz et al. 1985), the use of Simian virus 40-transformed cells, in which the presence of the viral genome causes translocations, deletions and mutations of the host genome (Marshak et al. 1975; Lübbe et al. 1982), possibly including the correcting repair gene. In our study, we attempted to overcome these difficulties by using nontransformed primary fibroblasts and a selection procedure that took into account the slower growth rate of FA cells compared with that of normal cells (Elmore and Swift 1976; Dutrillaux et al. 1982; Kaiser et al. 1982).

Primary skin fibroblast FA cell lines were cotransfected with pSV_2 *neo* plasmid

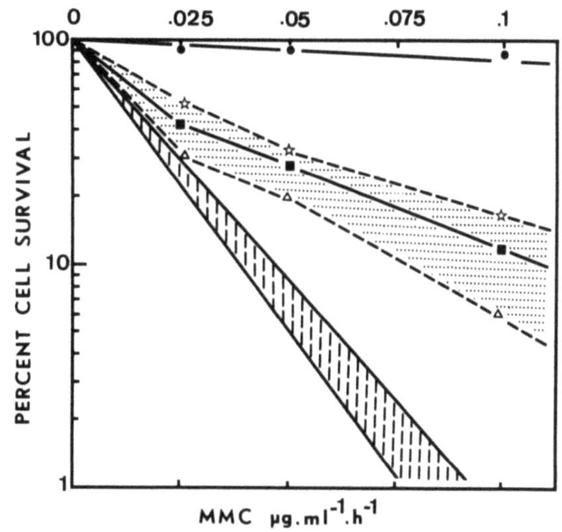

Fig. 6. Survival after MMC treatment of FA fibroblasts transfected with normal human DNA and reconstruction experiments. FA 150 cells were cotransfected with the pSV^2 *neo* plasmid and high molecular weight DNA from the TK6 MA cell line obtained from W. Thilly (MIT, Boston). Survival after MMC treatment was established 40 days after transfection either without MMC selection (■) or following selection with 0.025 μg/ml MMC for 1 h (●). The *hatched area* between *solid lines* corresponds to the range of survival of untransfected FA 150 cells, and FA 150 cells cotransfected with UV-treated pSV$_2$ *neo* plasmid and their own DNA, or UV-irradiated DNA from normal cells, or yeast or salmon sperm DNA, or mock-transfected (22 different survival curves). The *hatched area* between *broken lines* corresponds to reconstruction experiments. Normal cells (cell line 1 BR3 provided by C. Arlett, University of Sussex) and FA 150 cells were mixed in proportions ranging from 10^{-2} (☆) to 10^{-4} (△) and, after growth, exposed to different doses of MMC

and high molecular weight DNA from wild-type human cells. The restoration of normal cellular resistance to MMC (Fig. 6) as well as the recovery of a normal pattern of semiconservative DNA synthesis after treatment with 8-MOP plus UVA were observed, provided that several conditions were fulfilled. These included, firstly, the choice of an FA cell line suitable for DNA-mediated transformation (*neo* gene). Indeed, for some of the FA cell lines tested, we did not succeed in isolating G418-resistant transformants even in conditions which were optimal for other cell lines. Secondly, in accord with results obtained by others (Spivak et al. 1984; Van Duin et al. 1985), UV irradiation of the plasmid had a stimulatory effect, in that transformants were produced in cell lines FA 150 and FA 121. Thirdly, transformants of these FA cell lines were observed only after two rounds of transfection. The double transfection procedure was therefore systematically applied.

Survival after exposure to MMC was determined for the whole cell population at different times after gene transfer. Figure 6 shows that survival curves 40 days after transfection have a tailed shape, indicating the presence of an important fraction of MMC-resistant cells (MMC^R) in the population (30% at 40 days). After exposure to a dose of 0.025 μg/ml of MMC for 1 h, the surviving cells were grown for 40 days and subjected to various doses of MMC. The survival curves are then indicative of a homogeneous population of cells with a normal resistance to

MMC, the first MMC treatment having eliminated the MMC-sensitive cells (Fig. 6).

Control consisting of UV-irradiated pSV_2 *neo* plasmid and autologous DNA (FA 150 DNA transfected in the FA 150 cell line), salmon sperm DNA, yeast DNA, or heavily UV-irradiated DNA from normal cells never showed the presence of an MMC^R fraction. The same was true when FA 150 cells were subjected to the transfection procedure, but without DNA. In all cases, the survival curves obtained after treatment with MMC were within the range of that of an untransfected population (Fig. 6). These observations imply that neither the plasmid by itself nor the mock transfection favors the selection of putative MMC^R spontaneous mutants or confers MMC resistance to the population.

In order to understand how such a high proportion of MMC^R cells arises in the transfected population, reconstruction experiments were performed, mixing various proportions (10^{-2} to 10^{-4}) of normal and FA cells. The clonogenic cell survival of MMC treatment conditions mimicking a transfection experiment was determined. Tailed survival curves similar to those following transfection with normal DNA were obtained (Fig. 6). The proportion of MMC^R cells was estimated by extrapolation to the ordinate axis of the second part of survival curves. This fraction (30%–60%) was much higher than that expected from this experimentally mixed population (10^{-2} to 10^{-4}). The higher growth rate and plating efficiency of normal cells (MMC^R) seems to provide an explanation for this (Fig. 6). The presence of a diffusible factor produced by normal cells which would correct the defect in FA cells cannot explain this result. Cocultivation of FA and normal cells at a ratio much higher than the ratio in our study (1:2) led to an increase in chromosomal aberrations in the normal cells, while a reduction of MMC-induced chromosomal damage was found in FA cells (Zakrewski and Sperling 1980). However, the residual frequency of aberrations in cocultivated FA cells was significantly higher than the frequency in normal cells (Nordenson et al. 1980). Moreover, unless it is assumed that such a putative diffusible factor induces a genetically transmissible effect, it would be difficult to explain the persistence of the MMC^R phenotype in transfection experiments for more than ten generations.

Some characteristics of transfected FA 150 cells were determined (Diatloff-Zito et al. 1986). These included determination of HLA antigens in nontransfected cells and in MMC^R cells derived from a transfection experiment. The results of the determination of histocompatibility antigens excluded inadvertent contamination of FA 150 cells by a normal cell line. Determination, by alkaline elution, of the amount of cross-linked DNA in FA 150 and in the derived MMC^R population after transfection ruled out the possibility that the MMC^R phenotype of transfected cells was due to reduced uptake or accessibility to DNA of the drug. It should also be noted that MMC^R cells derived from transfection experiments have not only acquired resistance to MMC but also demonstrate a normal pattern of recovery of semiconservative DNA synthesis after 8-MOP photoaddition. Finally, the presence of exogenous pSV_2 *neo* DNA sequences in transfected cells was shown by Southern blot analysis. The blots indicated that both integrated copies of the *neo* gene into the genome and nonintegrated copies were present in MMC^R cells several generations after transfection. The presence of nonintegrated copies may reflect a recombinational activity in such cells. Cytogenetic analysis of MMC^R

cells in comparison with untransfected FA cells is under way. It has been established that FA cells show a higher frequency of spontaneous and induced chromosomal aberrations than normal cells (Schroeder 1982). Consequently, it is important to determine whether or not the MMC^R transformants have recovered a completely normal phenotype, including normal cytogenetic behavior, in addition to the restoration of resistance to MMC and the recovery of semiconservative DNA synthesis after 8-MOP photoaddition already demonstrated.

In order to be able to isolate and characterize the gene(s) involved in the correction of the FA defect, it was essential to demonstrate that gene transfer was possible in FA cells. In view of the difficulties in distinguishing foreign from endogenous DNA in this human system, other cloning strategies are currently being studied.

Conclusion

We have shown here that the two genetic complementation groups reported for FA correspond to two phenotypic classes identifiable by measurements of the rate of semiconservative DNA synthesis after 8-MOP photoaddition. Complementation group B is indistinguishable from normal cells and heterozygotes: the phase of inhibition of DNA synthesis is followed by recovery of a near-normal rate of semiconservative DNA synthesis. In contrast, the FA cells belonging to complementation group A show an abnormal pattern, in that such a recovery does not take place. This test allows a rapid classification of FA patients. Whether the clinical variability and degree of severity of the disease observed in FA patients correlates with the genetic and phenotypic classes reported here remains to be established.

In terms of clonogenic cell survival FA cells belonging to complementation group A were found to be twice as sensitive as normal cells to 8-MOP photoaddition. FA cells of complementation group B turned out to be slighly more resistant than group A cells. The response reflected the range of sensitivity:
FA(A) > FA(B) > heterozygote > normal.

The incision of photoinduced DNA cross-links was analyzed using the alkaline elution technique. After 24 h of posttreatment incubation, the elution rate of initially cross-linked DNA increased in normal and FA cell lines. However, differences in the kinetics were seen. FA fibroblasts and lymphoblasts from complementation group A showed slower incision kinetics than normal cells. Only half of the cross-links incised in normal cells were incised in FA cells after 6 h of posttreatment incubation. Complementation group B cells showed response, which lay between that of normal and FA group A cells. We conclude that although FA cells are able to incise DNA cross-links, their ability to process 8-MOP photoinduced cross-links is not the same as that of normal cells. All cells were analyzed while they were in the exponential phase of growth. It should be kept in mind that FA cells tend to accumulate in the G_2 phase, which generally favor recombinational repair. Thus, it may well be that the significance of DNA repair in FA is in fact overestimated because of this cell cycle disturbance. Analysis of S phase cells may provide an answer to this.

Finally, we showed that the correction of the FA defect by gene transfer with normal high molecular weight DNA can be achieved. It is now possible to envisage the cloning of the gene(s) involved. The development of molecular probes will certainly help in the diagnosis of this disease.

Acknowledgements. The technical assistance of F. Sangrado and C. Vivès is gratefully acknowledged.

References

Auerbach AD, Wolman SR (1976) Susceptibility of Fanconi's anemia fibroblasts to chromosome damage by carcinogens. Nature 261: 494-496

Billardon C, Moustacchi E (1986) Comparison of the sensitivity of Fanconi's anemia and normal fibroblasts to the induction of sister-chromatid exchanges by photoaddition of mono- and bifunctional psoralens. Mutat Res 174: 241-246

Boyland E, Williams K (1965) An enzyme catalysing the conjugation of epoxides with glutathione. Biochem J 94: 190-197

Claassen E, Kortbeek H, Arwert F (1986) Effects of mitomycin C on the rate of DNA synthesis in normal and Fanconi anemia cells. Mutat Res 165: 15-19

Cleaver JE (1968) Defective repair replication of DNA in xeroderma pigmentosum. Nature 218: 652-654

Diatloff-Zito C, Papadopoulo D, Averbeck D, Moustacchi E (1986) Abnormal response to DNA cross-linking agents of Fanconi anemia fibroblasts can be corrected by transfection with normal human DNA. Proc Natl Acad Sci USA 83: 7034-7038

Duckworth-Rysiecki G, Hulten M, Mann J, Taylor AMR (1984) Clinical and cytogenetic diversity in Fanconi's anemia. J Med Genet 21: 197-203

Duckworth-Rysiecki G, Taylor AMR (1985) Effects of ionizing radiation on cells from Fanconi's anemia patients. Cancer Res 45: 416-420

Duckworth-Rysiecki G, Cornich K, Clarke CA, Buchwald M (1985) Identification of two complementation groups in Fanconi's anemia. Somatic Cell Mol Genet 11: 35-43

Dutrillaux B, Aurias A, Dutrillaux AM, Buriot D, Prieur M (1982) The cell cycle of lymphocytes in Fanconi's anemia. Hum Genet 62: 327-332

Elmore E, Swift M (1976) Growth of cultured cells from patients with Fanconi's anemia. J Cell Physiol 87: 229-239

Fanconi G (1967) Familial constitutional panmyelopathy, Fanconi's anemia (FA). I. Clinical aspects. Semin Hematol 4: 233-240

Finkelberg R, Thompson MW, Siminovitch L (1978) Survival after treatment with EMS, X-rays and mitomycin C of skin fibroblasts from patients with Fanconi's anemia. Am J Hum Genet 26: 30A

Fornace AJ, Little JB, Weichselbaum RR (1979) DNA repair in a Fanconi's anemia fibroblast cell strain. Biochim Biophys Acta 561: 99-109

Friedberg EC (1985) DNA repair. Freeman, USA

Friedberg EC, Ehman UK, Williams JI (1979) Human diseases associated with defective DNA repair. Adv Radiat Biol 8: 85-174

Fujiwara Y, Tatsumi M, Sasaki MS (1979) Cross-link repair in human cells and its possible defect in Fanconi's anemia cells. J Mol Biol 113: 635-649

Fujiwara Y (1982) Defective repair of mitomycin C cross-links in Fanconi's anemia and loss in confluent normal human and xeroderma pigmentosum cells. Biochim Biophys Acta 699: 217-225

Glanz A, Fraser FC (1982) Spectrum of anomalies in Fanconi's anemia. J Med Genet 19: 412-416

Gruenert DC, Cleaver JE (1985) Repair of psoralen-induced cross-links and monoadducts in normal and repair-deficient human fibroblasts. Cancer Res 45: 5399-5404

Gruenert DC, Kapp LN, Cleaver JE (1985) Inhibition of DNA synthesis by psoralen-induced lesions in xeroderma pigmentosum and Fanconi's anemia fibroblasts. Photochem Photobiol 41: 534-550

Hama-Inaba H, Hieda-Shiomi N, Shiomi T, Sato K (1983) Isolation and characterization of mitomycin C-sensitive mouse lymphoma cell mutants. Mutat Res 108: 405-416
Hanawalt PC, Sarasin A (1986) Cancer-prone hereditary diseases with DNA processing abnormalities. Trends Genet 2: 124-129
Ishida R, Buchwald M (1982) Susceptibility of Fanconi's anemia lymphoblasts to DNA cross-linking and alkylating agents. Cancer Res 42: 4000-4006
Jaspers NGJ, Bootsma D (1982) Genetic heterogeneity in ataxia teleangiectasia studied by cell fusion. Proc Natl Acad Sci USA 79: 2641-2644
Kaiser TN, Lojewski A, Dougherty C, Juergens L, Sahar E, Latt SA (1982) Flow cytometric characterization of the response of Fanconi's anemia cells to mitomycin C. Cytometry 2: 291-297
Kaye J, Smith CA, Hanawalt PC (1980) DNA repair in human cells containing photoadducts of 8-methoxypsoralen of angelicin. Cancer Res 40: 696-702
Klocker H, Burtscher HJ, Auer B, Hirsch-Kauffmann M, Schweiger M (1985) Fibroblasts from patients with Fanconi's anemia are not deficient in excision of thymine dimer. Eur J Cell Biol 37: 240-242
Kohn KW, Erickson LC, Ewing RAG, Friedman CA (1976) Fractionation of DNA from mammalian cells by alkaline elution. Biochemistry 15: 4629-4637
Lam LH, Reynolds RJ (1986) Repair of closely opposed cyclobutyl pyrimidine dimers in UV-sensitive human diploid fibroblasts. Mutat Res 166: 199-205
Lehmann AR, Kirk-Bell S, Mayne L (1979) Abnormal kinetics of DNA synthesis in ultraviolet irradiated cells froms patients with Cockayne's syndrome. Cancer Res 39: 4237-4241
Lehmann AR (1982) Three complementation groups in Cockayne's syndrome. Mutat Res 106: 347-356
Lehmann AR (1985) Use of recombinant DNA techniques in cloning DNA repairs genes and in the study of mutagenesis in mammalian cells. Mutat Res 150: 61-67
Lübbe L, Strauss M, Schernek S, Geissler E (1982) The DNA tumor virus SV40 induces gene mutations in human cells. Reversion of HPRT deficiency. Hum Genet 61: 236-241
Marshak MA, Varshaner NB, Shapiro NI (1975) Induction of gene mutations and chromosomal aberrations by simian virus 40 in cultured mammalian cells. Mutat Res 30: 383-396
Mayne LV, Lehmann AR, Waters R (1982) Excision repair in Cockayne syndrome. Mutat Res 106: 197-189
Moustacchi E, Diatloff-Zito C (1985) DNA semi-conservative synthesis in normal and Fanconi anemia fibroblasts following treatment with 8-methoxypsoralen and near ultraviolet light or with X-rays. Hum Genet 70: 236-242
Moustacchi E, Papadopoulo D, Diatloff-Zito C, Buchwald M (1987) Two complementation groups of Fanconi's anemia differ in their phenotypic response to a DNA cross-linking treatment. Hum Genet 75: 45-47
Murnane JP, Painter RB (1982) Complementation of the defects in DNA synthesis in irradiated and unirradiated ataxia telangiectasia cells. Proc Natl Acad Sci USA 79: 1960-1964
Nordenson I, Björksten B, Lundt B (1980) Prevention of chromosomal breakage in Fanconi's anemia by cocultivation with normal cells. Hum Genet 56: 169-171
Painter RB (1977) Rapid test to detect agents that damage human DNA. Nature 265: 650-651
Painter RB (1986) Inhibition of mammalian cell DNA synthesis by ionizing radiation. Int J Radiat Biol 49: 771-781
Poll EHA, Arwert F, Kortbeek HT, Eriksson AW (1984) Fanconi anemia cells are not uniformly deficient in unhooking of DNA interstrand crosslinks by mitomycin C or 8-methoxypsoralen plus UVA. Hum Genet 68: 288-294
Pritsos CA, Sartorelli AC (1986) Generation of reactive oxygen radicals through bioactivation of mitomycin antibiotics. Cancer Res 46: 3528-3532
Royer-Pokora B, Haseltine WA (1984) Isolation of UV-resistant revertants from a xeroderma pigmentosum complementation group A cell line. Nature 311: 390-392
Rubin JS, Joyner AL, Bernstein A, Whitmore GF (1983) Molecular identification of a human DNA repair gene following DNA-mediated gene transfer. Nature 306: 206-208
Rubin JS, Prideaux VR, Willard HF, Dulhanty AM, Whitmore GF, Bernstein A (1985) Molecular cloning and chromosomal localization of DNA sequences associated with a human DNA repair gene. Mol Cell Biol 5: 398-405
Rudé JM, Friedberg EC (1977) Semi-conservative deoxyribonucleic acid synthesis in unirradiated

and ultraviolet-irradiated xeroderma pigmentosum and normal human skin fibroblasts. Mutat Res 42: 433-442

Sasaki MS, Tonomura A (1973) A high susceptibility of Fanconi's anemia to chromosome breakage by DNA-crosslinking agents. Cancer Res 33: 1829-1836

Schroeder TM, Tilgen D, Krüger J, Vogen F (1976) Formal genetics of Fanconi's anemia. Hum Genet 32: 257-288

Schroeder TM (1982) Genetically determined chromosome instability syndromes. Cytogenet Cell Genet 13: 119-132

Schulz RA, Barbis DP, Friedberg EC (1985) Studies on gene transfer and reversion to UV resistance in xeroderma pigmentosum cells. Somatic Cell Mol Genet 11: 617-624

Song PS, Tapley KJ (1979) Photochemistry and photobiology of psoralens. Photochem Photobiol 29: 1177-1197

Spivak G, Ganesan AK, Hanawalt PC (1984) Enhanced transformation of human cells by UV-irradiated pSV_2 plasmids. Mol Cell Biol 4: 1169-1171

Van Duin M, Westerveld A, Hoeijmakers JHJ (1985) UV stimulation of DNA-mediated transformation of human cells. Mol Cell Biol 5: 734-741

Van Duin M, De Wit J, Odijk H, Westerveld A, Yasui A, Koken MHM, Hoeijmakers JHJ, Bootsma D (1986) Molecular characterization of the human excision repair gene *ERCC-1:* cDNA cloning and amino acid homology with the yeast DNA repair gene *RAD10.* Cell 44: 913-923

Weksberg R, Buchwald M, Sargent P, Thompson MW, Siminovitch L (1979) Specific cellular defects in patients with Fanconi's anemia. J Cell Physiol 101: 311-324

Westerveld A, Hoeijmakers JHJ, Van Duin M, De Wit J, Odijk H, Pastnik A, Wood RD, Bootsma D (1984) Molecular cloning of a human DNA repair gene. Nature 310: 425-429

Wunder E, Fleischer B (1983) Response of lymphocytes from Fanconi's anemia patients and heterozygous relatives to 8-methoxypsoralen in a cloning survival test system. Hum Genet 64: 167-172

Zakrewski S, Sperling K (1980) Antagonistic effect of cocultivation on mitomycin C-induced aberration rate in cells of a patient with Fanconi's anemia and in Chinese hamster ovary cells. Hum Genet 56: 85-88

Part IV

Complementation Studies in Fanconi Anemia

Complementation Studies in Fanconi Anemia*

A. D. Auerbach, R. E. Koorse, R. Ghosh, V. S. Venkatraj, M. Zhang, and N. Chiorazzi

Introduction

Fanconi anemia (FA) was originally described as an autosomal recessive disorder characterized by a progressive pancytopenia, diverse congenital abnormalities, and an increased predisposition to the development of malignancy (Fanconi 1967; Schroeder et al. 1976). More recently, it has been recognized that the phenotype is so variable that diagnosis on the basis of clinical manifestations alone is difficult and often unreliable (Glanz and Fraser 1982; Alter and Potter 1983). The enormous clinical variation seen in FA suggests that there is likely to be an underlying genetic heterogeneity.

The molecular basis for FA is unknown, but several defects have been detected in cells cultured from FA patients, including increased chromosomal instability and hypersensitivity to a great variety of mutagenic and carcinogenic chemicals (Schroeder et al. 1964; Sasaki and Tonomura 1973; Auerbach and Wolman 1976; Ishida and Buchwald 1982). It has been suggested that the hypersensitivity to DNA cross-linking agents is caused by deficient DNA interstrand cross-link repair (Fujiwara et al. 1977), but other investigators have failed to confirm this hypothesis and have reported normal DNA repair after exposure of FA cells to a variety of mutagenic agents (Poll et al. 1984). In most of the cellular studies reported to date, analyses were done on cells from small numbers of patients, often using a single cell line from a cell bank. Conflicting results may be due to difficulties in accurate diagnosis and the possible existence of genetic subgroups.

Complementation analysis has proven to be an effective tool for the elucidation of the basis of genetic disease. Genetic heterogeneity has been demonstrated in cells from patients with a variety of metabolic disorders, after fusion of cultured skin fibroblasts from different patients to form heterokaryons (Lyons et al. 1973; Rattazzi et al. 1976). Complementation analysis has been used to demonstrate extensive heterogeneity in two syndromes which, like FA, are associated with chromosome instability or defective DNA repair: xeroderma pigmentosum and ataxia-

* This work was supported in part by Basil O'Connor Starter Research Grant No. 5-446 from the March of Dimes Birth Defects Foundation, by PHS Grants No. HL32987 and AI21061 from the National Institutes of Health, by a General Clinical Research Center Grant RR00102 from the National Institutes of Health to the Rockefeller University Hospital, and by support from the Pew Memorial Trust to the Laboratory for Investigative Dermatology.

T. M. Schroeder-Kurth A. D. Auerbach G. Obe (Eds.)
Fanconi Anemia, Clinical, Cytogenetic and Experimental Aspects

telangiectasia (Fischer et al. 1985; Murnane and Painter 1982; Jaspers and Bootsma 1982). In contrast to this, studies in FA have not shown extensive intergenic heterogeneity (Yoshida 1982; Zakrzewski and Sperling 1980, 1982; Zakrzewski et al. 1983). We feel that technical problems with these experiments may prevent them from reflecting an accurate picture of genetic heterogeneity in FA.

One of the difficulties encountered in performing complementation studies in FA results from the necessity of producing true hybrid cells capable of cell division. Because the cellular defect used as a marker for complementation in FA is correction of the abnormally high frequency of baseline and DNA cross-link-induced chromosomal breakage, metaphase spreads are needed for cytogenetic studies. The success of investigators in producing hybridomas by fusing mutagenized human lymphoblastoid cell lines (Epstein-Barr virus-transformed B cell lines) with peripheral blood lymphocytes (Chiorazzi et al. 1982) suggested to us that this may be a better approach to use for complementation studies in FA (Auerbach et al. 1985). The demonstration of complementation in hybrids constructed by fusion of two FA lymphoblastoid cell lines (Duckworth-Rysiecki et al. 1985) supports the validity of this type of approach to the problem. In this chapter we present results of our studies of complementation and gene dosage effects in FA.

Methods

Hypoxanthine-Guanine Phosphoribosyltransferase-Deficient Variant Cell Line

We routinely establish lymphoblastoid cell lines (LCLs) from blood samples received in our laboratory from FA patients and their parents (obligate heterozygotes). One of these FA cell lines, from a 4-year-old boy with aplastic anemia, short stature, microcephaly, microphthalmia, and café-au-lait spots, was chosen for use in complementation studies because it was exceedingly sensitive to DNA cross-linking agents in both cytogenetic and cell toxicity assays. Exponentially growing cells from this cell line were exposed for 20 h to a dose of ethyl methanesulfonate (EMS; 400 μg/ml), which permitted only 15%–20% cell survival. Hypoxanthine-guanine phosphoribosyltranserase (HGPRT)-deficient mutant cells were selected in medium containing 20 μg/ml 8-azaguanine, and cloned by limiting dilution methods. Mutant colonies were checked for HGPRT activity by determination of the uptake of ^{3}H-hypoxanthine (mutant cells should show a lack of incorporation). Maintenance of chromosomal instability and cross-link hypersensitivity in the mutant cells was also determined.

Cell Fusion

Peripheral blood samples from FA patients with demonstrated chromosomal instability and diepoxybutane (DEB) sensitivity (Auerbach, Ghosh, Pollio, and Zhang, this volume) were used for complementation studies. Ficoll-Hypaque-separated mononuclear cells were stimulated with pokeweed mitogen and then fused with cells from the FA HGPRT-deficient LCL described above, by a modification of the technique of Kennett et al. (1978). Mitogen-stimulated cells (10^7) and an equal number of LCL cells were incubated at room temperature with 0.5 ml 40% polyethelene glycol (PEG) (4000 MW, Merck) for 2 min with continuous swirling, and then centrifuged at 1800 rpm for 6 min. After washing with RPMI 1640 medium, 10^5 cells were dispersed in H-T medium in 96-well tissue culture plates (Linbro). H-T medium consists of RPMI 1640, 15% fetal bovine serum (FBS), penicillin (100 U/ml), streptomycin (100 μg/ml), 10^{-4} *M* hypoxanthine *(H)* and 5×10^{-5} *M* thymidine *(T)*. After 24 h, 10^{-7} *M* aminopterin *(A)* was added to each well. All wells were fed every 3rd day, for 3-6 weeks, with HAT medium. Unfused LCL cells died after a few days of exposure to HAT medium, and mitogen-stimulated lymphocytes did not grow in long-term culture. The hybrid cells were grown to mass culture.

Cells were harvested for cytogenetic studies, using standard methods, and analyzed with Q-banding (Caspersson et al. 1970) to confirm their hybrid status. Opposite-sex fusions were identified chromosomally as cells with a chromosome complement of 92, XXXY. Like-sex hybrids were verified by comparison of fluorescent chromosomal heteromorphisms in the hybrid to those found in the parental cell lines.

Hybrid status of cells was also confirmed by determining the class of human immunoglobulin light chain synthesized by the alleged hybridomas. Since the mutant FA cell line produced only lambda light chains, if putative hybrid cells synthesized or secreted kappa chains, then the gene for this chain must have been supplied by the other parental cell, thereby indicating that the cells were truly hybrid. The types of light chain produced by cells were determined in two ways: (a) by direct immunofluorescent staining of the cytoplasm of the fixed cells to visualize the types of light chain synthesized, and (b) by enzyme immunoassay to determine the types of light chain secreted by the cells into the culture medium. For both of these procedures, affinity-purified antibodies to human kappa or lambda light chains were employed. In the first instance, these antibodies were labeled with fluorescein isothiocyanate to allow visual detection by fluorescence microscopy; in the second instance, antibodies were labeled with horseradish peroxidase to allow reduction of aminoantipyrine substrate and detection at 490 nm. Specific details for these procedures have been published elsewhere (Chiorazzi et al. 1982; Giallongo et al. 1982).

The sensitivity of the hybrid cells to DNA cross-linking agents was then analyzed, using the methods described below. Both chromosomal breakage and growth inhibition assays were used. Persistence of the FA cellular phenotype indicated a lack of complementation, while correction of the defect in hybrid cells indicated that the parental lines belonged to different complementation groups.

Similar techniques were used for studies of the effects of gene dosage in hybrids between the mutant FA homozygous cell line and FA heterozygous and normal peripheral blood lymphocytes. Fusion of cells from an FA heterozygote with the HGPRT-deficient FA LCL resulted in hybrid cells with three copies of the FA gene, while fusion of the FA LCL normal cells produced hybrid cells with two copies.

Assays for DNA Cross-link Sensitivity

The DNA cross-link sensitivity of FA homozygous, FA heterozygous, normal control, and hybrid cells was assayed using two different endpoints. Growth inhibition studies and chromosomal breakage studies were performed as follows.

Growth Inhibition Studies
The method used for these studies was similar to that described by Ishida and Buchwald (1982). Exponentially growing LCLs or hybridomas were seeded in RPMI growth medium in 24-well tissue culture plates (Linbro) at a cell density of 5×10^4 cells/ml. Cells were incubated for a total of 7 days at 37 °C in a 5% CO_2 atmosphere at high humidity. Mitomycin C (MMC) at three different concentrations (1, 10, and 100 n*M*) was added to six replicate culture wells per concentration. Untreated cells served as controls. Cell counts were obtained using an electronic cell counter (Coulter Electronics) 1, 4, and 6 days after the addition of the genotoxic agent. Growth inhibition was determined by comparing the number of cells in the treated wells with the number of cells in the untreated wells. Dose response curves at 4 and 6 days post treatment and 7-day growth curves for each treatment condition were plotted for individual cell lines in each experiment.

Chromosomal Breakage Studies
Peripheral Blood Lymphocytes. These cells were tested for baseline and DEB sensitivity as previously described (Auerbach et al. 1981; Auerbach, Ghosh, Pollio, and Zhang, this volume). Cultures were harvested after 72 h, and chromosome preparations made following standard methods. Replicate cultures from each individual served as untreated controls.

Lymphoblastoid Cell Lines (LCLs) and Hybridomas. For these studies, cells were subcultured at 2.5×10^5 cells/ml. After 24 h, appropriate cultures were exposed to 0.1 µg/ml DEB. This concentration was chosen because it was relatively nontoxic to normal cells in growth inhibition studies. At higher concentrations, this agent induced sufficient chromosomal breakage in normal cells so that distinction between FA and normal cells became more ambiguous. Cells were harvested after an additional 24-48 h. Replicate cultures served as controls.

Analysis of Breakage. Analysis was performed on 100 Giemsa-stained metaphases from each preparation. To avoid bias in cell selection, consecutive metaphases which appeared unbroken with sufficiently well-defined chromosome morphology were selected for study on coded slides. Each cell was scored for the number of chromosomes and for the numbers and types of structural abnormalities. Achromatic areas less than a chromatid in width were scored as gaps, while exchange configurations, translocations, and dicentric and ring chromosomes were scored as rearrangements. Gaps were excluded in the calculations of chromosomal breakage frequency, and rearrangements were scored as two breaks.

Results

Isolation of Hybrid Clones

Our strategy for the isolation of hybrid cell lines was based on the use of a variant FA LCL that was HGPRT-deficient, and thus unable to grow in HAT medium, as one of the parental cell lines. An LCL derived in our laboratory from a male FA patient was mutagenized with 400 μg/ml EMS, and selected for growth in medium containing 8-azaguanine. Scintillation counting after growth of cells from the mutant cell line FA1-AG^r (RA022.4AG^r) in ^{3}H-hypoxanthine showed lack of uptake of this nucleotide, evidence that the cells were HGPRT-deficient. Failure of the mutant line to grow in HAT medium was demonstrated. Cells from this line were fused with normal female control peripheral blood lymphocytes, and antibody-secreting hybridoma cells isolated. Eleven rapidly dividing hybrid clones were propagated and studied. Cytogenetic analysis of Q-banded cells showed hybrid cells to have a chromosomal complement of 92,XXXY. Hybrid clones were comprised solely of tetraploid cells; no diploid cells from either parental line were found. The hybrid nature of the clones was further confirmed by analysis of immunoglobulin light chain production. The mutant FA cell line was positive for lambda light chain production. Each of the hybrid clones was shown to produce either (a) both kappa and lambda light chains or (b) a far greater amount of lambda light chains (when kappa was *not* produced) than the mutant cell line. Additional PEG-mediated cell fusions between the FA mutant cell line and peripheral blood lymphocytes from FA patients, FA heterozygotes, and normal controls resulted in the isolation of one or more hybrid clones from two FA patients, 12 FA heterozygotes, and a second normal individual.

Growth Inhibition Studies

In order to establish standards for studies of MMC-induced growth inhibition in hybrid cells, LCLs derived from FA homozygous, FA heterozygous, and normal individuals were screened for sensitivity to the DNA cross-linking agent MMC. Cells were exposed to MMC at three different concentrations (1, 10, and 100 n*M*), while untreated cells from each cell line served as controls. Dose-response curves at 4 and 6 days of exposure and growth curves at 10 n*M* and 100 n*M* MMC, were plotted for cell lines from 19 FA homozygotes, 16 FA heterozygotes, and six normal individuals. Twelve FA homozygous cell lines were hypersensitive to MMC, while seven FA lines exhibited an MMC-induced growth inhibition similar to that in normal cells (Fig. 1a). When the pooled data from each group were analyzed, there was no significant difference between normal and FA heterozygous cells (Fig. 1b). The difference between the sensitive FA cells and the other two groups was most pronounced at the lower concentrations of MMC studied. At the highest concentration (100 n*M*), all cells tested showed a marked inhibition of growth. This was consistent with our earlier cytogenetic studies showing that one could best discriminate between groups at relatively nontoxic concentrations of DEB.

All normal and heterozygous hybrid cell lines tested in the growth inhibition assay complemented the hypersensitivity to MMC seen in the FA mutant cell line

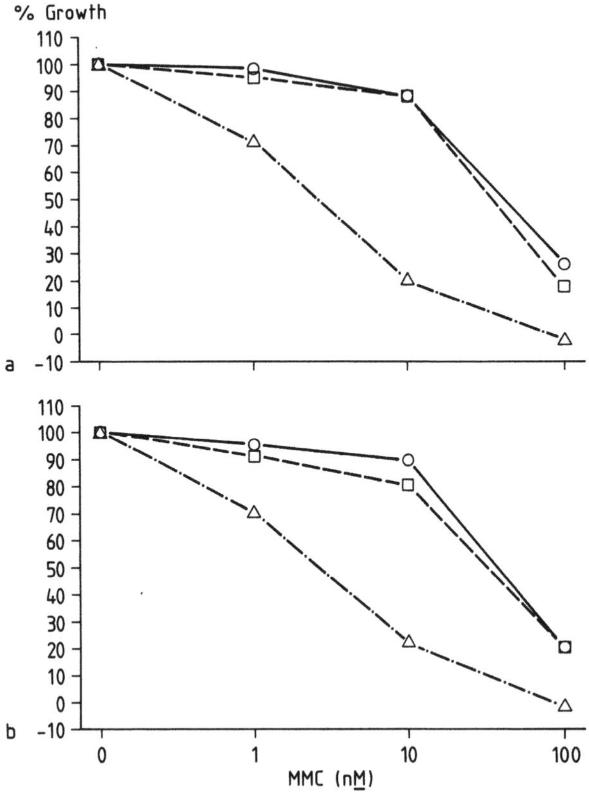

Fig. 1a, b. Mean growth of LCLs from 19 FA homozygotes, 16 FA heterozygotes, and 6 normal individuals. Percentage growth inhibition was calculated after 4 days of exposure to MMC. At the highest concentration of MMC (100 n*M*), all cells tested showed marked inhibition of growth. **a** LCLs derived from 12 of the FA patients showed marked hypersensitivity to low concentrations of MMC, while LCLs derived from seven of the FA patients showed normal sensitivity in this assay. ·—△—·, sensitive FA LCLs; —○—, nonsensitive FA LCLs; – □ –, normal LCLs. **b** There was no significant difference between normal and FA heterozygous cells, while LCLs derived from 12 FA patients showed marked hypersensitivity to low concentrations of MMC. ·—△—·, sensitive FA LCLs; – □ –, heterozygous LCLs; —○—, normal LCLs

(Fig. 2). Studies of inhibition of cell growth by MMC also showed complementation for cellular hypersensitivity to this agent in the two homozygous hybrid lines (Fig. 3).

Chromosomal Breakage Studies

Cytogenetic studies showed that at a concentration of 0.1 μg/ml DEB, which had no appreciable clastogenic effect on normal or FA heterozygous LCLs, cells from the mutant FA line maintained their high frequency of chromosomal breaks and exchanges (Fig. 4a). Most of the hybridomas constructed by fusion of the mutant FA cell line with lymphocytes from normal or FA heterozygous individuals

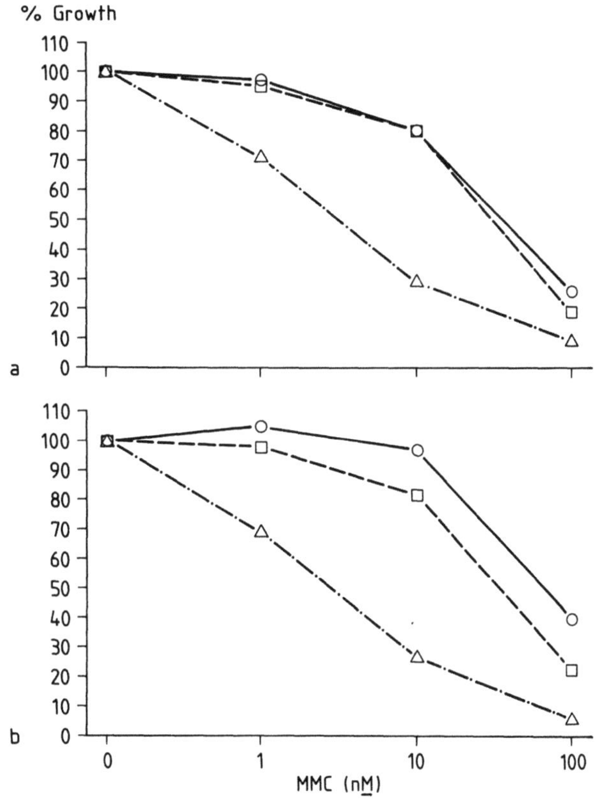

Fig. 2 a, b. Mean growth of cloned hybrid cell lines derived by fusion of the mutant FA cell line (FA1-AG^r) with pokeweed mitogen-stimulated peripheral blood lymphocytes from normal control and FA heterozygous individuals. Percentage growth inhibition was calculated after 4 days of exposure to MMC. **a** The MMC hypersensitivity of the FA cell line was complemented in the two hybrids constructed by fusion of the FA cells with cells from normal individuals. —○—, FA1-AG^r × normal hybrids; ·—△—·, FA1-AG^r; – □ –, normal LCLs; **b** The MMC hypersensitivity of the FA cell line was complemented in the 12 hybrids constructed by fusion of the FA cells with cells from FA heterozygous individuals. —○—, FA1-AG^r × heterozygote hybrids; ·—△—·, FA1-AG^r; – □ –, FA heterozygous LCLs

showed complementation of this DEB-induced chromosomal breakage (Fig. 4b, Table 1). One hybrid clone from each of three FA homozygote-FA heterozygote fusions showed an elevated frequency of DEB-induced chromosomal breakage compared with the rest of the clones of this genotype. Because of the inclusion of these three outliers, with breakage frequencies greater than 0.3, these data did not have a normal distribution. The distribution was skewed, with the majority of observations falling around the median of 0.04. The median of the chromosomal breakage data was basically the same for DEB-treated cell cultures with equal numbers of FA and normal genes (diploid FA heterozygous cells and hybrids constructed by fusion of the FA mutant cell line and normal control lymphocytes) as for the FA homozygote-FA heterozygote hybrids; the distribution of the former group falls within that of the latter.

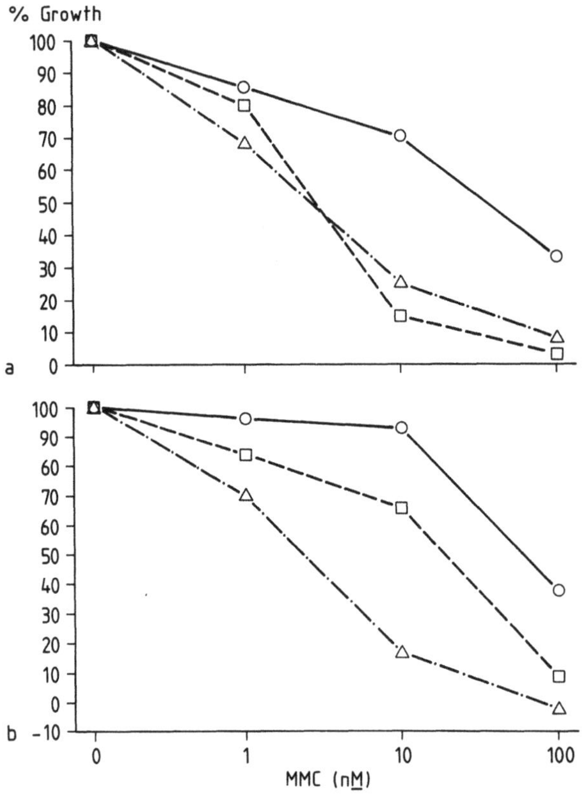

Fig. 3a, b. Mean growth of cloned hybrid cell lines derived by fusion of the mutant FA cell line (FA1-AG^r) with pokeweed mitogen-stimulated peripheral blood lymphocytes from two FA patients. Percentage growth inhibition was calculated after 4 days of exposure to MMC. The MMC hypersensitivity of the FA cell line was complemented in both hybrids. **a** —○—, FA1-AG^r × FA2 hybrid; ·—△—·, FA1-AG^r; – □ –, FA2 LCL. **b** —○—, FA1-AG^r × FA3 hybrid; ·—△—·, FA1-AG^r; – □ –, FA3 LCL

Cytogenetic studies of hybrid clones isolated after fusion of the FA mutant cell line with B cells from two FA patients showed complementation for the DEB-induced chromosomal breakage typical of FA cells. Attempted fusions of the mutant FA cell line with B cells from other FA patients failed to result in viable hybrid clones.

Discussion

Hypersensitivity of FA cells to DNA cross-linking agents was used as a cellular marker in complementation studies. The specific endpoints used were inhibition of cell growth by MMC, and induction of chromosomal breakage by DEB. Although in our experience DEB is a more effective agent than MMC for discrimination of the FA cellular phenotype, MMC was used in the growth inhibition

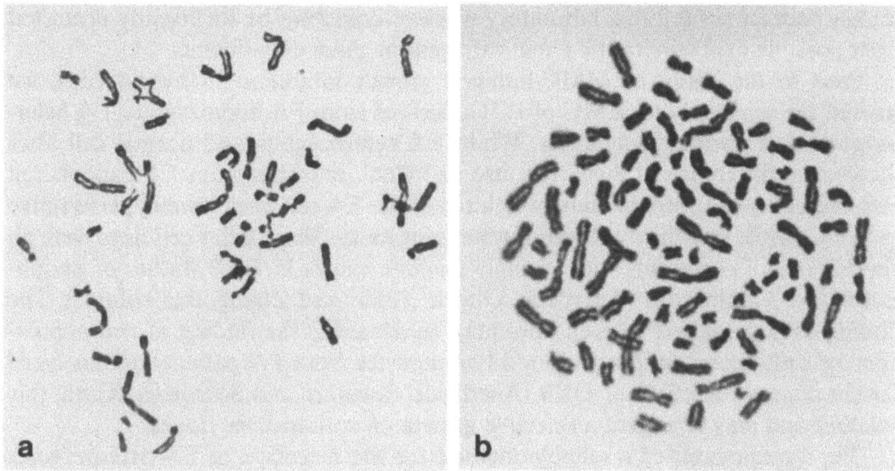

Fig. 4. a Part of a metaphase spread of a cell from the FA mutant cell line (FA1-AG[r]) after treatment with 0.1 μg/ml DEB for 48 h. Multiple chromatid breaks and exchange figures are seen. **b** Metaphase spread of a DEB-treated hybridoma cell, constructed by fusion of the FA mutant cell line with pokeweed mitogen-stimulated peripheral blood lymphocytes from a normal individual. Complementation of the FA cellular phenotype is seen

Table 1. Chromosomal breakage in DEB-treated hybrid cells

Cell Line	Chromosome no.	Genotype	Mean chromosomal breaks/cell	
			Clone 1	Clone 2
FA1-AG[r] × N1	92	+/+/fa/fa	0.08	0.08
FA1-AG[r] × N2	92	+/+/fa/fa	0.08	0.04
FA1-AG[r] × FA1H	92	+/fa/fa/fa	0.18	0.04
FA1-AG[r] × FA2H	92	+/fa/fa/fa	0.04	0.03
FA1-AG[r] × FA3H	92	+/fa/fa/fa	0.04	0.00
FA1-AG[r] × FA4H	92	+/fa/fa/fa	0.40[a]	0.02
FA1-AG[r] × FA5H	92	+/fa/fa/fa	0.02	0.00
FA1-AG[r] × FA6H	92	+/fa/fa/fa	0.40[a]	0.06
FA1-AG[r] × FA7H	92	+/fa/fa/fa	0.10	0.06
FA1-AG[r] × FA8H	92	+/fa/fa/fa	0.06	0.00
FA1-AG[r] × FA9H	92	+/fa/fa/fa	0.08	0.04
FA1-AG[r] × FA10H	92	+/fa/fa/fa	0.06	0.02
FA1-AG[r] × FA11H	92	+/fa/fa/fa	0.02	0.00
FA1-AG[r] × FA12H	92	+/fa/fa/fa	0.34[a]	-
FA1-AG[r]	46	fa/fa	5.32	
Normal controls (mean)	46	+/+	0.02	
FA heterozygotes (mean)	46	+/fa	0.03	

[a] These values cause the distribution for data in the table to be skewed to the left; if they are omitted a normal distribution is obtained. They are thus outliers and comprise a separate group.

studies because we felt that laboratory workers could not be sufficiently protected from possible exposure to the chemical agent in these experiments.

Prior to the study of MMC-induced growth inhibition in hybrid cells, we studied the sensitivity to MMC of LCLs derived from FA homozygous, FA heterozygous, and normal individuals. While FA heterozygous and normal cell lines showed no difference in their response to MMC, cell lines from FA patients fell into two groups. Approximately two-thirds of the FA cell lines were hypersensitive to MMC, while one-third showed normal sensitivity. These latter cell lines were all derived from FA patients with strongly positive results in DEB studies of peripheral blood lymphocytes (Auerbach, Ghosh, Pollio and Zhang, this volume). The finding of nonsensitive FA cell lines may be related to the finding of two populations of cells when peripheral blood lymphocytes from FA patients are analyzed for the clastogenic effect of DEB (Auerbach, Rogatko, and Schroeder-Kurth, this volume) and may represent a selective growth of nonsensitive clones.

The development of a reliable method for the detection of FA heterozygotes would be of great benefit to FA family members at risk of being gene carriers. Although the results of studies of DEB-induced chromosomal breakage in peripheral blood lymphocytes show that the mean chromosomal breakage is significantly higher in a group of FA obligate heterozygotes than in a group of normal controls, there is an overlap in individual breakage frequencies in the two groups (Auerbach et al. 1981). We performed gene dosage studies in hybrid cells in order to determine whether cells with only one normal allele at the FA locus (FA homozygote × FA heterozygote hybrids) could be distinguished from cells with two normal alleles (FA homozygote × normal hybrids). We found that in most cases the FA cell line was equally complemented by heterozygous or normal control cells. In a few cases hybrid cells with three FA genes and a single normal gene at the FA locus showed increased sensitivity to DNA cross-linking agents compared to cells with equal numbers of FA and normal genes. Further studies are needed to evaluate the significance of this finding, and its potential for use as a method for the detection of heterozygotes in families at risk.

Hybridoma cell lines derived by fusion of an HGPRT-deficient FA cell line with pokeweed mitogen-stimulated peripheral blood lymphocytes from two other FA patients showed complementation of the FA cellular phenotype. Thus the patient from whom our mutant cell line was derived may belong to a different complementation group than the other two patients studied. Alternatively, these lines may represent selective growth of cells with normal MMC sensitivity, in the same way that LCLs derived from some FA patients had normal cross-link sensitivity, even though these patients were diagnosed as affected with FA on the basis of clinical manifestations of the syndrome and typical hypersensitivity of peripheral blood lymphocytes to the clastogenic effect of DEB. Studies by Moustacchi and Diatloff-Zito (1985) have demonstrated two classes among FA cell lines, in an assay that measures recovery in the rate of semiconservative DNA synthesis after exposure of cells to 8-methoxypsoralen (8-MOP) plus near-UV radiation (UVA). These appear to correspond to the two complementation groups in FA demonstrated by Duckworth-Rysiecki et al. (1985) (Moustacchi et al. 1987). We are currently investigating this parameter in LCLs and hybridomas from our patients to see if the complementation of the defect in our FA × FA hybrids does in fact represent genetic heterogeneity in the patients, as demonstrated by another assay. So far, we have been unable to reproduce the results of Moustacchi et al. (1987).

Conclusion

Additional complementation studies of hybrids derived from different FA patients are needed to analyze the full extent of genetic heterogeneity in the syndrome. The extensive clinical heterogeneity seen in FA suggests the presence of genetic heterogeneity. However, the finding of patients in the same sibship with diverse clinical manifestations indicates that the phenotypic variation in FA cannot be accounted for by genetic heterogeneity alone, but may result from gene interaction or from environmental causes. A full understanding of genetic heterogeneity in FA awaits the isolation and molecular characterization of the FA gene or genes. Although human genes for the excision repair of DNA have been cloned by transfection of human DNA into UV-sensitive rodent cell lines (Westerveld et al. 1984; Rubin et al. 1985; van Duin et al. 1986), it is unlikely that the UV- and MMC-sensitive Chinese hamster ovary (CHO) lines developed by Thompson and coworkers (Thompson et al. 1981; Thompson and Carrano 1983) will be suitable for the isolation of the FA gene. The defect in these cell lines does not appear to be analogous to the defect responsible for the DNA crosslink sensitivity found in FA (Hoy et al. 1985). The strategy for complementation used in these experiments should be applicable to human cells from any of the recessively inherited diseases for which there is a selectable assay. However, except for a recent report of successful transfer of MMC resistance to FA cells by transfection with normal human DNA (Diatloff-Zito et al. 1986), the results of such experiments have been disappointing, since the resistant clones isolated have been revertants rather than true transformants (Royer-Pokora and Haseltine 1984; Schultz et al. 1985; M. Buchwald, personal communication). Hopefully, the development of methods that will improve transfection frequencies will alleviate the problems encountered in these experiments, and will lead to the isolation and characterization of the FA gene or genes.

References

Alter BP, Potter NU (1983) Long term outcome in Fanconi's anemia: description of 26 cases and review of the literature. In: German J (ed) Chromosome mutation and neoplasia. Liss, New York, pp 43-62

Auerbach AD, Wolman SR (1976) Susceptibility of Fanconi's anaemia fibroblasts to chromosome damage by carcinogens. Nature 261: 494-496

Auerbach AD, Adler B, Chaganti RSK (1981) Prenatal and postnatal diagnosis and carrier detection of Fanconi anemia by a cytogenetic method. Pediatrics 67: 128-135

Auerbach AD, Venkatraj VS, Chiorazzi N, Carter DM (1985) Isolation of a human-human hybridoma showing complementation of a gene for hypersensitivity to clastogens. Environ Mutagen 7 (Suppl 3): 47-48

Caspersson T, Zech L, Johansson C, Modest EJ (1970) Identification of human chromosomes by DNA-binding fluorescing agents. Chromosoma 30: 215-227

Chiorazzi N, Wasserman RL, Kunkel HG (1982) Use of Epstein-Barr virus-transformed B cell lines for the generation of immunoglobulin-producing human B cell hybridomas. J Exp Med 156: 930-935

Diatloff-Zito C, Papadopoulo D, Averbeck D, Moustacchi E (1986) Abnormal response to DNA crosslinking agents of Fanconi anemia fibroblasts can be corrected by transfection with normal human DNA. Proc Natl Acad Sci USA 83: 7034-7038

Duckworth-Rysiecki G, Cornish K, Clarke CA, Buchwald M (1985) Identification of two complementation groups in Fanconi anemia. Somatic Cell Mol Genet 11: 35-41

Fanconi G (1967) Familial constitutional panmyelocytopathy, Fanconi's anemia (FA). I. Clinical aspects. Semin Hematol 4: 233-240

Fischer E, Keijzer W, Thielmann HW, Popanda O, Bohnert E, Edler L, Jung EG, Bootsma D (1985) A ninth complementation group in xeroderma pigmentosum, XP I. Mutat Res 145: 217-225

Fujiwara Y, Tatsumi M, Sasaki MS (1977) Cross-link repair in human cells and its possible defect in Fanconi's anemia cells. J Mol Biol 113: 635-649

Giallongo A, Kochoumian L, King TP (1982) Enzyme- and radioimmunoassays for specific murine IgE and IgG with different solid-phase immunosorbents. J Immunol Methods 52: 379-393

Glanz A, Fraser FC (1982) Spectrum of anomalies in Fanconi anaemia. J Med Genet 19: 412-416

Hoy CA, Thompson LH, Mooney CL, Salazar EP (1985) Defective DNA cross-link removal in chinese hamster cell mutants hypersensitive to bifunctional alkylating agents. Cancer Res 45: 1-7

Ishida R, Buchwald M (1982) Susceptibility of Fanconi's anemia lymphoblasts to DNA-crosslinking and alkylating agents. Cancer Res 42: 4000-4006

Jaspers NGJ, Bootsma D (1982) Genetic heterogeneity in ataxia telangiectasia studied by cell fusion. Proc Natl Acad Sci USA 79: 2641-2644

Kennett RH, Denis KA, Tung AS, Klinman NR (1978) Hybrid plasmacytoma production: fusions with adult spleen cells, monoclonal spleen fragments, neonatal spleen cells and human spleen cells. Curr Top Microbiol Immunol 81: 77-91

Lyons LB, Cox RP, Dancis J (1973) Complementation analysis of maple syrup urine disease in heterokaryons derived from cultured human fibroblasts. Nature 243: 533-535

Moustacchi E, Diatloff-Zito C (1985) DNA semi-conservative synthesis in normal and Fanconi anemia fibroblasts following treatment with 8-methoxypsoralen and near ultraviolet light or with X-rays. Hum Genet 70: 236-242

Moustacchi E, Papadopoulo D, Diatloff-Zito C, Buchwald M (1987) Two complementation groups of Fanconi's anemia differ in their phenotypic response to a DNA cross-linking treatment. Hum Genet 75: 45-47

Murnane JP, Painter RB (1982) Complementation of the defects in DNA synthesis in irradiated and unirradiated ataxia-telangiectasia cells. Proc Natl Acad Sci USA 79: 1960-1963

Poll EHA, Arwert F, Kortbeek HT, Eriksson AW (1984) Fanconi anaemia cells are not uniformly deficient in unhooking of DNA interstrand crosslinks, induced by mitomycin C or 8-methoxypsoralen plus UVA. Hum Genet 68: 228-234

Rattazzi MC, Brown JA, Davidson RG, Shows TB (1976) Studies on complementation of hexosaminidase deficiency in human GM2 ganliosidosis. Am J Hum Genet 28: 143-154

Royer-Pokora B, Haseltine WA (1984) Isolation of UV-resistant revertants from a xeroderma pigmentosum complementation group A cell line. Nature 311: 390-392

Rubin JS, Prideaux VR, Willard HF, Dulhanty AM, Whitmore GF, Bernstein A (1985) Molecular cloning and chromosomal localization of DNA sequences associated with a human DNA repair gene. Mol Cell Biol 5: 398-405

Sasaki MS, Tonomura A (1973) A high susceptibility of Fanconi's anemia to chromosome breakage by DNA cross-linking agents. Cancer Res 33: 1829-1836

Schroeder TM, Anschütz F, Knopp A (1964) Spontane Chromosomenaberrationen bei familiärer Panmyelopathie. Humangenetik 1: 194-196

Schroeder TM, Tilgen D, Krüger J, Vogel F (1976) Formal genetics of Fanconi's anemia. Hum Genet 32: 257-288

Schultz RA, Barbis DP, Friedberg EC (1985) Studies on gene transfer and reversion to UV resistance in xeroderma pigmentosum cells. Somatic Cell Mol Genet 11: 617-624

Thompson LH, Carrano AV (1983) Analysis of mammalian cell mutagenesis and DNA repair using in vitro selected CHO cell mutants. In: Friedberg EC, Bridges BR (eds) Cellular responses to DNA damage, UCLA symposium on molecular and cellular biology, new series, vol 11. Liss, New York, pp 125-143

Thompson LH, Busch DB, Brookman K, Mooney CL, Glaser DA (1981) Genetic diversity of UV-sensitive DNA repair mutants of Chinese hamster ovary cells. Proc Natl Acad Sci USA 78: 3734-3737

van Duin M, de Wit J, Odijk H, Westerveld A, Yasui A, Koken MHM, Hoeijmakers JHJ, Bootsma D (1986) Molecular characterization of the human excision repair gene ERCC-1: cDNA cloning and amino acid homology with the yeast DNA repair gene RAD10. Cell 44: 913-923

Westerveld A, Hoeijmakers JHJ, van Duin M, de Wet J, Odijk H, Pastink A, Wood RD, Bootsma D (1984) Molecular cloning of a human DNA repair gene. Nature 310: 425-429

Yoshida MC (1982) The absence of genetic heterogeneity in Fanconi's anemia in five patients demonstrated by somatic cell hybridization. Cytogenet Cell Genet 32: 329-330

Zakrzewski S, Sperling K (1980) Genetic heterogeneity of Fanconi's anemia demonstrated by somatic cell hybrids. Hum Genet 56: 81-84

Zakrzewski S, Sperling K (1982) Analysis of heterogeneity in Fanconi's anemia patients of different ethnic origin. Hum Genet 62: 321-323

Zakrzewski S, Koch M, Sperling K (1983) Complementation studies between Fanconi's anemia cells with different DNA repair characteristics. Hum Genet 64: 55-57

Complementation and Gene Transfer Studies in Fanconi Anemia*

M. Buchwald, C. Clarke, J. Ng, G. Duckworth-Rysiecki, and R. Weksberg

Introduction

Fanconi anemia (FA) is an autosomal recessive disorder characterized by pancytopenia, a complex assortment of congenital malformations and an increased incidence of cancer (Fanconi 1967; German 1972). At the cellular level, FA shows an increased sensitivity to DNA cross-linking agents (Arlett and Lehmann 1978). The increased incidence of cancer and increased susceptibility to DNA damaging agents is chracteristic of "DNA repair disorders" such as xeroderma pigmentosum (XP), ataxia-telangiectasia (AT) and Bloom's syndrome (BS) (Setlow 1978). In the cases of XP, AT, and FA, it has been possible to use somatic cell genetic techniques to demonstrate the existence of multiple complementation groups (Cleaver 1984; Jaspers et al. 1985; Duckworth-Rysiecki et al. 1985, this volume).

However, in spite of considerable effort, it has not been possible to identify the aberrant biochemical step in any of the above diseases (Cleaver 1984). The development of DNA transfer techniques has provided an alternative approach to the identification of the defects in these diseases. To date, at least one human DNA repair gene has been isolated using Chinese hamster ovary (CHO) mutant cells as recipients for human DNA (Westerveld et al. 1984; Rubin et al. 1985). Attempts to use XP and AT cells in similar experiments have so far been unsuccessful (Royer-Pokora and Haseltine 1984; Schultz et al. 1985; Green et al. 1985; Lehmann et al. 1986). In this paper we review our evidence for the existence of at least two FA complementation groups and our attempts to show, by means of DNA transfer techniques, that wild-type DNA can be used to correct the cellular phenotype in FA cells.

Materials and Methods

Complementation Studies

Cell Lines. The lymphoblast cell lines used to define the complementation groups have been described elsewhere (Ishida and Buchwald 1982; Duckworth-Rysiecki et al. 1985). Four additional cell lines are reported in this paper. Two were isolated

* This research was supported by grants from the Medical Research Council of Canada and the Jagade Kartmer Fund.

T. M. Schroeder-Kurth A. D. Auerbach G. Obe (Eds.)
Fanconi Anemia, Clinical, Cytogenetic and Experimental Aspects

from sibs of the donor of the GM1309 fibroblast cell line (NIGMS Human Genetic Mutant Cell Repository, Institute for Medical Research, Camden, NJ) and are called FA 5 and FA 6 (Duckworth-Rysiecki et al. 1986). The other two were from previously unreported patients with FA (FA 7 and FA 8). All cells were cultured in medium containing 15% fetal calf serum in a humidified incubator in 5% CO_2 at 37 °C. Cells were tested periodically for the presence of mycoplasma and found negative.

Cell Fusions. The techniques for demonstrating complementation among FA lymphoblast cell lines have been fully described (Duckworth-Rysiecki et al. 1985). In brief, two selectable markers (resistance to ouabain and 6-thioguanine) were introduced into an FA cell line. This cell line was then used as a "universal parent" in somatic cell hybridization experiments. Following fusion of this cell line with another unmarked FA cell line, true hybrids between the two FA lines were selected in ouabain, which killed the unmarked cell line and its homokaryons, and hypoxanthine, amethopterin, thymidine (HAT), which killed the marked parent and its homokaryons. Cells able to grow in ouabain and HAT were tetraploid and had chromosomes derived from both parental cell lines. These cells were then tested for the three cellular FA phenotypes: growth sensitivity to mitomycin C (MMC, Sigma) spontaneous chromosome breakage, and MMC-induced chromosome breakage.

Tests for Complementation. The sensitivity of lymphoblasts to MMC was measured by growth inhibition tests (Ishida and Buchwald 1982). Briefly, cells were seeded into 24-well plates and different concentrations of MMC added to each well. After 72 h, the cells in each well were counted and the extent of growth inhibition determined by comparison with the number of cells in untreated wells. The effect of MMC was quantitated by plotting the number of cells vs. the logarithm of the drug concentration and by determining the concentration of MMC which caused 50% inhibition of growth (EC_{50}).

Levels of both spontaneous and MMC-induced chromosome breakage were determined for the parental and hybrid cell lines. In each instance a minimum of 50 mitoses were analyzed and all abnormalities scored.

Gene Transfer

Cell Lines. The Simian virus (SV) 40-transformed cell line used for DNA transfer studies (GM 6914) has been described elsewhere (Duckworth-Rysiecki et al. 1986) and corresponds to complementation group A. The untransformed parental fibroblast cell line is GM 1309. Two different SV 40-transformed control cell lines were used (GM 637 and GM 1468). All of these are available from the Institute for Medical Research, Camden, N.J. The CHO cell line used to obtain CHO DNA was provided by Dr. Peter Ipp from the same institute. Both the SV 40-transformed human and the CHO cell lines were cultured in medium with 10% fetal calf serum and were passaged by trypsinization.

Survival and Reconstruction Experiments. The sensitivity of cells to MMC was determined by survival experiments (Weksberg et al. 1979; Duckworth-Rysiecki et al. 1986). Briefly, exponentially growing cells were exposed to a specific concentration of MMC for 1 h, washed, and replated at the appropriative density. The plates were stained after 2 weeks and all colonies with more than 50 cells were counted. The D_{10} value was determined by interpolation from a plot of the logarithm of the survival (relative to untreated cells) vs. the concentration of the drug. Reconstruction experiments to establish selection conditions were performed as the survival experiments, except that mixtures of GM 6914 and control cells were plated separately and together in the appropriate concentration of MMC. Staining and counting of colonies were done as described above.

Transfer of DNA and Selection of Resistant Colonies. DNA was introduced into GM 6914 cells by the $CaPO_4$ coprecipitation method of Graham and Van der Eb (1973). In brief, partly confluent cells were exposed to a precipitate of DNA and $CaPO_4$ for a period of 8 h. The precipitate was then removed and the cells washed.

To isolate cells that had taken up DNA, the experiments were performed by cotransfecting with a mixture of genomic DNA and plasmid DNA (pRSVneo, carrying the bacterial *neo* gene; Southern and Berg 1982). Transfected cells were selected by adding 400 μg/ml of G-418 (Geneticin, Gibco) to the culture medium 48 h after transfer. The cells were refed twice weekly for 2 weeks, when all control plates (mock-transfected cells) had no cells. The resulting colonies were then cultured in medium containing 15 n*M* MMC and fed twice weekly for 4 weeks. At this time only a few colonies remained. These were expanded in the presence of absence of MMC and then tested for their sensitivity to MMC.

Molecular Techniques. The plasmid containing *neo* and the methods for the preparation of plasmid and genomic DNA have been described elsewhere (Duckworth-Rysiecki et al. 1986; Breitman et al. 1982; Tsui et al. 1982). Blot analysis of DNA was done according to the method of Southern (1975).

Results

Complementation Studies

Demonstration of Genetic Complementation. A summary of the relevant physical and laboratory findings which led to the clinical diagnosis of FA in the four patients used for the initial complementation studies is given in Table 1 A (Finkelberg 1976). Cells from all four patients were sensitive to MMC and other DNA crosslinking drugs as determined by both cell toxicity and chromosome breakage measurements (Table 1 B; Weksberg et al. 1979; Ishida and Buchwald 1982; Duckworth-Rysiecki et al. 1985). These four patients fall into two complementation groups. Group A consists of FA 1 and FA 4, since these cells do not complement each other (Fig. 1 A), while FA 2 and FA 3 are in complementation group B, since they complement FA 1 (Fig. 1 B). Until further complementation tests are done, more than one complementation group may be represented by the patients

Table 1. Clinical characteristics of patients with FA and properties of cells from these patients

	FA 1	FA 2	FA 3	FA 4	FA 5	FA 6	FA 7	FA 8	Normal
A. Clinical characteristics									
Age of onset (years)	9	2	3	7	13	10	12	4	–
Birth weight (g)	2000	1800	3000	2350	–	–	–	–	3300
Stature (percentile)	5	<3	<3	50	25	<3	<3	50	
Abnormal pigmentation	–	–	+	+	+	+	+	+	–
Hand abnormalities	+	+	–	+	+	–	–	+	–
Kidney abnormalities	+	–	+	+	+	–	–	+	–
Bone marrow failure	+	–	+	+	+	+	–	+	–
Chromosome breakage (%); (lymphocytes)	30	10	>5	<1	6	8	32	18	<1
B. Properties of cells									
D_{10} MMC (μg/ml; fibroblasts)	1.0	7.0	3.3	3.0	–	–	–	–	20–24
EC_{50} MMC (n*M*; lymphoblasts)	1.4	6.9	2.9	1.7	1.3	0.4	6.8	1.1	30–50

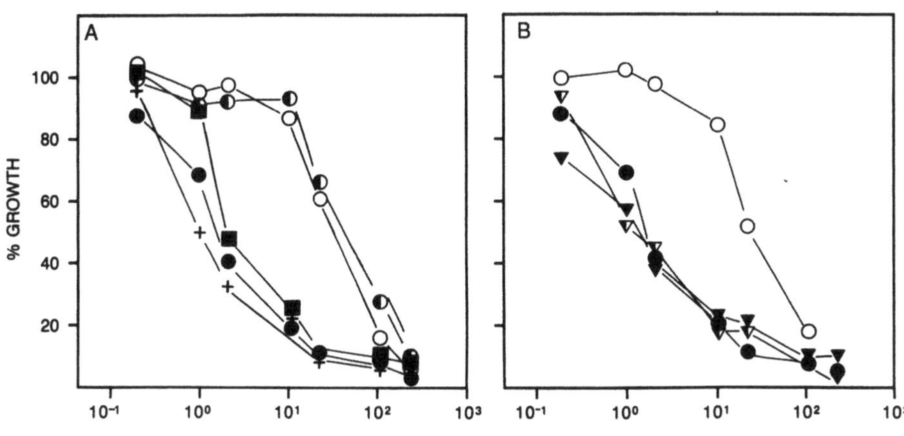

Fig. 1 A, B. Growth inhibition following treatment of normal (N) or FA cells with MMC. **A** illustrates a typical experiment in which complementation was observed. ●, FA 1; ■, FA 3; ○, N 1; ◐, FA 1/FA 3a; +, a well in which equal numbers of FA 1 and FA 3 cells were cocultivated without fusion. **B** illustrates an experiment in which complementation was not observed. ●, FA 1; ▼, FA 4; ○, N 3; ▽, FA 1/FA 4a; (Redrawn from Duckworth-Rysiecki et al. 1985)

provisionally placed in group B. Analysis of the data in Table 1 shows that no single clinical feature or group thereof correlates with the complementation groups. The two complementation groups cannot be distinguished on the basis of cellular sensitivity to MMC, as is the case with some of the XP complementation groups. However, a more detailed analysis will require a larger number of patients from each complementation group.

Further Complementation Studies. Since the initial studies, we have analyzed four other FA lymphoblast cell lines. Two of these (FA 5 and FA 6) came from the brothers of the patient with FA who was the donor of GM 1309, and belong to group A (Duckworth-Rysiecki et al. 1986). These patients were seen originally by Dr. M. Swift (Chapel Hill, NC). Unlike the first four patients analyzed, this family is black. Thus, complementation group A does not seem to be restricted to Caucasians. We also analyzed two other patients (FA 7 and FA 8). Both had some clinical features of FA (Table 1). The cells of FA 7 demonstrated an intermediate sensitivity to MMC (EC_{50} = 6.8 n*M*) and to several other DNA cross-linking agents, similar to that shown by FA 2 cells (R. Ishida and M. Buchwald, unpublished experiments). FA 8 cells were highly sensitive, with an EC_{50} of 1.1 n*M* MMC. Both of these cell lines complemented FA 1 and were placed in group B. Experiments to establish whether there is a further group C are in progress. We have constructed a doubly marked FA 3 cell line and are using this to perform complementation experiments with all cell lines that are currently in group B. As described in more detail by Moustacchi et al. (this volume), it has been possible to demonstrate the existence of two types of FA cells by biochemical assays (Moustacchi and Diatloff-Zito 1985). Using cells from the four original patients (FA 1-FA 4), our two groups have shown that these two biochemical phenotypes correlate with the two genetic complementation groups (Moustacchi et al. 1987). Whether this biochemical assay can ultimately be used as a substitute for the genetic experiments is still to be determined.

Gene Transfer Studies

The biochemical defect in FA is not known and it is therefore not possible to identify the FA gene by its gene product. Several genes were isolated, however, by complementation of a cellular phenotype of the cells of interest via DNA-mediated gene transfer (DMGT). In FA, the cellular phenotype of interest is MMC sensitivity. We therefore attempted to demonstrate that the introduction of normal DNA can correct the MMC sensitivity of FA cells. Since the long-term goal is to clone the FA gene, we chose to use cells with an unlimited growth potential. These cells, a line of SV 40-transformed FA fibroblasts (GM 6914), have been fully characterized by us and shown to belong to complementation group A (Duckworth-Rysiecki et al. 1986).

Establishment of Selection Conditions. In order to select MMC-resistant cells from a background of MMC-sensitive FA cells, we determined conditions under which FA cells would be selectively killed while control cells would not. Examination of the survival of GM 6914 cells following a single dose of MMC (Duckworth-Rysiecki et al. 1986), indicated that concentrations of MMC necessary to kill 10^5 to 10^6 FA cells would also kill a significant number of control cells. Since the number of recipient cells with the normal phenotype was likely to be small, a strategy involving a single dose of MMC might also have killed the desired recipients. We therefore chose instead to use a dose of MMC which would allow the survival of a significant number of control cells, and to use this dose as a chronic treatment. Figure 2 shows the effect of the chosen concentration of MMC (15 n*M*) on the

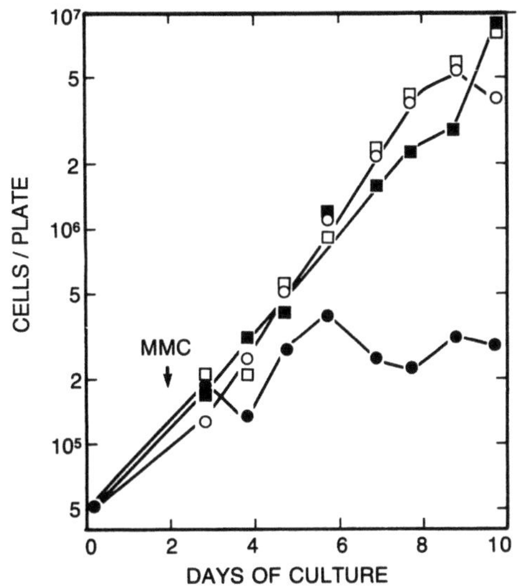

Fig. 2. Growth of cells in MMC. Normal (□, ○, GM 637) and FA (■, ●, GM 6914) cells were grown in the presence (○, ●) or absence (□, ■) of 15 n*M* MMC

Table 2. Isolation of MMC-resistant (MMC^R) Colonies

Source of DNA	CHO	Human	
Genotype	–	N	FA
Experiments *(n)*	4	2	5
Cells selected with G 418 ($\times 10^6$; *n*)	36	15	26
G 418^R colonies selected with MMC ($\times 10^3$; *n*)	25	3.6	12
MMC^R colonies *(n)*	9	1	5
Frequency of G 418^R colonies ($\times 10^{-4}$)	6.9	2.4	4.5
Overall frequency of MMC^R colonies ($\times 10^{-7}$)	2.5	0.7	1.9

N, normal cells

growth of FA and control cells. As can be seen, at this dose of MMC, the growth of normal cells is unaltered while the growth of FA cells is markedly decreased.

In order to verify that these selection conditions could in fact allow normal cells to proliferate while killing FA cells, we performed several reconstruction experiments. When plated in the presence of 15 n*M* MMC, the survival of a small number of normal cells in the presence of a large number of FA cells was close to 100%. No FA cells survived this treatment. The results of the reconstruction experiments confirmed that the conditions that we had chosen could be used to select for recipients undergoing complementation of MMC sensitivity in the DMGT experiments.

Results of DMGT experiments. The selection for recipients which were MMC resistant was done in two stages. First, cells which had taken up foreign DNA were selected for the presence of the *neo* gene by growing cells in G-418. Colonies were obtained at a frequency in the range of $2\text{-}8 \times 10^{-4}$ (Duckworth-Rysiecki et al. 1986), a value similar to that seen for several other SV 40-transformed cell lines

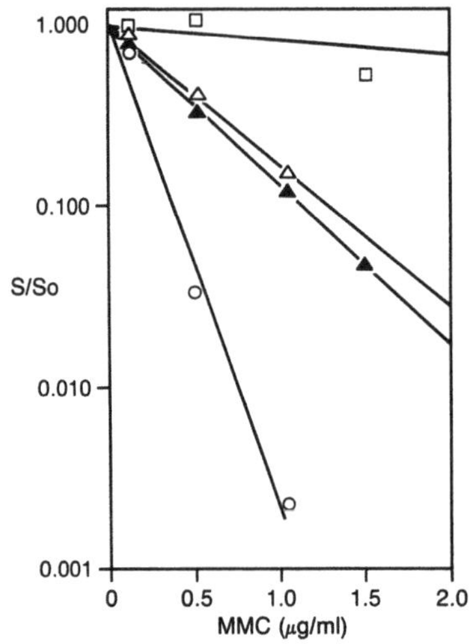

Fig. 3. Survival of MMC-resistant cells. Cells were treated with MMC for 1 h and plated to determine their survival. GM 637 (□), GM 6914 (○) A 18 was cultured in the presence (▲) or absence (△) of 15 n*M* MMC before determination of survival

(Mulligan and Berg 1980; Gorman et al. 1983; Royer-Pokora et al. 1984; Protic-Sabljic et al. 1985). These colonies were then exposed to 15 n*M* MMC. A summary of the results of five experiments in which either normal human, FA, or CHO DNA was introduced into GM 6914 cells is presented in Table 2. As can be seen, MMC-resistant colonies were obtained in all three cases and the frequencies were approximately the same, in the range of 2×10^{-7}. This represents the combined frequency of cells able to take up the *neo* plasmid and that of the G-418-resistant cells which survived the MMC selection.

Characterization of the MMC-Resistant Cells. Several colonies derived from independent DMGT experiments were isolated and characterized. We first determined the survival of the cells with respect to MMC. As is shown in Fig. 3 the sensitivity of cells from one of the colonies (A 18, from a CHO transfer) was between that of GM 6914 and that of normal cells. In order to establish whether this intermediate phenotype represented the acquisition of resistance to MMC through an alternative mechanism, we also tested the cells for their resistance to two other DNA-cross-linking agents [nitrogen mustard (NM) and diepoxybutane (DEB)]. Unlike MMC, NM and DEB do not require cellular activation to produce cross-links (Szybalski and Iyer 1967; Fox and Scott 1980). In addition, NM and MMC are transported into cells by different mechanisms (Byfield and Calabro-Jones 1981). A 18 cells also have an intermediate phenotype when tested with NM and DEB (data not shown). Thus, the intermediate phenotype is probably related to the ability of cells to repair the cross-links introduced by the chemical agents and not to a difference in their ability to metabolize or activate MMC. Colonies arising from several other experiments also showed an intermediate phenotype when tested for survival with MMC. The fact that such colonies arise, even when FA DNA is introduced, suggests that we are either selecting for partial revertants or that the DMGT protocol causes some alteration in the ability of cells to deal with cross-links.

Discussion

In this paper, we have discussed two aspects of complementation in FA. The first is the unequivocal demonstration of the existence of two complementation groups in FA. The isolation of somatic cell hybrids has allowed us to examine several different cellular properties of FA cells and to show that complementation is complete. All three features of FA cells - growth inhibition by MMC, spontaneous chromosome breakage, and MMC-induced chromosome breakage - are corrected in the complementing hybrids (Duckworth-Rysiecki et al. 1985). It has also been possible to show that the two complementation groups can be correlated with two biochemical phenotypes of FA cells, lending support to genetic heterogeneity of the two groups (Moustacchi et al. 1987, this volume). The genetic technique is the only unequivocal method of establishing complementation groups in FA, since it is not possible to determine in advance whether new complementation groups will share the known biochemical phenotypes (Moustacchi and Diatloff--Zito 1985). The correlation of these genetic classes with clinical phenotypes is a long-term project, since a significant number of patients in each class must be accumulated. However, on the basis of the clinical descriptions of the patients described in this paper, it seems unlikely that the multiple congenital malformations characteristic of FA will be clearly separable into genetically determined groups.

The second aspect of complementation presented in this paper is an attempt to use DMGT to complement the cellular phenotype of FA cells. Using the protocols described here, we were not able to show complementation successfully through DMGT. This result is the same as reported elsewhere in the case of XP and AT. Using SV 40-transformed cells, several groups have been unable to reproduce the original results of Takano et al. (1982), who claimed to be able to complement group A XP cells using wild-type DNA. UV-resistant colonies were obtained, but these represent revertants rather than true transformants (Royer-Pokora and Haseltine 1984; Schultz et al. 1985). The frequency of these revertants (10^{-7}) is similar to that obtained by us. In the case of AT, Green et al. (1985) have used DMGT to isolate a derivative of AT which has a partially reverted phenotype. The cells show a wild-type radioresistance but an AT-like inhibition of DNA synthesis (Lehmann et al. 1986).

While these experiments were in progress, Diatloff-Zito et al. (1986) reported the successful complementation of FA with DNA from normal human cells. These experiments were performed using untransformed fibroblasts and were based, in part, on the exploitation of the faster growth of normal fibroblasts compared to that of FA fibroblasts. If these experiments can be reproduced, they may allow the cloning of the FA gene using DMGT and molecular cloning techniques.

Acknowledgements. We thank Drs. M. Swift and T. Holbrook for providing the clinical data on patients FA 5 and FA 6.

References

Arlett CF, Lehmann AR (1978) Human disorders showing increased sensitivity to the induction of genetic damage. Annu Rev Genet 12: 95-115

Breitman ML, Tsui LC, Buchwald M, Siminovitch L (1982) Introduction and recovery of a selectable bacterial gene from the genome of mammalian cells. Mol Cell Biol 2: 966-976

Byfield JE, Calabro-Jones PM (1981) Carrier-dependent and carrier-independent transport of anti-cancer alkylating agents. Nature 294: 281-283

Cleaver JE (1984) Defective DNA repair and cancer-prone disorders of man. In: Bishop JM, Rowley JD, Greaves M (eds) Genes and Cancer. Liss, New York, pp 117-135

Diatloff-Zito C, Papadopoulo D, Averbeck D, Moustacchi E (1986) Abnormal response to DNA crosslinking agents of Fanconi anemia fibroblasts can be corrected by transfection with normal human DNA. Proc Natl Acad Sci USA 83: 7034-7038

Duckworth-Rysiecki G, Cornish K, Clarke C, Buchwald M (1985) Identification of two complementation groups in Fanconi anemia. Somatic Cell Mol Genet 11: 35-41

Duckworth-Rysiecki G, Toji L, Ng J, Clarke C, Buchwald M (1986) Characterization of a Simian virus 40-transformed Fanconi anemia fibroblast cell line. Mutat Res 166: 207-214

Fanconi G (1967) Familial constitutional panmyelocytopathy, Fanconi's anemia I. Clinical aspects. Semin Hematol 4: 233-240

Finkelberg R (1976) Studies on patients with Fanconi anemia. Ph D thesis, University of Toronto, Toronto, Canada

Fox M, Scott D (1980) The genetic toxicology of nitrogen and sulphur mustard. Mutat Res 75: 131-165

German J (1972) Genes which increase chromosomal instability in somatic cells and predispose to cancer. Prog Med Genet 8: 61-101

Gorman C, Padmanabhan R, Howard BH (1983) High efficiency DNA-mediated transformation of primate cells. Science 221: 551-553

Graham FL, van der Eb AJ (1973) A new technique for the assay of infectivity of human adenovirus 5 DNA. Virology 52: 456-467

Green MHL, Lowe JE, James MR, Arlett CF (1985) An attempt to transfer radiation resistance to an ataxia-telangiectasia cell line. In: Gatti RA, Swift M (eds) Ataxia-telangiectasia: genetics, neuropathology and immunology of a degenevative disease of childhood. Liss, New York, pp 173-179

Ishida R, Buchwald M (1982) Susceptibility of Fanconi's anemia lymphoblasts to DNA-crosslinking and alkylating agents. Cancer Res 42: 4000-4006

Jaspers NGJ, Painter RB, Paterson MC, Kidson C, Inoue I (1985) Complementation analysis of ataxia-telangiectasia. In: Gatti RA, Swift M (eds) Ataxia-telangiectasia: genetics, neuropathology and immunology of a degenerative disease of childhood. Liss, New York, pp 147-162

Lehmann AR, Arlett CF, Burke JF, Green MHL, James MR, Lowe JE (1986) A derivative of an ataxia-telangiectasia (A-T) cell line with normal radiosensitivity but A-T-like inhibition of DNA synthesis. Int J Radiat Biol 49: 639-643

Moustacchi E, Diatloff-Zito C (1985) DNA semi-conservative synthesis in normal and Fanconi's anemia fibroblasts following treatment with 8-methoxypsoralen and near ultraviolet light or X-rays. Hum Genet 70: 236-242

Moustacchi E, Papadopoulo D, Diatloff-Zito C, Buchwald M (1987) Two complementation groups of Fanconi's anemia differ in their phenotypic response to a DNA crosslinking treatment. Hum Gen 75: 45-47

Mulligan RC, Berg P (1980) Expression of a bacterial gene in mammalian cells. Science 209: 1422-1427

Protic-Sabljic M, Whyte D, Fagan J, Howard BH, Gorman CM, Padmanabhan R, Kraemer KH (1985) Quantification of expression of linked cloned genes in a Simian virus 40-transformed xeroderma pigmentosum cell line. Mol Cell Biol 5: 1685-1693

Royer-Pokora B, Haseltine WA (1984) Isolation of UV-resistant revertants from a xeroderma pigmentosum complementation group A cell line. Nature 311: 390-392

Royer-Pokora B, Peterson WD, Haseltine WA (1984) Biological and biochemical characterization of an SV 40-transformed xeroderma pigmentosum cell line. Exp Cell Res 151: 408-420

Rubin JS, Prudeaux VR, Willard HF, Dulhanty AM, Whitmore GF, Bernstein A (1985) Molecular

cloning and chromosomal localization of DNA sequences associated with a human DNA repair gene. Mol Cell Biol 5: 398-405
Schultz RA, Barbis DP, Friedberg EC (1985) Studies on gene transfer and reversion to UV resistance in xeroderma pigmentosum cells. Somatic Cell Mol Genet 11: 617-624
Setlow RB (1978) Repair deficient human disorders and cancer. Nature 271: 713-717
Southern EM (1975) Detection of specific sequences among DNA fragments separated by agarose gel electrophoresis. J Mol Biol 98: 503-515
Southern PJ, Berg P (1982) Transformation of mammalian cells to antibiotic resistance with a bacterial gene under control of the SV 40 early region promoter. J Mol Appl Genet 1: 327-341
Szybalksi W, Iyer VN (1967) The mitomycins and porfiromycins. In: Gottlieb D, Shaw PD (eds) mechanisms of action, Springer-Verlag. pp 211-245 (Antibiotics, vol I)
Takano T, Noda M, Tamura T (1982) Transfection of cells from a xeroderma pigmentosum patient with normal human DNA confers UV resistance. Nature 296: 269-270
Tsui LC, Breitman ML, Siminovitch L, Buchwald M (1982) Persistence of freely replicating SV 40 recombinant molecules carrying a selectable marker in permissive Simian cells. Cell 30: 499-508
Weksberg R, Buchwald M, Sargent P, Thompson MW, Siminovitch L (1979) Specific cellular defects in patients with Fanconi anemia. J Cell Physiol 101: 311-324
Westerveld A, Hoeijmakers JHJ, van Duin M, deWit J, Odijk H, Pastink A, Bootsma D (1984) Molecular cloning of a human DNA repair gene. Nature 310: 425-429

Complementation Studies in Fanconi Anemia Using Cell Fusion and Microinjection of mRNA*

M. Digweed, S. Zakrzewski-Lüdcke, and K. Sperling

Introduction

In medical genetics, it has frequently been found that a well-known clinical syndrome, once believed to be a single genetic entity, actually represents a collection of genetically distinct disorders (intergenic heterogeneity). On the other hand, it is also clear that a single defective gene can lead to strikingly different phenotypes. If constant phenotypic differences are found between afflicted members from different families, these may be attributable to different allelic mutations (interallelic heterogeneity). If however, clinical variability is found within affected families, this must be due to the remaining genetic background and/or epistatic factors.

The analysis of genetic heterogeneity in man can be performed at different levels with varying reliability, beginning at the phenotype level and ending with the analysis of the molecular architecture of the gene itself (for a review see Sperling 1983). In the case of Fanconi anemia (FA), in which the primary defect is still unknown, even correct diagnosis carries some uncertainty. Whilst progressive pancytopenia and malformations are characteristic, but not always present, the only symptom which must be present for diagnosis of FA is hypersensitivity to polyfunctional alkylating agents such as mitomycin C (MMC) (Auerbach et al. 1981; Cervenka et al. 1981). The importance of family history is clear in this connection.

Further biochemical investigations indicate that the basic defect must be related to a defect in repair of DNA damage causing a disturbed progression through the cell cycle (Poon et al. 1974; Latt et al. 1982). In such studies, considerable quantitative and qualitative variability has been observed which might indicate, but cannot prove, intergenic or interallelic heterogeneity.

Two experimental methods are available for directly analyzing the phenomenon of intergenic heterogeneity in FA; both are based on the normalization of the characteristic hypersensitivity of FA cells to cross-linking agents. In the first technique, somatic cells from different patients with FA are fused and the resulting hybrids are analyzed cytogenetically with respect to their sensitivity to MMC. If there is intergenic heterogeneity, then complementation should lead to "normal" - certainly not increased - levels of chromosomal damage. In the second approach, "transient" complementation of the defect is achieved after the injection of either

* This research was supported by the Deutsche Forschungsgemeinschaft.

T. M. Schroeder-Kurth A. D. Auerbach G. Obe (Eds.)
Fanconi Anemia, Clinical, Cytogenetic and Experimental Aspects

primary transcripts (mRNA) or primary gene products (proteins) isolated from other FA or normal cells.

While the first approach is merely descriptive, although of great value in estimating the degree of intergenic heterogeneity among patients with FA, the second approach offers the additional possibility of eventually identifying the defective gene and its abnormal product. In this chapter, we will first describe the FA cells used in our studies, with special reference to indirect biochemical and cytogenetical evidence of heterogeneity. Then we will present a critical evaluation of our experiments, which analyzed intergenic heterogeneity through cell hybrids. Finally, we will describe our microinjection system and its application to the study of transient complementation in FA, together with our preliminary results.

Characterization of FA Cell Lines

Most experiments were performed on skin fibroblast cultures taken from FA patients who were chosen for the following reasons:

1. They represent a wide spectrum of clinical variability.
2. They cover a range of ethnic origins and therefore possibly different mutational events.
3. The cells have been characterized biochemically, particularly with respect to DNA repair (see Table 1 for details).

The case histories of patients A, B, and C exemplify the extremes of the disease. Patient A had no skeletal anomalies but did show other typical features of FA: growth retardation, microcephaly, and hyperpigmentation. Pancytopenia was observed at the age of 6 and the patient died 5 years later from acute leukemia. Patient B was a "more typical" FA patient, with growth retardation, skeletal deformities, including thumb and radial aplasia, and pancytopenia from the age of 3. Patient C was suffering from a milder form of FA; pancytopenia started at the age of 24, although the high frequency of chromosomal breakage observed in his lymphocytes had already led to the diagnosis of FA (Schroeder et al. 1964). He had no skeletal anomalies but did have hyperpigmented areas of skin. An older brother also suffered from FA and he too had late onset of pancytopenia (Schroeder et al. 1976).

Chromosomal breakage in cells from these patients, several other FA cell lines, and a control fibroblast line is shown in Fig. 1. There is obviously considerable variation in the extent of chromosomal breakage both with and without MMC treatment. Such variation in response to clastogens is often found in FA fibroblasts. In survival assays, different FA cells were found to be between 3.1 and 27.5 times as sensitive to MMC as control cells (Latt et al. 1982). It should be noted that cells from the mother of patient B, who is therefore heterozygous for FA, showed no increased chromosomal breakage. This is important, since only when this is the case can a significant reduction in chromosomal breakage be expected from complemented hybrid cells.

Table 1. Characteristics of FA cell lines

Cell line	Characteristics	References/Source
FA A (lab. no. 1424)	No skeletal deformities	Sperling et al. (1975)
	Early onset of disease	
	German origin	Kunze (1980)
	Reduced DNA-ligase activity	Hirsch-Kaufmann et al. (1978)
	Reduced double-strand break repair	Coquerelle and Weibezahn (1981)
	Deficient cross-link repair	Gruenert and Cleaver (1985)
FA B (lab. no. 3557)	Severe skeletal deformities	Zakrzewski and Sperling (1980)
	Early onset of disease	
	Reduced double-strand break repair	Coquerelle and Weibezahn (1981)
FA C	No skeletal deformities	Schroeder et al. (1976)
	Late onset of disease	
	Normal double-strand break repair	Coquerelle and Weibezahn (1981)
FA D (lab. no. 3519)	Some skeletal deformities	Zakrzewski (1981)
	Early onset of disease	
FA E (lab. no. 4157)	Turkish origin	Zakrzewski and Sperling (1982)
	Early onset of disease	
GM 368	Black African origin	Institute for Medical Research Camden, New Jersey
GM 1746	Arabic origin	as above
GM 62 (CCL122, HG 261)	Reduced γ-ray and UV excision repair	as above
		Poon et al. (1974)
		Remsen and Cerutti (1976)
CRL 1196	Normal double-strand break repair	American Type Culture Collection
		Coquerelle and Weibezahn (1981)
CA 178	Anomalous cellular distribution of DNA topoisomerase I	Wunder et al. (1981)

We noted that two cell lines illustrated in Fig. 1 showed relatively low sensitivity to MMC in comparison with the other FA cells, namely FA C and CRL 1196. These cells showed 4.6 and 3.9 times the number of MMC-induced breaks found in control cells. In contrast, the other cells were 6.5–12.6 times as sensitive as control cells. Furthermore, after γ-irradiation these two cell lines showed normal DNA double-strand break repair kinetics while FA A and FA B were significantly impaired in this respect (Coquerelle and Weibezahn 1981). This finding suggests a deficiency in the process of DNA ligation in the FA A and FA B cells, which is

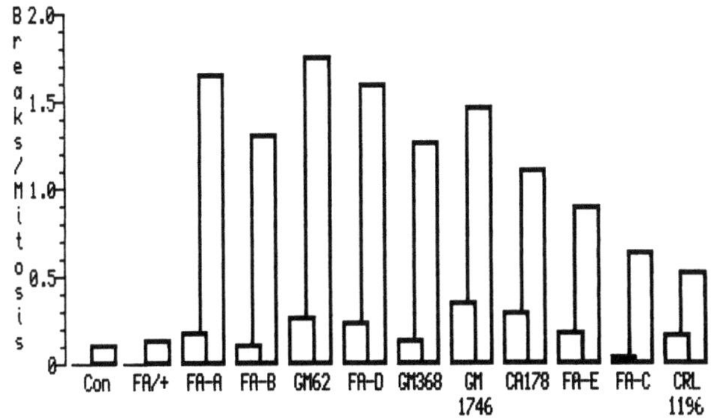

Fig. 1. Spontaneous and MMC-induced chromosomal breakage in FA, heterozygote, and control fibroblasts. Chromosomal breaks were counted in mitotic cells after cultivation for 24 h in normal medium *(left columns)* or in medium with 0.04 μg/ml MMC *(right columns)*. Details of the cells are given in Table 1 and in the text. The number of cells analyzed for each line was: Control (con), 150 (spontaneous breaks) and 150 (MMC-induced breaks); FA/+, 150,175; FA A, 150,110; FA B, 150,100; GM 62, 7,33; FA D, 50,18; GM 368, 116,77; GM 1746, 66,63; CA 178, 50,11; FA E, 150,91; FA C, 125,125; CRL 1196, 150,150

supported by earlier data for the FA A line. Pulse-labeling (Hirsch-Kaufmann et al. 1978) revealed that there was a slower shift of radioactivity from small to larger DNA fragments in FA A cells than in normal cells. This apparent reduction in DNA ligase activity was further tested by following the circularization of labeled poly(dAdT) in cell homogenates. FA A extracts showed only 44.3% of the activity found in control fibroblasts. With lymphocyte homogenates, a reduction to 25% of the normal level of activity was found in the patient and to 55% in his heterozygous mother. This loss of DNA ligase activity in the heterozygote contrasts with the chromosomal breakage in the heterozygote shown in Fig. 1. Presumably the 55% activity is sufficient for normal repair under these in vitro conditions. The examination of DNA ligation activity has unfortunately not been extended to other cells; however, a recent paper demonstrating a DNA ligase I deficiency in lymphoid B cell lines from patients with Bloom's syndrome reported no abnormality in the DNA ligase I and II activity of the FA cell line examined (Willis and Lindahl 1987). Of course, the deficiency in DNA ligation found in FA A cells does not necessarily originate in a defective DNA ligase as such, but rather in other components of the ligation machinery. DNA ligase is activated by adenosine diphosphate (ADP) ribosylation, catalyzed by the nicotinamide adenine (NAD^+)-dependent enzyme ADP ribosyltransferase (ADPRT). The consumption of free NAD^+ was shown to be reduced in FA fibroblasts after UV treatment, even though thymine dimers were efficiently excised (Klocker et al. 1983). Examination of nuclear extracts showed that several FA cell lines (including FA A) had significantly reduced ADPRT activity.

To summarize all the cytogenetical and biochemical evidence, FA A and FA B cells share a number of common characteristics which distinguish them from the cell lines FA C and CRL 1196, which themselves appear to be rather similar. Clinically, the patients FA A and FA B showed an early onset of the disease, while patient C had late onset of pancytopenia. The relevance of these observations for genetic heterogeneity can be tested by complementation analysis as discussed below.

Analysis of Heterogeneity by Somatic Cell Hybrids

As has already been pointed out, normalization of the hypersensitivity of FA cells to cross-linking agents is a reliable criterion for complementation in cell hybrids. This assay, however, depends on the selection of proliferating hybrid cells from unfused parental cells and homologous fusions. This raises serious technical problems, since proper selective media for human diploid cells are available for only a few specific problems. We sought to overcome this difficulty by transforming our FA A cell line with Simian virus (SV) 40 into a permanent line and by using a semiselective technique.

The new cell line, FA A', had the typical altered morphology of transformed cells, proliferated rapidly, and was no longer contact inhibited. After transformation, the average number of chromosomes rose to over 70. The transformed cells were cloned and one clone was used for all fusion experiments. The distribution of chromosome number in FA A' cells is shown in Fig. 2; there is clearly considerable variation, the average being 72. Karyotype analysis showed that the majority of chromosomes had retained their original morphology but the number of copies varied. While FA A cells were of the karyotype 46,XY, no Y chromosomes were found in FA A' cells. Chromosome rearrangements were constantly observed (see Table 2). They resulted in dicentric and tricentric chromosomes and acentric chromosome fragments, none of which were found in the original FA A cells, even after MMC treatment.

At the chromosome level, FA A' cells were essentially as sensitive to MMC as FA A cells with, respectively, 0.0246 and 0.0303 chromatid breaks per chromosome (Table 2). Chromosome-type aberrations in FA A' cells did not occur more frequently after MMC treatment; however, the proportion of acentric fragments per metaphase did rise from 28% to 47%. This may have been due to MMC-

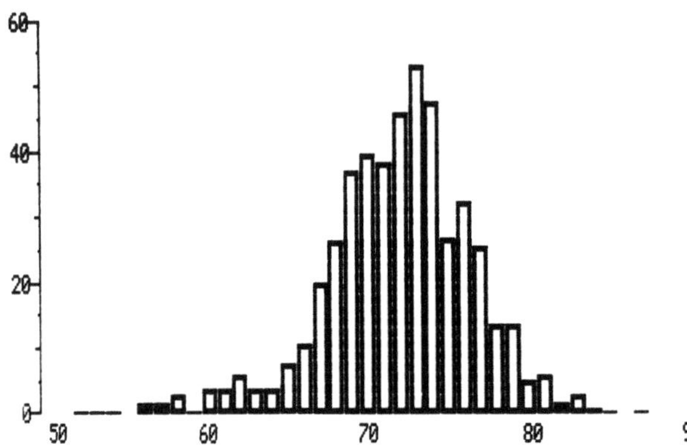

Fig. 2. Distribution of chromosome number in FA A' cells. x-axis, number of chromosomes/cell; y-axis, number of cells. Chromosomes of 500 mitotic cells were counted, giving an average of 71.8

induced isochromatid breaks which, however, cannot be distinguished from the spontaneously occurring acentric fragments, typical of transformed cells. These considerations made it expedient to count only chromatid breaks and translocations and to ignore dicentric, tricentric, ring, and acentric chromosomes in the fusion experiments. At the molecular level, FA A' cells were shown to be unable to excise DNA cross-links produced by treatment with 8-methoxypsoralen plus UVA (Gruenert and Cleaver 1985).

The strategy chosen for our hybridization experiments is shown schematically in Fig. 3. Criteria for the selection of hybrid cells against parental cells were the diethyl-pyrocarbonate (DEP)-induced death of the FA A' cells and the continued proliferation of hybrid cells after the diploid parent was already contact inhibited.

Table 2. Comparison of chromatid and chromosome breaks in FA A and FA A'

Line	MMC	Cells counted	B	RB	Ring	DIC	TRIC	ACE	Breaks/ mitosis	Breaks/ chromosome
FA A	–	250	42	–	–	–	–	–	0.1825	0.00397
FA A'	–	250	61	2	–	197	3	70	0.2375	0.00332
FA A	+	90	115	6	–	–	–	–	1.4	0.03030
FA A'	+	100	168	5	2	54	–	47	1.78	0.02460

The cells were grown for 24 h in the presence of 0.04 μg/ml MMC. FA A, diploid fibroblasts from patient A; FA A', SV40-transformed cells derived from FA A; B, chromatid breaks; RB, chromatid translocations; Ring, ring chromosomes; DIC, TRIC, ACE, dicentric, tricentric, and acentric chromosomes, respectively. For calculation of breakage rates, translocations were counted as two breaks, and rings, dicentrics, tricentrics, and acentrics were ignored. Data from Zakrzewski (1981).

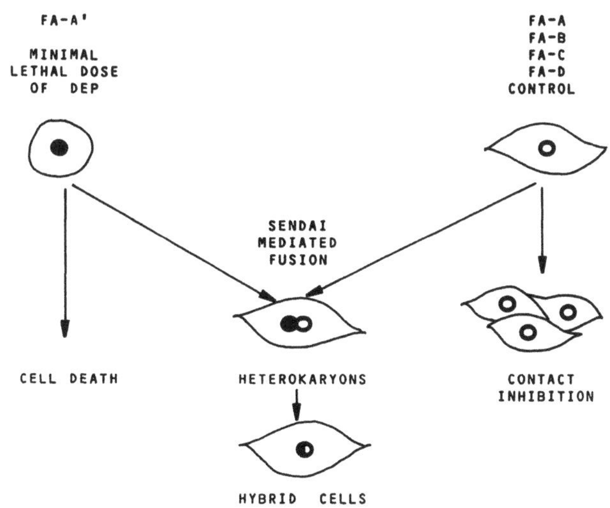

Fig. 3. The strategy for cell fusion in the study of complementation in FA fibroblasts. DEP, diethyl-pyrocarbonate

The cells were then isolated by gentle trypsinization and their rate of chromosomal aberrations after MMC treatment was analyzed (Zakrzewski and Sperling 1980).

Since the strategy employed was not fully selective and some contamination of hybrids with parental cells or homologous fusions might have been expected, the heterogeneous nature of the hybrids was confirmed in two other ways. Firstly, the number of chromosomes in hybrid cells could be expected to be the sum of that in the parental cells, that is about 118 chromosomes (FA A', 72 chromosomes; diploid fibroblasts, 46). However, since the number of chromosomes in FA A' is so variable (see Fig. 2), only cells with between 80 and 129 chromosomes were considered to be hybrids. Secondly, the FA A' cells have a high number of dicentric and acentric chromosomes as discussed above, but, despite their origin, no Y chromosome. Most of the other FA cells used were from male patients so that the simultaneous presence of a Y chromosome and dicentric or acentric chromosomes indicated the heterologous nature of a hybrid cell.

In the first series of experiments, the parental cells were taken from FA patients who exhibited considerable differences in phenotypic expression (FA A-FA D). The results are illustrated in Figure 4 A. Clearly, the FA A'/FA C hybrid cells were much less sensitive to MMC than the FA A'/FA A hybrids. The picture was similar when spontaneous breakage was measured. Thus the FA A' and FA C cells complemented each other, and consequently represent members of two distinct forms of FA. Obviously, no complementation is observed between FA A' and FA B or FA D cells. Initially, the same seemed to be true for all the other fusions in which the parental cells differed with respect to either their ethnic origin (Fig. 4 B) or repair characteristics (Fig. 4 C). As expected, a significant reduction in the aberration rate was observed in hybrids between FA A' and control cells.

Surprisingly, these hybrids still have a higher sensitivity to MMC than that normally found in control cells and those of heterozygotes, even more than in the heterologous FA cross, FA A'/FA C. This sensitivity in FA A'/control cells was repeatedly observed and casts doubt on the validity of the test system. In this respect, it must be noted that considerable chromosome loss was observed with passage number in all the hybrids and this was accompanied in some cases by an increase in chromosomal breakage (Fig. 5). It is difficult to compensate for this effect, since the time between cell fusion and the first experimental analysis differed considerably among the various hybrids. Moreover, one must consider that since chromosome loss occurs more or less randomly, the hybrids may also differ in the number not only of repair-related genes and integrated SV40 genomes, but also of those genes involved in the uptake, activation, and degradation of MMC, which must surely affect their MMC sensitivity.

In the face of these findings, the importance of comparison with the homologous FA A'/FA A fusion becomes evident. We have now reexamined the hybrids with CRL 1196 cells (Fig. 4 C), since, although these differed significantly from the FA A'/control hybrids, they were also considerably different from the FA A'/FA A hybrids. The replicate measurements of chromosomal breakage in FA A'/FA A and FA A'/CRL 1196 hybrids were analyzed using the Kolmogorow-Smirnow test and the Bonferroni method for multiple testing. Since no significant difference could be found between independent measurements in the individ-

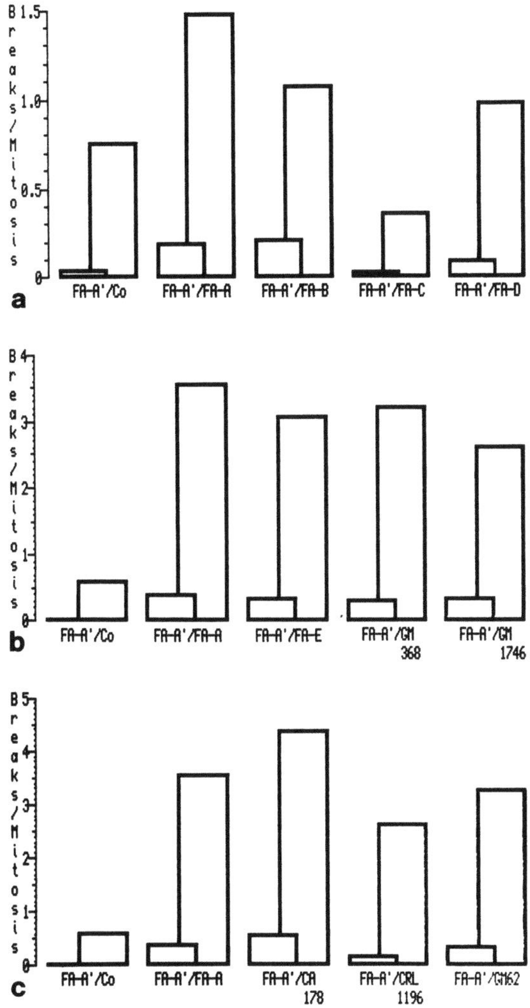

Fig. 4a–c. Spontaneous and MMC-induced chromosomal breakage in hybrids of FA fibroblasts. Hybrid cells were cultivated in normal medium *(left columns)* or medium with MMC *(right columns)* for 24 h, and mitotic cells were collected over 4 h with colcemid and breaks scored as discussed in the text. **a** Fibroblasts from patients showing phenotypic heterogeneity. Cells scored: FA A'/Co,150 (spontaneous), 150 (MMC-induced); FA A'/FA A, 150,150; FA A'/FA B, 150,150; FA A'/FA C, 150,150; FA A'/FA D, 100,100. **b** Fibroblasts from patients of different ethnic origin. Cells scored: FA A'/Co, 245,136; FA A'/FA A, 194,143; FA A'/FA E, 250,92: FA A'/GM 368, 110,4; FA A'/GM 1746, 225,139. **c** Fibroblasts with different biochemical characteristics. Cells scored: FA A'/Co, 245,136; FA A'/FA A, 194,143; FA A'/CA 178, 137,40; FA A'/CRL 1196, 225,134; FA A'/GM 62, 10,10. Data are taken from Zakrzewski and Sperling (1980, 1982) and Zakrzewski et al. (1983)

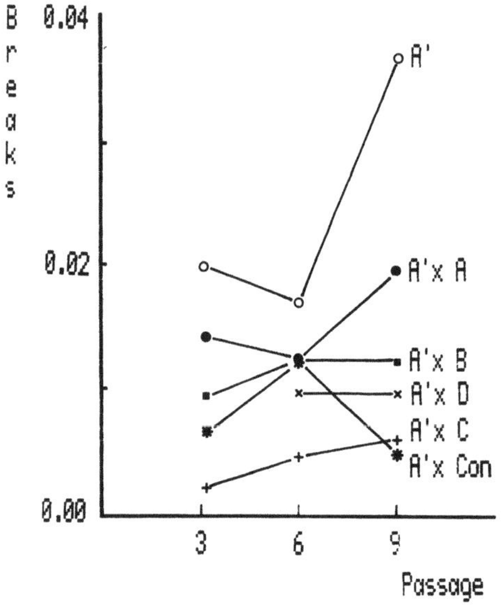

Fig. 5. Chromosomal breakage in hybrids after continued cultivation. Chromosomal breakage after 24 h in medium containing 0.04 μg/ml MMC was scored at the 3rd, 6th, and 9th passages. The results are expressed as breaks/chromosome. Each point represents at least 50 mitotic cells

ual hybrids, these could then be compared. The distributions of the number of breaks per mitosis of the two hybrid cell lines were compared and found to be significantly different ($p < 0.001$). Thus, CRL 1196 cells formed hybrids with FA A' cells which were significantly different to both FA A'/FA A and FA A'/control hybrids. This finding possibly represents a second genuine complementation event. We have no evidence to suggest that FA C and CRL 1196 belong to distinct groups.

We have interpreted our results to suggest that intergenic heterogeneity is less extensive in FA than in other hereditary diseases, for example, xeroderma pigmentosum (XP), where fusion studies rapidly established nine complementation groups. In our studies, complementation was found twice amongst nine hybrid cells, indicating the existence of at least two complementation groups. One of these is a large group comprising cells from patients of different ethnic origin, cells with different biochemical lesions, and cells from patients with and without the skeletal anomalies often found in FA. The second complementation group is represented by the cells from FA C, which differ from the cells of the other group in the age of onset of pancytopenia in the patient and in the clinically associated symptoms. On the basis of our fusion studies, the cell line CRL 1196 probably also belongs to this second group.

In vitro, these two groups may be distinguishable by several phenotypic traits, although it must be emphasized that most examinations have only been carried out with individual cell lines. The first group seems to be more sensitive to MMC than the second, as shown for chromosomal breakage (Fig. 1) and for cell-cycle blocking in FA A, FA B (first group), and FA C (second group; see Fig. 11). In their fusion studies using lymphoblastoid cells, Duckworth-Rysiecki et al. (1985) also found two complementation groups among four patients and these too differed somewhat in their MMC sensitivity (50% inhibition of growth,

EC_{50} = 2.0 n*M* and 1.7 n*M* in one group, 6.9 n*M* in the other). To further define the complementation groups, their ability to ligate DNA may be significant, since reduced ligation activity is indicated for two members of the first group (FA A and FA B; Coquerelle and Weibezahn 1981; Hirsch-Kaufmann et al. 1978) compared with the normal activity in the two members of the second group (FA C and CRL 1196; Coquerelle and Weibezahn 1981).

Finally, cells from these two groups differ in their response to a cross-linking challenge. CRL 1196 cells recover normal semiconservative DNA synthesis rates 10 h after treatment with psoralen and UVA, as do normal fibroblasts (Moustacchi and Diatloff-Zito 1985). The alternative response, a permanent repression of the DNA synthesis rate, is shown by FA A and FA B cells, whilst FA C cells recover normal synthesis rates (see below and Digweed et al. 1988). A correlation between MMC sensitivity and response to psoralen/UVA is shown by three cell lines used by Moustacchi and Diatloff-Zito (1985) and Diatloff-Zito et al. (1986); lines FA 150 and FA 121 have 40 times the control cell sensitivity to MMC and do not recover normal DNA synthesis rates, while the cell line FA 109 has lower MMC sensitivity (11 times control) and does recover from psoralen/UVA treatment. That the phenotypic response to psoralen/UVA treatment correlates with complementation groups has been demonstrated for both sets of genetically characterized cells (Digweed et al. 1988; Moustacchi et al. 1987).

Complementation of FA Cells by Microinjection of mRNA

Figure 6 shows diagrammatically the strategy for examining complementation by microinjection of mRNA. An active mRNA preparation is needed, and this is extracted from cells grown in suspension or by monolayer culture using standard techniques. A crude cytoplasmic extract is phenolized to extract the RNA and the 2%-3% of mRNA present in this extract can be isolated by oligo(dT) affinity chromatography.

The instrumentation used for microinjection is shown in Fig. 7. Microinjection is carried out under a Leitz Fluovert inverted microscope with the microcapillary maneuvered by a motor-driven micromanipulator. Due to their high viscosity, microinjection of mRNA solutions can be difficult. The RNA must be centrifuged immediately before use in order to pellet any debris and RNA aggregates, which are readily formed. For delivery of the sample into the cells we use compressed air precisely controled by the ECET system (Eppendorf, FRG). Fibroblasts were plated out onto 18 mm × 18 mm coverslips in small petri dishes. The coverslips were marked with a grid to enable injected cells to be found after the assay.

Before use, we check that the mRNA is active in protein biosynthesis. This can be done in vitro using extracts from rabbit erythrocytes or wheat germ, or in vivo after injection into oocytes or somatic cells. We test mRNA by injecting it into mouse or human fibroblasts with specific nucleotide metabolism defects, and assay for complementation by following the uptake and incorporation of ^{3}H-labeled nucleotide bases. Cells from patients with adeninephosphoribosyl transferase (APRT) deficiency are not normally able to incorporate ^{3}H-adenine. Thus $APRT^-$ cells incubated for several hours in medium containing ^{3}H-adenine and subse-

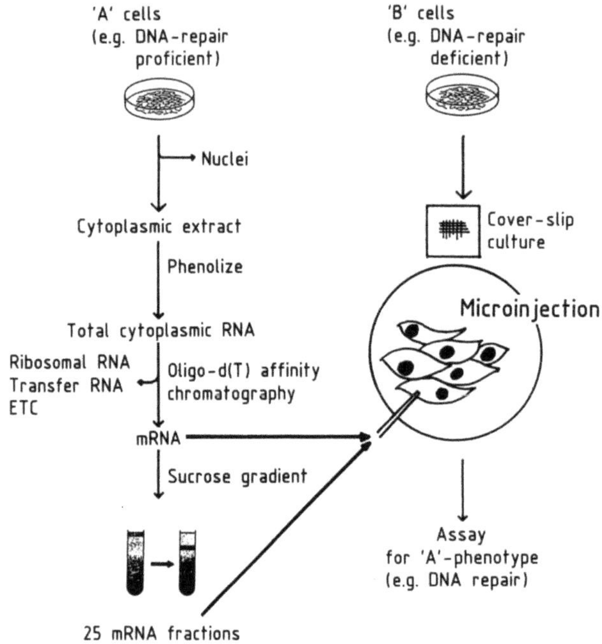

Fig. 6. Strategy for examining complementation through microinjection of mRNA

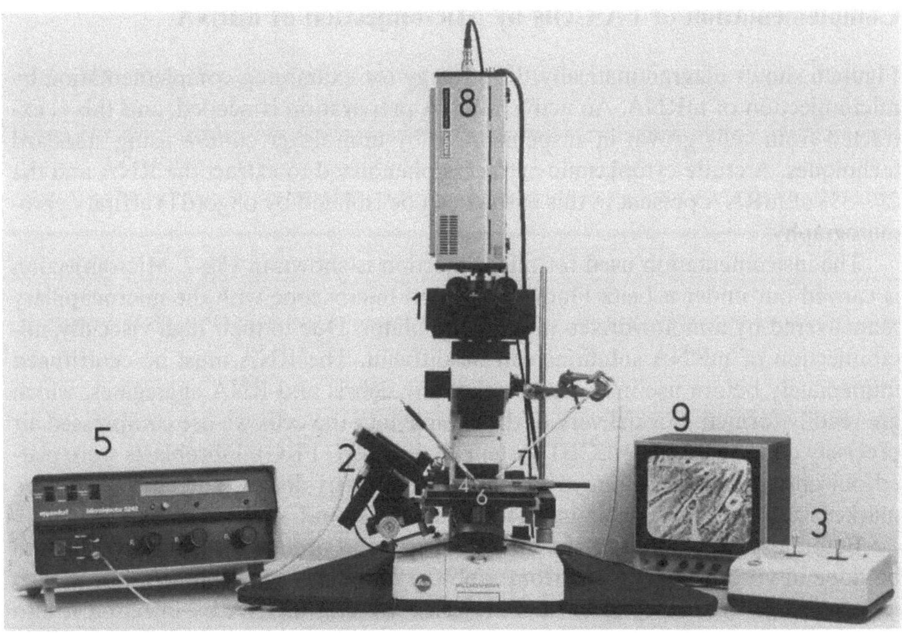

Fig. 7. The microinjection system. The system consists of a Leitz Fluovert invertoscope *(1)* with micromanipulator *(2)* controled by a pair of joysticks *(3)*. The microcapillary *(4)* is connected to the ECET injector *(5)*. A stream of sterile CO_2 is projected onto the cells *(6)* from the pipette *(7)* to maintain an optimal pH value. A video camera *(8)* and monitor *(9)* allow filming and observation of the injection procedure

quently autoradiographed, show essentially no silver grains above their nuclei, as shown in Fig. 8a. After injection of HeLa mRNA and 20 h cultivation, $APRT^-$ cells are able to incorporate ^{3}H-adenine (Fig. 8b), indicating that mRNA is active in protein synthesis and has provided the missing enzyme. In a typical assay, He-La mRNA at 0.8-1.2 mg/ml is able to transiently complement over 70% of injected cells. Since the individual molecular species in a cellular mRNA population differ in three basic properties - length, secondary structure, and base composition - they may be separated from one another and the individual fractions tested for presence of a particular mRNA by monitoring complementation after microinjection. Figure 9 shows the absorption profiles of sucrose gradients loaded with HeLa $poly(A)^+$ and $poly(A)^-$ RNA. The fraction leading to maximal complementation of $APRT^-$ cells is shaded. Using the $poly(A)^-$ RNA profile to calibrate the gradient, we estimate that fraction 18 contains mRNA 1120 ($\pm$80) nucleotides in length. Assuming 300 of these nucleotides are the poly(A) tail, we would expect a cDNA copy of the APRT mRNA to be about 820 nucleotides long, which agrees excellently with the actual length found by Dush et al. (1985). As an example of mRNA-mediated complementation in a human DNA repair deficient cell line, Fig. 10 shows the complementation of XP (complementation group A) fibroblasts after injection of HeLa mRNA. The assay is for unscheduled DNA synthesis (UDS) and measures repair synthesis of DNA as a response to exposure to UV light. In the population of 183 injected cells, mRNA injection allows 43% of the

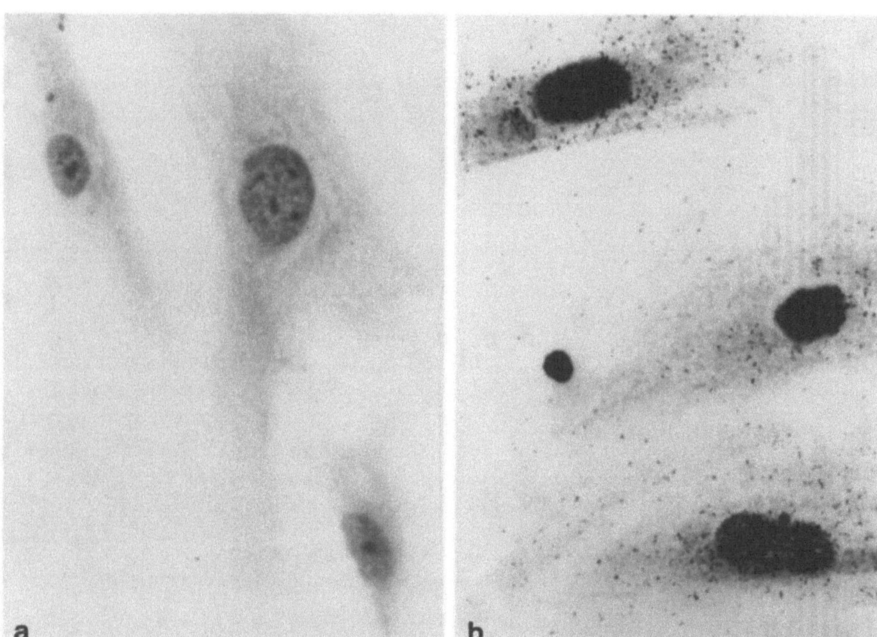

Fig. 8 a, b. Complementation of $APRT^-$ cells by mRNA microinjection. **a** $APRT^-$ cells, cultivated in ^{3}H-adenine (40 µCi/ml) for 3 h and subsequently processed for autoradiography and exposed for 3 days. **b** $APRT^-$ cells, labeled as described above, 24 h after injection of 1.2 mg/ml total HeLa mRNA

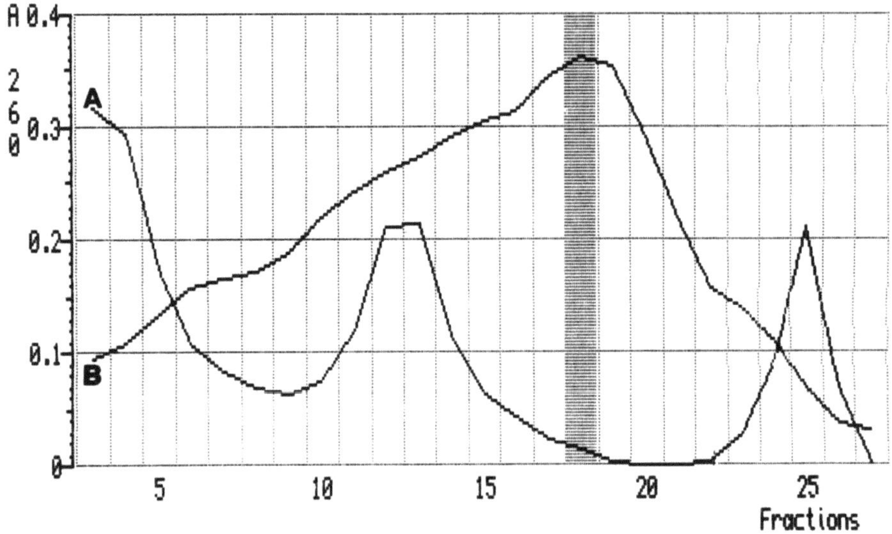

Fig. 9. Fractionation of poly(A)$^+$ mRNA. Absorption profile at 260 nm of a 15%–30% sucrose gradient loaded with *(A)* 200 μg poly(A)$^-$ and *(B)* 200 μg poly(A)$^+$ HeLa RNA. Centrifugation was at 35 000 rpm for 17 h. Fractions (0.5 ml) were collected and used to microinject APRT$^-$ cells. The fraction giving the highest complementation (99%) is *shaded*. The poly(A)$^-$ RNA peaks are, from left to right, 26S, 18S and 5S rRNA

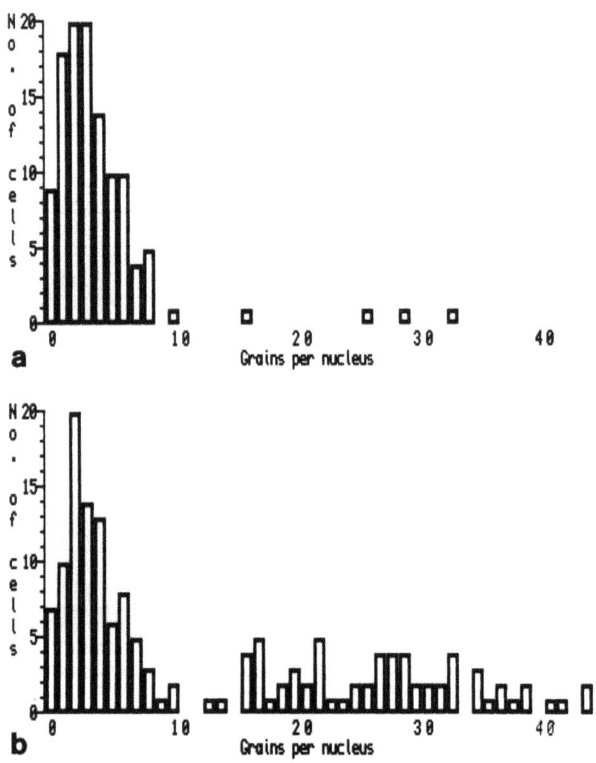

cells to show the same UDS level found in normal fibroblasts. Examination of complementation by microinjection in FA fibroblasts depends upon the availability of an assay as reliable as the UDS assay for XP cells. We have concentrated on the two assays described below.

One effect of clastogens on FA cells is to block the cell cycle, resulting in a reduction of the number of cells in mitosis (Kaiser et al. 1982). We examined this in our FA cells by exposing them to increasing concentrations of MMC for 30 h of cultivation and then collecting mitotic cells over 10 h by colcemid arrest (Fig. 11). The molarity of MMC required to reduce the mitotic index by 50% (D_{50}) was 70 n*M* for control cells but 6 n*M* for FA A and FA B cells and 20 n*M* for FA C cells, reflecting their unusual sensitivity to this chemical.

As an assay for complementation after microinjection of mRNA, this method is particularly attractive since it involves little manipulation of the cells and has the advantage that chromosomal breakage may be measured in the fixed mitoses. Pilot experiments with buffer injection have shown that this alone has little effect on the mitotic index at least.

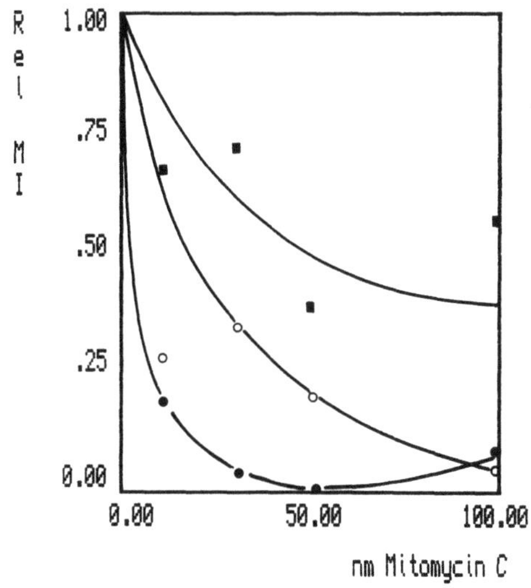

Fig. 11. The effect of MMC on mitotic index in FA fibroblasts. Fibroblasts were cultured for 24 h in medium containing increasing concentrations of MMC and mitotic cells were collected by the addition of colcemid for a further 10 h. After this, the coverslip cultures were gently fixed and the mitotic index determined for 500 cells. The results are presented relative to untreated control cultures for FA A cells (●), FA C cells (○), and control cells (■)

Fig. 10a, b. Unscheduled DNA synthesis in xeroderma pigmentosum fibroblasts. Fibroblasts from XP complementation group A were exposed to 15 J/m^2 UV light and then incubated in ^3H-thymidine (10 μCi/ml) for 2 h. **a** Histogram of grains/nucleus for 115 cells (average, 4.1 grains/nucleus). **b** Histogram of grains/nucleus for a field of 183 cells which were injected with HeLa mRNA (1.2 mg/ml) 19 h prior to the UV treatment; two populations were found with averages of 3.3 and 26.4 grains/nucleus; the complemented population represented 43% of the total cells. Control fibroblasts had 23.9 grains/nucleus in this particular experiment (data not shown)

As reported by Moustacchi and Diatloff-Zito (1985), FA and normal fibroblasts respond to psoralen and intermediate doses of long-wave UV with a rapid reduction in their rate of semiconservative DNA synthesis. The normal rate of synthesis is regained in normal and some FA fibroblasts after a 10-h recovery period. Other FA cell lines do not recover normal DNA synthesis rates. The rate of DNA synthesis can be readily estimated in single cells by autoradiography after incorporation of ^{3}H-thymidine. Twelve hours after treatment with 8-methoxypsoralen and UVA, FA A cells show a lower synthesis rate than sham-irradiated FA A cells (Fig. 12a; Digweed et al. 1988). FA A cells apparently belong to the group of FA fibroblasts which do not recover normal synthesis rates. This is clearly in full agreement with the lack of cross-link removal in psoralen/UVA-treated FA A' cells found by Gruenert and Cleaver (1985). In contrast, FA C cells belong to the class which does recover normal DNA synthesis rates (Fig. 12b). These results show that FA A cells are also suitable for microinjection experiments using this assay for complementation. Figure 12c shows the distribution profiles for FA A cells injected with HeLa mRNA 24 h prior to cross-linking treatment with psoralen/UVA. In the distribution of injected cells, there is a clear shift to a higher level of thymidine incorporation than in neighboring, uninjected cells, as would be expected when complementation has occurred. The two distributions differ significantly in the Kolmogorow-Smirnow test ($p = 0.10$). The complementing mRNA has been localized to gradient fraction 21 (mRNA of 640 ± 80 nucleotides in length); cells injected with these mRNA fractions have a DNA synthesis rate nearly twice that of uninjected cells ($p < 0.01$ in the Kolmogorow-Smirnow test). With reasonable assumptions on poly(A) tail and 5'-noncoding sequence lengths, we estimate that this fraction of mRNA codes for polypeptides with a molecular mass of 18($\pm$3) kilodaltons. This assay has also been successfully exploited by Gök and Wunder (1987) to demonstrate complementation in FA cells after injection of protein extracts (see elsewhere in this volume).

The Way to the Gene

A typical mammalian fibroblast cell contains about 400000 molecules of mRNA composed of about 11500 different molecular species, which are present in differing abundance, as shown in Table 3. We must assume that the FA and XP mRNAs belong to the scarce mRNAs, a class which represents 46% of the total cellular mRNA. The fraction of total cytoplasmic, poly(A)$^{+}$ mRNA which a single

Table 3. The mRNA of a mammalian fibroblast

Class	Copies/cell	Different sequences	Total
1	12000	4	48000
2	300	500	150000
3	15	11000	165000

After Hastie and Bishop (1976)

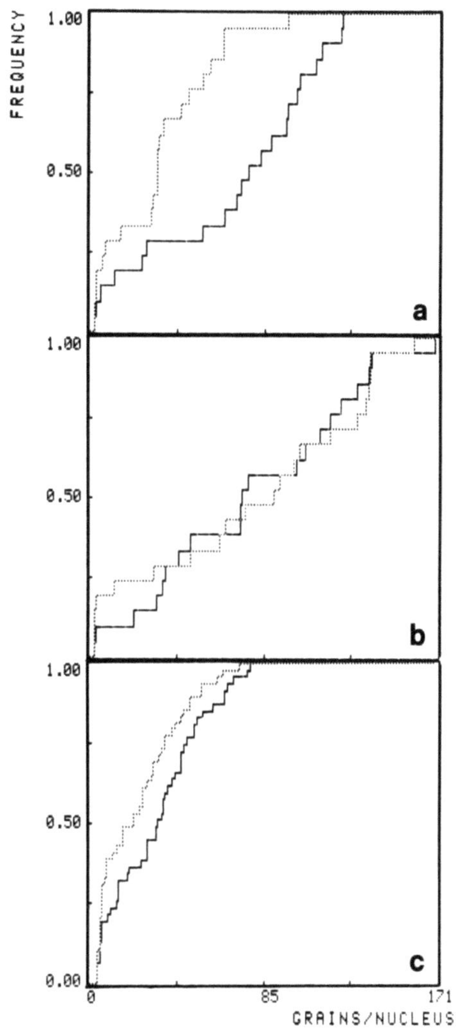

Fig. 12a–c. Semiconservative DNA synthesis in FA fibroblasts after 8-methoxypsoralen (8-MOP) and UVA treatment. Coverslip cultures of FA A and FA C cells were incubated for 10 min in 0.1 μg/ml 8-MOP and either irradiated with 365 nm UV light for 20 min (·····) or left in the dark at room temperature for the same length of time (——). Ten hours later, all cultures were labeled for 10 min with ^{3}H-thymidine (0.1 μCi/ml). After autoradiography, grains/nucleus were counted for at least 30 cells and the proportional cumulative frequency diagrams drawn. **a** FA A cells in which the difference between irradiated and control cells was found to be significant (Kolmogorow-Smirnow test $p < 0.001$). **b** FA C cells. **c** Grain distributions for FA A cells injected with HeLa mRNA (——) and uninjected cells (·····), treated as above. Of the 173 cells injected, 47 were in the S phase (> 3 grains/nucleus) at labeling. As a control, 49 uninjected S phase cells from neighboring fields were scored. Cells from a parallel but sham-irradiated culture were scored and showed a distribution which was essentially the same as that in **a.** Note that the injected cells incorporated more ^{3}H-thymidine, indicating complementation

scarce mRNA represents is 1/24000. This frequency is readily detected in microinjection assays for both XP and FA.

In order to clone these molecules they may be converted into cDNA and then inserted into a mammalian/bacterial expression vector. The frequency of plasmids containing the mRNA of interest remains 1/24000. However, due to sampling variation and preferential cloning of some sequences, the actual number of bacterial clones required to ensure that every scarce mRNA is represented in the library is given by the following formula, taken form Clarke and Carbon (1976):

$$N = [ln(1-P)]/[ln(1-1/n)]$$

where N is the number of clones required, P is the probability desired (0.99), and n is the fractional proportion of a scarce mRNA, 1/24000. The number of clones required turns out to be about 110000, a reasonably practicable number obtainable from relatively small amounts of mRNA using standard cDNA cloning techniques.

Starting not with total mRNA but with a fraction enriched for the mRNA sought dramatically improves the situation. Fraction 21 is enriched for the FA-correcting mRNA by a factor of 24, so that this sequence should be contained in a partial cDNA bank of just 5000 recombinants. This is fortunate, since the identification system, namely the human fibroblast cell, is particularly unwilling to take up naked DNA. For example, only about 0.1% of a cell population is able to take up high-molecular-weight DNA in calcium phosphate-mediated transfection experiments. Furthermore, given the extremely small proportion of genomic DNA that a single-copy gene represents, the frequency of transformants with a particular gene will be something like 1 cell in 10^7-10^8. This is an uncomfortable frequency to work with, particularly since spontaneous reversion can occur at even higher frequencies.

A more efficient way to the gene may be through transient expression of an mRNA fraction library in an appropriate vector after microinjection. Injecting the thymidine kinase gene into mouse LA TK^- cells led to 50%-100% transient expression of the enzyme activity (Capecchi 1980). Since the desired mRNA is already detectable in the mRNA fraction, and subsequent cloning can only improve its frequency, it should be possible to identify a complementing clone through library partition. One approach to expression of the cDNAs in injected cells is to use a eukaryotic expression vector which carries the SV40 replication origin and transcription enhancer sequences 5' to the cloning site. The mRNAs are cloned directly, and in correct orientation, into the vector, using the differential tailing technique for vector preparation described by Oberbäumer (1986). In an alternative strategy, the cells are injected with mRNA synthesized in vitro from cDNA recombinants in vectors carrying the SP6 polymerase promoter.

The use of microinjection as described here can perhaps be extended to other hereditary diseases which can be characterized at the cytological level. For example, the rate of DNA synthesis is not reduced in cells from patients with ataxia-telangiectasia and related syndromes (complementation groups V1 and V2; Jaspers et al. 1987) after bleomycin treatment, which contrasts with the response of normal control fibroblasts. After microinjection of fibroblasts assigned to complementation group V2 with HeLa mRNA, and subsequent bleomycin treatment, measurement of DNA synthesis showed that a proportion of the injected cells had reduced their semiconservative DNA synthesis rates.

In conclusion, the phenomenon of heterogeneity in genetic disorders in which the primary defect is unknown, but which show characteristic cellular response, may be studied through cell fusion and microinjection of mRNA. These two approaches complement one another and offer a way to search for the genes themselves.

Acknowledgements. We thank Dr. H. Neitzel for stimulating discussions and Dr. R. Plätke for advice on the statistical tests.

References

Auerbach AD, Adler B, Chaganti RSK (1981) Prenatal and postnatal diagnosis and carrier detection of Fanconi's anaemia by a cytogenetic method. Pediatrics 67: 128-135

Capecchi MR (1980) High efficiency transformation by direct microinjection of DNA into cultured mammalian cells. Cell 22: 479-488

Cervenka J, Arthur D, Yasis C (1981) Mitomycin C test for diagnostic differentiation of idiopathic aplastic anemia and Fanconi's anemia. Pediatrics 67: 119-127

Clarke L, Carbon J (1980) A colony bank containing synthetic ColE1 hybrid plasmids representative of the entire *E. coli* genome. Cell 9: 91-99

Coquerelle TM, Weibezahn KF (1981) Rejoining of DNA double-strand breaks in human fibroblasts and its impairement in one ataxia telangiectasia and two Fanconi strains. J Supramol Struc Cell Biochem 17: 369-376

Diatloff-Zito C, Papadopoulo D, Averbeck D, Moustacchi E (1986) Abnormal response to DNA crosslinking agents in Fanconi anemia fibroblasts can be corrected by transfection with normal human DNA. Proc Natl Acad Sci USA 83: 7034-7038

Digweed M, Zakrzewski-Lüdcke S, Sperling K (1988) Fanconi's anaemia: correlation of genetic complementation group with Psoralen/UVA response. Hum Genet 78: 51-54

Duckworth-Rysiecki G, Cornish K, Klarke CA, Buchwald M (1985) Identification of two complementation groups in Fanconi anemia. Somatic Cell Mol Genet 11: 35-41

Dush MK, Sikela JM, Khan SA, Tischfield JA, Stambrook PJ (1985) Nucleotide sequence and organisation of the mouse adenine phosphoribosyltransferase gene. Proc Natl Acad Sci USA 82: 2731-2735

Gök MM, Wunder E (1987) Microinjection of normal cell extracts into Fanconi anemia fibroblasts corrects their scheduled DNA synthesis rate after 8-methoxypsoralen plus UVA treatment. Hum Genet 75: 350-355

Gruenert DC, Cleaver JE (1985) Repair of psoralen-induced cross-links and monoadducts in normal and repair-deficient human fibroblasts. Cancer Res 45: 5399-5404

Hastie ND, Bishop JO (1976) The expression of three abundance classes of mRNA in mouse tissues. Cell 9: 761-774

Hirsch-Kauffmann M, Schweiger M, Wagner EF, Sperling K (1978) Deficiency of DNA ligase activity in Fanconi's anemia. Hum Genet 45: 25-32

Jaspers NGJ, Taalman RDF, Baan C (1988) Patients with an inherited syndrome characterized by immunodeficiency, microcephaly and chromosomal instability: genetic relationship to ataxia telangiectasia. Am J Hum Genet 42: 66-73

Kaiser TN, Lojewski A, Dougherty C, Juergens L, Sahen E, Latt SA (1982) Flow cytometric characterisation of the response of Fanconi's anemia cells to mitomycin C treatment. Cytometry 2: 291-927

Klocker H, Auer B, Hirsch-Kaufmann M, Altmann H, Burtscher HJ, Schweiger M (1983) DNA repair dependent NAD+ metabolism is impaired in cells from patients with Fanconi's anemia. EMBO J 2: 303-307

Kunze J (1980) Estren-Dameshek-Anämie mit myelomonocytärer Leukämie (Subtyp der Fanconi Anämie?). In: Tolksdorf M, Spranger J (eds) Klin Genetik in der Pädiatrie. Thieme, Stuttgart, p 213

Latt SA, Kaiser TN, Lojewski A, Dougherty C, Juergens L, Brefach S, Sahar E, Gustashaw K, Schreck RR, Powers M, Lalande M (1982) Cytogenetic and flow cytometric studies of cells from patients with Fanconi's anemia. Cytogenet Cell Genet 33: 133-138

Moustacchi E, Diatloff-Zito C (1985) DNA semi-conservative synthesis in normal and Fanconi anemia fibroblasts following treatment with 8-methoxypsoralen and near UV-light or X-rays. Hum Genet 70: 236-242

Moustacchi E, Papadopoulo D, Diatloff-Zito C, Buchwald M (1987) Two complementation groups of Fanconi's anemia differ in their phenotypic response to a DNA-crosslinking treatment. Hum Genet 75: 45-47

Oberbäumer I (1986) New pUC-derived vectors for rapid construction of cDNA libraries. Gene 49: 81-91

Poon PK, O'Brien RL, Parker JW (1974) Defective DNA repair in Fanconi's anemia. Nature 250: 223-225

Remsen JF, Cerutti PA (1976) Deficiency of gamma-ray excision repair in skin fibroblasts from patients with Fanconi's anemia. Proc Natl Aced Sci USA 73: 2419-2423

Schroeder TM, Anschütz F, Knopp A (1964) Spontane Chromosomenaberrationen bei familiärer Panmyelopathie. Humangenetik 1: 194-196

Schroeder TM, Drings P, Beiler P, Buchinger G (1976) Clinical and cytogentic observations during a six-year period in an adult with Fanconi's anemia. Blut 34: 119-132

Sperling K, Wegner RD, Riehm H, Obe G (1975) Frequency and distribution of sister chromatid exchanges in a case of Fanconi's anemia. Humangentik 27: 227-230

Sperling K (1983) Analisi dell'eterogenetica nell'uomo. Prospettive Pediatria 49: 53-66

Willis AE, Lindahl T (1987) DNA ligase I deficiency in Bloom's syndrome. Nature 325: 355-357

Wunder E, Burghardt U, Lang B, Hamilton L (1981) Fanconi's anemia: anomaly of enzyme passage through the nuclear membrane? Hum Genet 58: 149-155

Zakrzewski S, Sperling K (1980) Genetic heterogeneity of Fanconi's anemia demonstrated by somatic cell hybrids. Hum Genet 56: 81-84

Zakrzewski S (1981) Analyse der Heterogenie eines menschlichen Erbleidens (Fanconi anämie) an Somazellhybriden. Inaugural dissertation, Freie University of Berlin

Zakrzewski S, Sperling K (1982) Analysis of heterogeneity in Fanconi's anemia patients of different ethnic origin. Hum Genet 62: 321-323

Zakrzewski S, Koch M, Sperling K (1983) Complementation studies between Fanconi's anemia cells with different repair characteristics. Hum Genet 64: 55-57

Part V

Fanconi Anemia: The Family's Point of View

Fanconi Anemia: The Family's Point of View

D. Frohnmayer and L. Frohnmayer

Fanconi anemia does not happen very often, but it happens to real people. They have names, families, hopes and plans. Fanconi anemia will affect them profoundly and forever. The experience is almost certain to be devastating and rarely has any obvious redeeming features.

Denial occurs first. "It isn't happening; it can't happen. A lethal, childhood illness isn't part of our plans." If it is not simply a bad dream or a false diagnosis, there must be a quick fix. Health foods and exotic vitamins (callers by the dozens offer them), more sleep, a new diet - all might regenerate marrow cells. Medicine ... prayer ... flight (physical or psychological) ... In some combination, all might cause the disease to go away.

You feel *shock*. The relief of hearing a physician say "It's not leukemia!" is replaced by the slowly growing knowledge that this diagnosis is worse. We are people accustomed routinely to news reports of medical miracles. Diagnosis of childhood illness is nearly equivalent to promise of cure. Then, painfully, you learn that every single cell of your child's body does not respond as it should, because it is not, and never will be quite normal. But no one, yet, can quite explain why.

Helplessness accompanies this news. Your fate is in the hands of medical professionals - experts who themselves do not have answers. Sometimes they may seem less informed than you quickly have become. Perhaps you, as many FA families relate, endure years of medical misdiagnoses until chromosomal breakage analysis ties heterogeneous symptoms together and confirms the real problem. There is no present cure. Now you know. Yet your child is still alive, but threatened. Where do you turn?

You probably experience deep, profound *anger*. You are outraged by the visitation of an undeserved and unanticipated lethal condition. There was no warning, and, really, no possibility of one. You had other plans for your life. You still do. How can you be expected to cope? Down the line, how will you cope with what, almost certainly, will continue to get worse?

Guilt feelings may be profound, though not always near the surface. You, together with your spouse, unknowingly passed on this disease, poisonously hidden deep within your genes, to a wonderful, happy, blessed, and innocent child. No matter that it's no one's "fault," that it is rare, and that it cannot routinely be detected by the unsuspecting. The knowledge of genetic responsibility lies deep in the subconscious, but it can weigh heavily on the soul.

T. M. Schroeder-Kurth A. D. Auerbach G. Obe (Eds.)
Fanconi Anemia, Clinical, Cytogenetic and Experimental Aspects

Isolation overwhelms almost all FA families. No one you know, usually not even experts, treats this disease routinely; some have never even heard of it. There is no one else to share the anguish, the occasional hopes and the peaks and troughs of crisis after crisis. Your child will not be taken by a sudden accident, horribly scarring as that always is. The outcome is usually predictable and the knowledge of this will torture you and dominate your thoughts indefinitely.

Isolation has two other aspects. First, your problems are different in quality and dimension from those of other parents. A friend worries understandably about behavior problems, or frets that her child's grades will not be competitive for entrance to a top college. Another shares her youngster's pain at not being invited to a birthday party. Your concern is whether the last platelet count is telling you that the downward spiral has continued, that your child may not live long enough to experience a single year of college, in fact that there may not *be* another birthday, and whether health insurance - if there is any - will enable you to secure every possible lifeline of hope.

The second aspect is your own potential victimization. You are apart, and people sense it. The wisest of them ask and help, but sometimes even the most sensitive of friends is at a loss for words. You both know it, and without anybody meaning it to happen, this can wrench you from your community roots and family support.

Grief and *sadness* are a continuing part of your life from the start. We would happily trade places with our children because we've had our chance. There is some completeness in our lives, joys, tragedies, and experiences of life-fulfillment. How cruel that a child, bright with talent and promise, does not posses the genetic constitution to know and learn about this vast and wonderful world, to make the choices that shape life, and to experience at least the fleeting moments of mature reflection that most of us have known. Any parent wants to be his child's companion and share the experiences of a child's maturity. It wrenches. "You cry for them, and you cry for yourself," one FA parent remarked.

But there are helpful ways to cope. Treatment professionals should be aware of and sensitive to these avenues:

1. Take things one day at a time and one step at a time. One blood count does not necessarily tell a disastrous story. Counts can ebb and flow, sometimes unpredictably. This disease runs a course, usually a long course (and the more FA is studied, the longer it seems to be). A journey of a thousand miles begins with a single step, as the saying tells us. Plan tasks to deal with this illness in small, manageable doses. Do not project tomorrow into today.
2. Fight back. This is the strongest, most helpful attitude and reaction we can advise. Do not yourself become a "victim," even though forces pushing you in that direction seem irresistable. Ongoing research should lead to a greater understanding of the mechanisms of this disease, and hence its possible therapies. Bone marrow transplant techniques are not yet available for all victims, but they are for some, and they are improving on all fronts. Raising funds to promote research is a positive way to fight back. You can also fight back by learning more. Even discovering the many conflicting medical opinions can help your own understanding.

3. Do not accept blame or guilt. Every person carries lethal genes. This disease was not predictable, and neither parent is at fault. Marriages have been needlessly damaged because one spouse did not understand or accept the autosomal recessive genesis of this disease.
4. Work with and talk to other FA families. This network, more than anything, can break down isolation and help relieve grief.
5. Retain optimism. Children do this better than adults. Remember that these conditions are hard on all family members, not just those who are ill. Stress and depression can be contagious; the family needs to concentrate on the positives. Set up occasions that reinforce normal family life. To the extent that it's medically advisable, treat your child as a normal child who is capable of enjoying a wide range of activities. Enjoy each and every day to the fullest.

Live with the knowledge that the future is uncertain, but still might be happy. A healthy 12-year-old brother of two sisters with FA told his parents: "The girls are doing fine, now. They are enjoying this time. You need to enjoy it, too. Don't ruin the good time by being depressed and fearful about the future. It's not here yet, and you don't know for sure what it will hold."

It's good advice. We try to live by it.

Anybody who would like to be in touch with other families affected by FA and receive an irregularly published newsletter can contact the FA Support Group, c/o Dave and Lynn Frohnmayer, 2875 Baker Blvd., Eugene, Oregon 97403, USA.

Subject Index

MIX
Papier aus verantwortungsvollen Quellen
Paper from responsible sources
FSC® C105338

If you have any concerns about our products,
you can contact us on
ProductSafety@springernature.com

In case Publisher is established outside the EU,
the EU authorized representative is:
Springer Nature Customer Service Center GmbH
Europaplatz 3, 69115 Heidelberg, Germany

Printed by Libri Plureos GmbH
in Hamburg, Germany